Minimally Invasive Thyroidectomy

Dimitrios Linos • Woong Youn Chung
Editors

Minimally Invasive Thyroidectomy

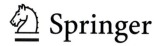

Editors

Dimitrios Linos, M.D., Ph.D.
Professor of Surgery,
St. George's University of London
Medical School at the University of Nicosia
Nicosia, Cyprus

Woong Youn Chung, M.D., Ph.D.
Department of Surgery
Yonsei University College of Medicine
Seoul, South Korea

ISBN 978-3-642-23695-2   e-ISBN 978-3-642-23696-9
DOI 10.1007/978-3-642-23696-9
Springer Heidelberg Dordrecht London New York

Library of Congress Control Number: 2012933428

© Springer-Verlag Berlin Heidelberg 2012

This work is subject to copyright. All rights are reserved, whether the whole or part of the material is concerned, specifically the rights of translation, reprinting, reuse of illustrations, recitation, broadcasting, reproduction on microfilm or in any other way, and storage in data banks. Duplication of this publication or parts thereof is permitted only under the provisions of the German Copyright Law of September 9, 1965, in its current version, and permission for use must always be obtained from Springer. Violations are liable to prosecution under the German Copyright Law.

The use of general descriptive names, registered names, trademarks, etc. in this publication does not imply, even in the absence of a specific statement, that such names are exempt from the relevant protective laws and regulations and therefore free for general use.

Product liability: The publishers cannot guarantee the accuracy of any information about dosage and application contained in this book. In every individual case the user must check such information by consulting the relevant literature.

Printed on acid-free paper

Springer is part of Springer Science+Business Media (www.springer.com)

To my wife Athena and our children Katerina and Stavros, Eleni and Pete, Natalia and Paul, Elizabeth and George, and Constantinos

Dimitrios Linos

Foreword

Today an operation on the thyroid gland, when performed by well-trained surgeons, is one of the safest procedures in the modern day surgical armamentarium. This was not always so.

In 1866, Samuel Gross condemned surgeons who dared to operate on the thyroid gland stating, rather bluntly: "lucky will it be for him if his victim lives long enough to survive his hard butchery." Couple this admonition with the 40% operative mortality for thyroidectomy experienced by the father of thyroid surgery Theodor Kocher in the early 1900s to realize just how far we have come.

Evidence-based data supports this safety evolution. Leigh Delbridge from Sydney has reported on more than 5,000 thyroidectomies with an operative mortality and complication rates of less than 1%. That is the current gold standard and should be achieved by all thyroid surgeons.

The inherent surgical drive for perfection is readily evident in this contribution to the surgical literature. Who would have imagined an entire book dealing with minimally invasive approaches to the thyroid gland? Certainly not I.

The advantages of the minimally invasive approach to most organs, including the thyroid gland, are self-evident and well proven. Despite this evidence, this approach has not been uniformly accepted by the surgical community. The reasons for this are manyfold and complex indeed. In today's surgical world, all surgeons need to have an open mind and be flexible enough to perhaps change what they have been doing for a long time. This contribution will help those who are unsure as to what they should do in their own practices, whether they should embrace the conventional, the endoscopic, or the robotic approaches via various routes. This difficult decision should be carefully weighed and must be based on surgical experience and maturity, training obtained in this new technology, and availability of support systems.

Regardless of which approach is ultimately chosen, the basic principles of surgery, whether they be for benign or malignant disease, should never be violated or sacrificed to the popular idol of new technology. This is nondebatable.

Having had the privilege of knowing Dr. Linos (and many of his contributors) for many decades, I feel confident that he/they shall not let this principle be violated and that they shall ALWAYS keep what is best for each patient foremost in their minds and in their actions. That is the way it should be for all of us as well.

Jon van Heerden, M.B., Ch.B.

Foreword

It is an honor for me to write a foreword for this impressive, comprehensive, and informative book titled *Minimally Invasive Thyroidectomy* by Doctors Dimitrios Linos and Woong Youn Chung. These experienced minimally invasive endocrine surgeons have recruited an outstanding group of internationally recognized authors from many countries with expertise in both minimally invasive and endocrine surgery. The book begins with a chapter by Professor Bertil Hamberger about Theodor Kocher and illustrates Kocher's initial, almost vertical, incision that paralleled the sternocleidomastoid muscle for thyroid operations. Kocher subsequently changed to a transverse or "collar" (Kocher) incision, which had initially been introduced by Jules Boeckel of Strasbourg in 1880 (Welbourn, R.B., *The History of Endocrine Surgery*, Praeger, New York, 1990, p. 35). Theodor Kocher was chair of the Department of Surgery in Bern, Switzerland, for 45 years and received the Nobel Prize for "his works on the physiology, pathology and surgery of the thyroid gland" (Welbourn 3). Kocher would undoubtedly have been interested in the various minimally invasive procedures or in more invasive procedures with no scar visible on the neck.

The book's subsequent chapters include: local anesthesia for thyroid and parathyroid procedures, video-assisted thyroidectomy, transaxillary and robotic thyroidectomy, as well as transoral and "face-lift" thyroidectomies. All endocrine and head and neck surgeons will benefit from reading this book as they become familiar with the authors' suggestions for a variety of approaches for thyroidectomy and parathyroidectomy that have been used effectively for many patients. It is an exciting time in endocrine surgery, and new approaches for thyroidectomy are described in this clearly written book.

To conclude, I would like to share an anecdote from the late 1960s when I was a surgical resident. At the time, many surgeons suggested that "big surgeons" make "big incisions." Now, in the age of rapid transfer of information and well-informed patients, I would suggest that surgeons who make big incisions will not have any patients, especially when the same operation can be done safely via a smaller incision.

Orlo Clark, M.D., FACS

Preface

Thyroid surgery attracts skilled surgeons interested in both technical precision as well as holistic patient care. Despite the excellent outcomes of the traditional thyroidectomy using the Kocher incision, the visibility of a long neck scar has led to potentially poor patient satisfaction. The answer to this problem is minimally invasive thyroid surgery. Unlike the established success of abdominal minimally invasive surgery, this is a relatively new field in thyroid surgery, and no single established method has become the gold standard yet.

Several surgeons have worked very creatively on alternative approaches to the traditional long Kocher neck scar. These include performing smaller neck incisions and varying the position of these for minimal scar visibility, as well as approaching the thyroid from the breast, the axilla, postauricular, or even through the mouth where the scars are effectively hidden. In this book, you will find detailed analyses of each of these techniques by the pioneers who have designed and optimized them. You will also find the basics including preoperative ultrasound, fine needle aspiration, traditional and more modern techniques, as well as postoperative pathology.

This is a very exciting time for thyroid surgery. I am extremely honored to be coediting this book in addition to Prof. Chung, with the input of so many internationally renowned surgeons and specialists. However, this is simply the beginning and we still have a long way to go. We need reliable science examining both clinical outcomes as well as patient reported outcomes of each of these surgical approaches. Furthermore, at a time of rising healthcare costs, it is crucial that the cost-effectiveness of each of these techniques is evaluated carefully. Patient safety and health is paramount, and this must never be compromised simply for the sake of a novel technique or a better cosmetic outcome.

Dimitrios Linos, M.D., Ph.D.
Professor of Surgery,
St. George's University of London
Medical School at the University of Nicosia,
Nicosia, Cyprus

Contents

1. **History of Thyroid Surgery: The Kocher Incision** 1
   Bertil Hamberger

2. **Surgical Anatomy in Minimally Invasive Thyroidectomy** 7
   Andreas Kiriakopoulos and Dimitrios Linos

3. **Thyroid Ultrasound** 17
   Irini S. Hadjisavva and Panayiotis A. Economides

4. **Fine-Needle Aspiration of Thyroid** 37
   Sofia Tseleni-Balafouta

5. **Thyroid Pathology** 59
   Zubair W. Baloch and Virginia A. LiVolsi

6. **Energy Devices in Minimally Invasive Thyroidectomy** 95
   Pier Francesco Alesina and Martin K. Walz

7. **Local Anesthesia in MIT** 105
   Leon Kushnir and William B. Inabnet

8. **Endoscopic Thyroidectomy in the Neck** 113
   Konstantinos P. Economopoulos and Dimitrios Linos

9. **Minimally Invasive Video-Assisted Thyroidectomy** 119
   Paolo Miccoli and Gabriele Materazzi

10. **Minimally Invasive Video-Assisted Thyroidectomy** 127
    Pier Francesco Alesina and Martin K. Walz

11. **Minimally Invasive Non-Endoscopic Thyroidectomy:
    The MINET Approach** 133
    Dimitrios Linos

12. **Endoscopic Transaxillary Thyroidectomy** 141
    Simon K. Wright

13. **Endoscopic Thyroidectomy Using the Gasless
    Transaxillary Approach** 149
    Dimitrios Linos

14. **Robotic Gasless Transaxillary Thyroidectomy** 155
    Woong Youn Chung

15	**Robotic Lateral Neck Node Dissection for the Thyroid Cancer via the Transaxillary Approach**............................. Sang-Wook Kang and Woong Youn Chung	161
16	**Bilateral Axillo-Breast Approach (BABA) Endoscopic and Robotic Thyroid Surgery**... June Young Choi, Kyu Eun Lee, and Yeo-Kyu Youn	169
17	**Other Minimally Invasive Thyroidectomy Techniques Using Remote Skin Incision Outside of the Neck**............................. Sang-Wook Kang and Woong Youn Chung	183
18	**Robotic Facelift Thyroidectomy**............................... David J. Terris and Michael C. Singer	191
19	**Trans-oral Endoscopic Thyroidectomy**......................... Thomas Wilhelm	199
20	**Intraoperative Nerve Stimulation in Minimally Invasive Thyroidectomy**.. Michal Mekel and Gregory W. Randolph	221
21	**Complications of Minimally Invasive Thyroidectomy**............. David Soonmin Kwon and Nancy Dugal Perrier	229
22	**Minimally Invasive Thyroidectomy for Thyroid Carcinoma**........ Roy Phitayakorn	235
23	**Conventional Thyroidectomy Versus MIT: An Outcome Analysis**.. Raymon H. Grogan and Quan-Yang Duh	247
Index	....	253

History of Thyroid Surgery: The Kocher Incision

Bertil Hamberger

1.1 Early Thyroid Surgery

Goiter has been known and described in the art for several centuries, but thyroid surgery was not frequent and, when performed was linked with high mortality. Reports on thyroid surgery are available starting from the seventeenth century. The technique was to tie the patient properly and often use vertical incisions. The procedures started with ligation of the vessels and then removal of part or whole of the thyroid with finger or knife. The wound was left open to suppurate and hopefully heal during the coming months, but bleeding and sepsis were common. The morbidity and mortality was very high and often more than 50% of the patients died.

1.2 The Surgical Revolution

The surgical revolution started in three major fields of progress from the middle of the nineteenth century. These three were anesthesia, knowledge about bacteria and antisepsis, and finally effective hemostasis. The last 30 years of the nineteenth century saw a rapid development in the safety and efficiency of several surgical procedures including thyroid surgery.

Theodor Kocher (Fig. 1.1) was the surgeon to start modern thyroid surgery. At an age of 31 years, he was in 1872 appointed professor and chairman of the

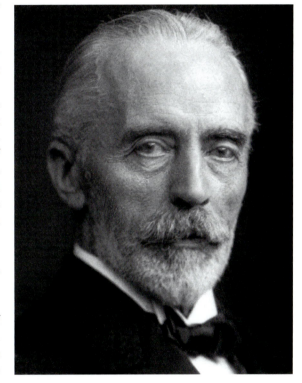

Fig. 1.1 Theodor Kocher (1841–1917), Professor of Surgery in Berne, Switzerland. Nobel Laureate in Medicine 1909 "for his work on the physiology, pathology and surgery of the thyroid gland" (Courtesy of Nobelprize.org)

Department of Surgery in Berne, Switzerland. Kocher applied the new knowledge of antisepsis and could perform his operations with low and declining mortality. This was due to his precise surgical technique with good visualization and no bleeding. Many surgeons from all over the world visited him, not only for his thyroid surgery but also for the whole spectrum of

B. Hamberger
Department of Molecular Medicine and Surgery,
Karolinska Institutet, Karolinska University
Hospital Solna L1:03,
Stockholm 171 76, Sweden
e-mail: bertil.hamberger@ki.se

surgical techniques including gunshot wounds and hernia. He always reported the results of his operations in great details. Before 1900s, his mortality for goiter had become very low, below 1%, and he also removed goiter for cosmetic reasons. In total, he performed up to his death more than 5,000 operations, in addition to a large number of operations in the whole surgical field.

The initial incision used by Kocher was lateral along the anterior border of the sternomastoid muscle or vertical midline (Fig. 1.2), sometimes with angulation for better access. Ligation of the superior and inferior thyroid arteries was commonly done to reduce bleeding in combination with removal of the thyroid lobes. In the last decade of the nineteenth century, he mainly used the collar incision today known by endocrine surgeons to be the Kocher incision (Fig. 1.3) as he recognized that this incision gave the best cosmetic results. Also, an oblique incision made in the right upper abdomen classically used for open cholecystectomy is called a Kocher incision. Kocher described in detail how to proceed with thyroidectomy. Anatomical details were well described (Fig. 1.4) including all vessels and the recurrent laryngeal nerve.

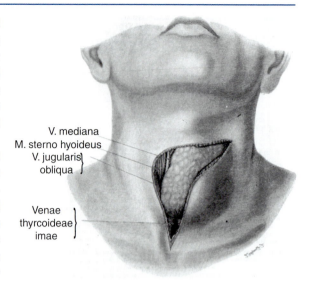

Fig. 1.2 Kocher's vertical incision with lateral extension (From Kocher (1894))

Although Theodor Billroth started with thyroid surgery already in 1861 when appointed professor of surgery in Zurich, but he soon stopped as his mortality was 40% mainly due to sepsis. He resumed thyroid surgery in 1877 when he had used antisepsis for

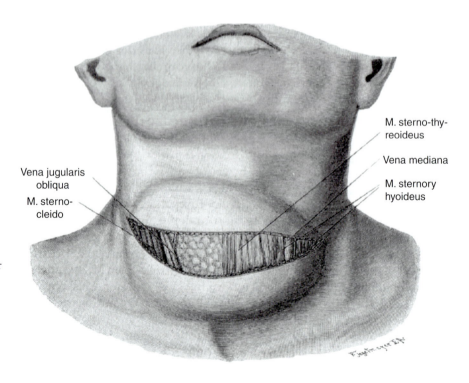

Fig. 1.3 The classic Kocher incision (German Kragenschnitt), was by Kocher considered to be the best cosmetic incision. The straight neck muscles could easily be divided when needed.

1 History of Thyroid Surgery: The Kocher Incision

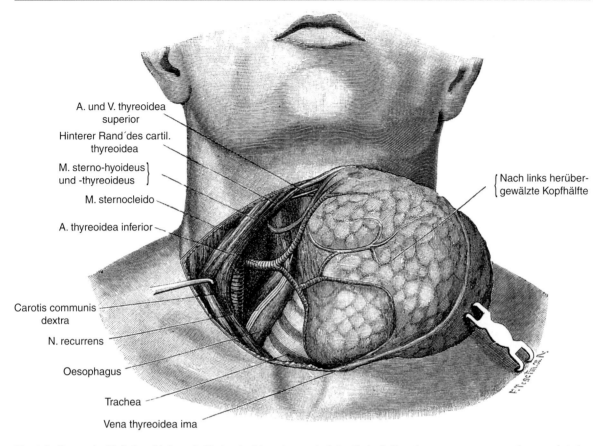

Fig. 1.4 Removal of left thyroid through Kocher incision. Anatomical details including the recurrent nerve can be seen, but the parathyroids are not recognized at this time (Kocher 1894)

some years for other procedures and was considered a leading thyroid surgeon together with Kocher.

1.3 Total or Less Than Total Thyroidectomy

Kocher's first series of total thyroidectomy seemed successful, but after some years it turned out that some patients were severely affected with physical and mental retardation.

Kocher's studies on one of his patients, who was operated on in 1874, led to this discovery. This 11-year-old girl had a successful removal of her thyroid, but afterward she became very tired, showed no signs of initiative, and became cretinoid. She remained small and had an ugly and idiotic appearance in contrast to her sister (Figs. 1.5 and 1.6).

This prompted Kocher to reinvestigate all his thyroid patients. Almost all of them, particularly the children, had evident symptoms of hypothyroidism, which he named "cachexia strumipriva." However, at this time, Kocher did not until later understand that this was due to the removal of the thyroid gland but ascribed it to tracheal injury. These data made Kocher decide not to remove the whole gland in his future patients. After description of the myxedema condition, transplantation and injection of extracts of thyroid tissue was tried. The studies "on the physiology, pathology and surgery of the thyroid gland" was the contributions that rendered Theodor Kocher the Nobel Prize 1909.

A significant early contribution to thyroid surgery was made by Thomas Dunhill in Melbourne, Australia. He particularly worked with patients with Graves's disease who had a very high mortality in the beginning of the twentieth century. He advised operation on both

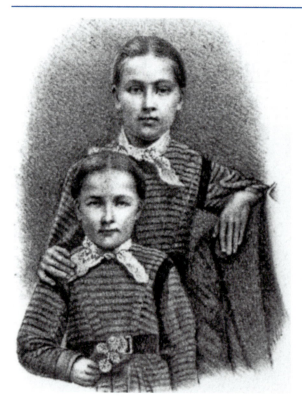

Fig. 1.5 The Kocher patient Marie, 11 years old, together with her younger sister before she was operated with total thyroidectomy for goiter. The patient was then taller than her little sister (From Kocher (1883))

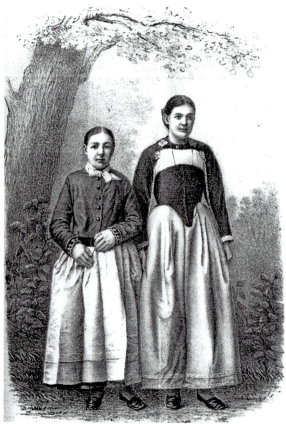

Fig. 1.6 Nine years after the operation. The patient had stopped growing, and her sister was now taller. She had also become cretinoid (From Kocher (1883))

lobes and performed total lobectomy and less than total on the other side. With precise surgical technique, he managed to press down the mortality in Grave's patients to 3% already in 1912.

1.4 Other Complications

Also, at this time, other complications were recognized, particularly damage to the recurrent laryngeal nerve, causing hoarseness. It was soon known that it was important to preserve this nerve. The discussion whether or not to identify the nerve went on for 100 years. Both Kocher and Billroth advocated the nerve should not be identified as this increased the risk of injury. Identification of the recurrent nerve became more common in the beginning of the twentieth century. Local anesthesia was by some surgeons considered safer as the patient's voice could be recorded, and if affected by a surgical clamp, the nerve could recover after removal of the clamp. The principle that "if you have seen the nerve it is hurt" became completely abandoned during the 1960s, and identification of the nerve has become routine in all centers.

The complications of tetany and hypoparathyroidism were not initially understood by Kocher and Billroth. However, Kocher in contrast to Billroth had a very neat and precise operating technique and worked in a relatively bloodless field. Probably because of this, he had less problems with postoperative tetany than Billroth. When the cause of tetany was recognized, various techniques were used to preserve the parathyroids. It was found important to dissect preserving the thyroid capsule posteriorly. The discussion on techniques for preserving parathyroid function is still today an important issue.

1.5 Future Development

The progress in thyroid surgery spread, and three American surgeons who visited Europe started successfully thyroid surgery in the USA. These were William Halsted in Baltimore, Charles Mayo in Rochester, and George Crile in Cleveland. Halsted and Kocher visited each other at several occasions exchanging experiences and progress in thyroid surgery.

In general, not much has happened after the establishment of surgical principles for the thyroid in the early part of the twentieth century. Surgical instruments have improved, anesthesia developed, and safety of surgery increased to allow procedures also on fragile patients. The big challenge of thyroid surgery came again when endoscopic procedures widely entered into surgery around 1990, which will be described in this book.

Suggested Readings

Dunhill TP (1912) Partial thyroidectomy under local anaesthesia, with special reference to exophthalmic goitre. Joint Meeting with the Medical Section and Section of Anaesthetics. 13 February 1912. Proc R Soc Med 5:70–130

Halsted WS (1920) The operative story of goitre. Johns Hopkins Hosp Rep 19:71–257

Kocher T (1883) Ueber Kropfexstirpation und ihre Folgen [von Langenbeck's]. Arch klin Chir 29:254–337

Kocher T (1894) Chirurgische Operationslehre. Jena, Zweite Auflage Verlag von Gustav Fischer

Nobelprize.org

Welbourn RB (1990) The thyroid. In: The history of endocrine surgery. Praeger, New York, pp 19–87

Surgical Anatomy in Minimally Invasive Thyroidectomy

2

Andreas Kiriakopoulos and Dimitrios Linos

2.1 Anatomical Position of the Thyroid

The normal thyroid gland weighs 11–25 g. It is a butterfly-shaped organ that lies over the anterior trachea wrapping around the upper tracheal rings just deep to the sternothyroid and sternohyoid muscles. It consists of a centrally located isthmus that covers the second and third tracheal rings and two lobes that extend lateral and posterior to the trachea. A pyramidal lobe may exist that extends from the isthmus up to the hyoid bone occasionally as a persistent thyroglossal duct. The thyroid gland is situated on the upper trachea. The isthmus usually lies inferior to the cricoid cartilage between the second and fourth tracheal rings, and its upper part is fixed to the upper trachea rings in the form of the ligament of Berry (Fig. 2.1). The superior pole of the thyroid lobe may extend past the inferior border of the thyroid cartilage, whereas the inferior pole normally extends to the sixth tracheal ring posteriorly.

A. Kiriakopoulos, M.D. (✉)
Department of Surgery, Hygeia Hospital,
4 Erythrou Stavrou St. and Kifissias Ave., 15123
Marousi, Athens, Greece
e-mail: kirian@ontelecoms.gr

D. Linos, M.D., Ph.D.
Professor of Surgery,
St. George's University of London Medical School
at the University of Nicosia, Nicosia, Cyprus

Department of Surgery, Hygeia Hospital,
7 Fragoklisias St., Marousi, Athens 15125, Greece
e-mail: dlinos@hms.harvard.edu

2.2 Muscles

The thyroid is covered by several muscles (Figs. 2.2 and 2.3). Of surgical interest for the thyroidectomy are the strap muscles. These are four pairs of muscles that create a double-layered plane in the anterior cervical triangle. These consist of the sternohyoid, sternothyroid, omohyoid, and thyrohyoid muscles:

- The *sternohyoid muscle* runs between the sternum and the hyoid bone, and it is the most superficial muscle (Figs. 2.2 and 2.3).
- The *thyrohyoid muscle* is short and runs between the greater horn of the hyoid bone and the oblique line of the thyroid cartilage (Figs. 2.2 and 2.3).
- The *sternothyroid muscle* continues the path of the thyrohyoid muscle from the thyroid cartilage to the sternum lying deep to the sternohyoid muscle (Figs. 2.2 and 2.3).
- The *omohyoid muscle* has two bellies: the *superior belly* that originates from the hyoid bone and descends vertically to the central tendon and the *inferior belly* that runs horizontally from the central tendon, passes deep to the SCM, and enters the posterior triangle to attach to the scapula (Figs. 2.2 and 2.3).

Another muscle that is encountered during thyroidectomy is the cricothyroid muscle. The cricothyroid muscle is attached to the cricoid and the inferior cornu and lower edge of the thyroid cartilage, tilting the thyroid cartilage forward and tensing the vocal cords (Fig. 2.4). It is the only laryngeal muscle that is not supplied by the recurrent laryngeal nerve but by the external branch of the superior laryngeal nerve.

Fig. 2.1 Anatomy of the thyroid

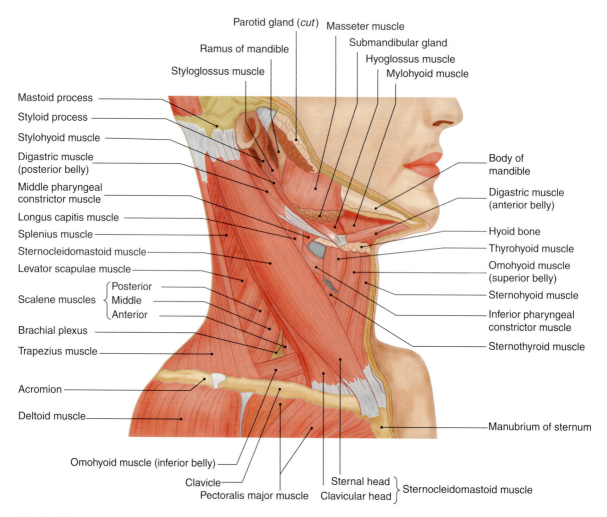

Fig. 2.2 Muscles of the thyroid – lateral view

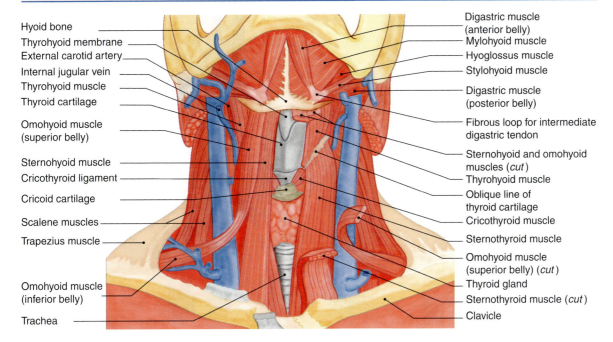

Fig. 2.3 Muscles of the thyroid – front view

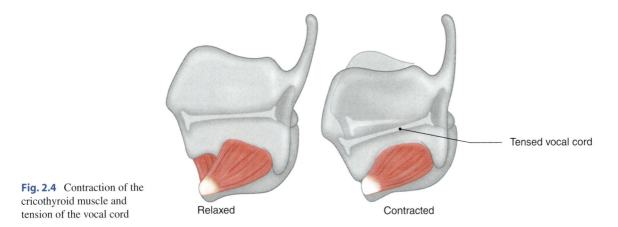

Fig. 2.4 Contraction of the cricothyroid muscle and tension of the vocal cord

2.3 Blood Supply

The blood supply of the thyroid gland is rich. The superior and inferior arteries are derived as pairs from the external carotid arteries and the thyrocervical trunks respectively. Occasionally, an unpaired third vessel named ima artery may exist, arising from the innominate artery or the aorta. It ascends in front of the trachea entering into the lower border of the isthmus. Its 10% of reported frequency occurrence is considered an overestimation by most. The veins are more variable than the arterial supply and may reach enormous sizes in vastly enlarged glands. They communicate freely among themselves, and they form a capillary network that is fragile and prone to hemorrhage. The veins always include paired superior and inferior pedicles and a highly variable middle thyroid vein.

2.4 Arterial Supply

The *superior thyroid artery* arises as the first branch of the external carotid artery just above the thyroid cartilage (Fig. 2.5). After giving off the superior laryngeal artery, it descends on the surface of the inferior constrictor of the pharynx. It enters the upper pole of the thyroid and then gives off two or sometimes three branches: a large anterior branch to the pyramidal lobe and

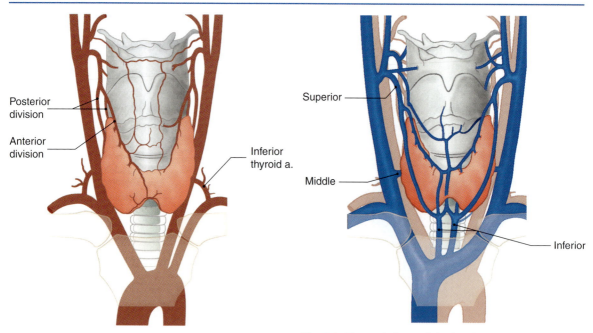

Fig. 2.5 Arterial supply of the thyroid

Fig. 2.6 Venous drainage of the thyroid and parathyroid glands

isthmus, a posterior branch that descends posteriorly on the gland feeding the superior parathyroid gland, and other additional branches that course over the anterior surface of the gland. The surgical significance of the superior thyroid artery derives from its close proximity to the external branch of superior laryngeal nerve that serves as the motor nerve to the cricothyroid muscle. In 6–18% of cases, the external branch of the superior laryngeal nerve runs with or around the superior thyroid artery or its branches. Thus, it is highly vulnerable during the ligation of the superior thyroid artery.

The *inferior thyroid artery* is the largest branch of the thyrocervical trunk (Fig. 2.5). It courses behind the carotid sheath and loops medially and downward to the level of the inferior pole of the thyroid before running upward to enter the gland at its middle portion. It divides into several glandular branches: inferior, posterior, and internal. These branches anastomose with branches of superior thyroid artery and give off branches to the parathyroid glands.

2.5 Venous Drainage

The *superior thyroid vein* that courses parallel to the superior thyroid artery drains directly or indirectly into the internal jugular vein (Fig. 2.6). The *middle veins* vary greatly in number. The *inferior thyroid veins* may be multiple as they leave off the lower poles and the isthmus of the thyroid gland and frequently form a plexus. They empty directly into the internal jugular vein. A potential point of recurrent laryngeal nerve injury lies in this point, and careful identification of the nerve is mandatory before the ligation of the most lateral inferior thyroid vein.

2.6 Lymphatic Drainage

The thyroid gland is richly endowed with lymphatics, and the flow may drain in many directions from the gland. There is an extensive intraglandular lymphatic network beneath the thyroid capsule that crosscommunicate through the isthmus with the contralateral thyroid lobe.

The regional lymph nodal stations of the thyroid gland include two zones:
- The visceral zone (compartment) of the neck that includes the prelaryngeal, the pretracheal, and the paratracheoesophageal lymph nodes
- The nodes of the lateral cervical region (the upper, middle, and lower jugular nodes), the anterosuperior mediastinal nodes, and the retropharyngeal and esophageal nodes

The *prelaryngeal lymph nodes* lie superior to the isthmus and join the lymphatic vessels of the superior

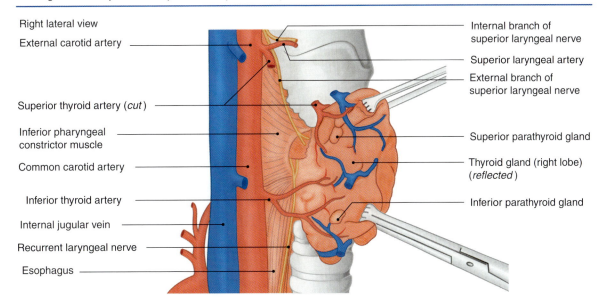

Fig. 2.7 Right lateral view of the thyroid. The external branch of the superior laryngeal nerve and the recurrent laryngeal nerve are depicted

pole of the thyroid to drain into the lymph nodes of the lateral cervical region. Lymph nodes found in the midline just above the isthmus are called *Delphian nodes*. The *pretracheal nodes* lie inferior to the isthmus and drain inferiorly into the anterosuperior mediastinal nodes. The *paratracheoesophageal lymph nodes* are found across the lateral and posterior borders of the thyroid along the course of recurrent laryngeal nerves. The normal flow direction of the central and lower parts of the neck is toward the tracheoesophageal and upper mediastinal lymph nodes. The upper neck drains directly to the lateral neck nodes. Therefore, the central neck area constitutes the primary zone of metastatic lymph node involvement in cases of thyroid cancer.

2.7 The Nerves

Two of the nerves that require special attention during the thyroidectomy are: the recurrent laryngeal nerve (RLN) and the external branch of the superior laryngeal nerve (EBSLN) (Fig. 2.7).

2.7.1 Right Recurrent Laryngeal Nerve

The right RLN arises from the vagus nerve at the point of crossing with the first portion of the subclavian artery. It then passes posterior to the subclavian artery and ascends lateral to the trachea (Figs. 2.7 and 2.8).

At the level of the inferior thyroid artery, the nerve is closer to the trachea. The RLN junction with the inferior thyroid artery is one of the most vulnerable areas for injury mainly because of the extremely variable nerve-artery relations. The relation is unpredictable because the nerve may be anterior, posterior, or between the arterial trunk branches (Fig. 2.9). Identification of the inferior thyroid artery and careful ligation of its branches close to the thyroid gland are excellent techniques for nerve injury prevention. In rare cases, the RLN may divide into one or more branches at the level of crossing with the inferior thyroid artery, so every effort to preserve them is absolutely necessary.

The RLN continues upward, and in the middle of the neck it runs behind the posterior surface of the thyroid gland 1–2 cm lateral to the tracheoesophageal groove. At the two upper tracheal rings, the nerve passes posterior or even transverses (25%) the Berry's ligament, where it frequently branches before entering the larynx (Figs. 2.7 and 2.8). At this point, the nerve cannot be identified until the most lateral posterior extension of the thyroid lobe, which is called the *tubercle of Zuckerkandl*, has been rotated medially. This point constitutes the most vulnerable site for RLN injury. In rare cases (0.63%), the right inferior laryngeal nerve does not recur. Nonrecurrence of the right laryngeal nerve may be associated with aplasia of the innominate artery and presence of aberrant subclavian artery (arteria lusoria syndrome).

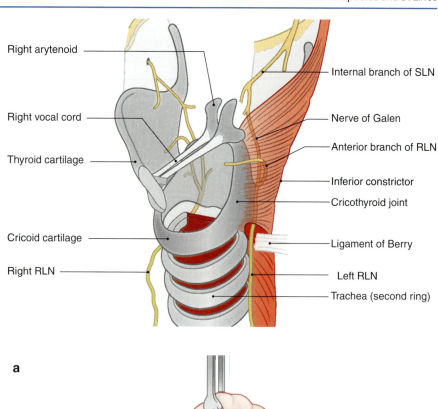

Fig. 2.8 Left and right recurrent laryngeal nerve

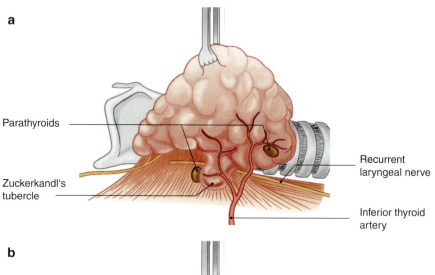

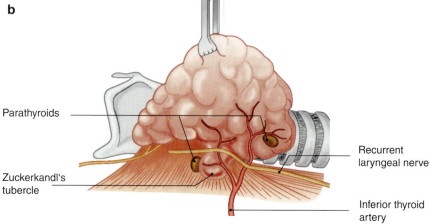

Fig. 2.9 The recurrent laryngeal nerve and the inferior thyroid artery. The nerve may be (**a**) posterior, or (**b**) anterior or between the arterial trunk branches

2.7.2 Left Recurrent Laryngeal Nerve

The left recurrent laryngeal nerve arises from the vagus nerve winding around the arch of the aorta behind the attachment of ligamentum arteriosum. It passes inferior and medial to the aorta and ascends usually in the left tracheoesophageal groove. The ascending course of the left recurrent laryngeal nerve is more medial than the right laryngeal nerve. Nonrecurrent left laryngeal nerve is exceedingly rare.

2.7.3 Injury to the Inferior Laryngeal Nerves

Injury to the laryngeal nerve is involved in most claims regarding complications of thyroid surgery. Thorough knowledge of the anatomy and the variable courses of the recurrent laryngeal nerves are mandatory. The risk of injury to the recurrent nerve is increased in situations such as:
- In large goiters and extensive thyroidectomies
- In patients with thyroid malignancy
- In reoperative thyroid cases

The recurrent laryngeal nerve is the motor nerve to the intrinsic muscles of the larynx. Postoperative hoarseness may be caused by several mechanisms:
- If it occurs early, it may be attributed to edema in the operative field that usually has a benign course.
- Stretching of the nerve may also cause nerve injury by forceful damage of its axons. This injury usually does not last over 6 months, is self-limited, and is mostly influenced by the regenerative process of axonic growth, which is usually 1 mm/day.

Injury to the recurrent laryngeal nerve results in paralysis of the vocal cord on the ipsilateral side. The cord may either remain in paramedian position or may be abducted to the midline. When the paralyzed cord is approximated by the functioning contralateral cord, the patient may have a normal although weakened voice. When the vocal cord is paralyzed in an abducted position, closure is prevented and a severely impaired voice and ineffective cough result.

Bilateral recurrent laryngeal nerve injuries have dramatic clinical presentation either with a complete loss of voice or, even worse, with complete airway obstruction requiring emergency intubation or tracheostomy. If both vocal cords are paralyzed in an abducted position, airway obstruction is delayed until contraction gradually makes them approach to the midline. In these cases, upper respiratory infection may necessitate an emergency operation to restore airway patency.

2.7.4 The External Branch of the Superior Laryngeal Nerve

The *superior laryngeal nerve* originates from the vagus nerve at the caudal end of the nodose ganglion above the hyoid bone. It passes deep to the carotid arteries onto the middle constrictor and at the level of the hyoid bone divides into two branches:
- The larger internal branch that is purely sensory and pierces the thyrohyoid membrane before innervating the larynx. It curves medially and perforates the thyrohyoid membrane above the superior laryngeal artery, where it divides into terminal branches. This branch provides sensory innervation of the base of the tongue, the inferior surface of the glottis and the subglottic region, and the vocal folds. It also conveys taste fibers from the epiglottis and provides the afferent limb of the cough reflex.
- The smaller external branch takes a more caudal course and descends on the surface of the inferior constrictor to innervate only the cricothyroid muscle. It runs in close proximity to the medial aspect of the superior thyroid artery and, just cranial to the upper thyroid pole, curves medially to innervate the cricothyroid muscle. This nerve is the motor nerve for the cricothyroid muscle, which produces tension of the vocal cords and makes possible the production of high-pitched sounds (Fig. 2.10).

Because this nerve accompanies the main trunk of the superior thyroid artery to its terminal branching (15%) or even courses between these branches (6%), superior thyroid artery ligation must be performed as near as possible to the thyroid capsule avoiding its en masse blind division (Fig. 2.11). A classification system regarding the relation of the external branch to the superior thyroid artery has been proposed by Cernea:
- Cernea type 1 (30% of cases): the nerve crosses medially into the cricothyroid membrane >1 cm cranially to the upper thyroid pole
- Cernea type 2 (30% of cases): distance <1 cm from the upper thyroid pole with subdivisions type a

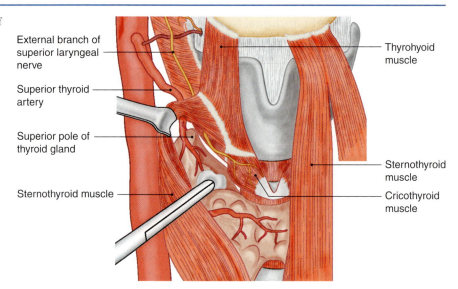

Fig. 2.10 External branch of the superior laryngeal nerve

symptoms than the damage of the recurrent nerve. The course of the internal branch is positioned cephalad to the dissection area of the thyroidectomy, therefore it is infrequently involved in standard thyroid surgery. Injury to the internal branch of the superior thyroid nerve presents as episodes of aspiration of food and drink on swallowing caused by the defective coordination of the glottis. Injury to the external branch of the superior thyroid nerve is manifested with mild hoarseness, voice weakness or fatigue, loss of voice range, and lower voice volume. In cases of bilateral injuries, the swallowing problems are greater and make patients vulnerable to aspiration pneumonias.

2.8 The Parathyroids

Normally, humans have four parathyroid glands. Supernumerary glands are found in 2.5–22% of cases. Their average weight is 40 mg (range 10–70), their average size is about $5 \times 3 \times 1$ cm, and they have a particular affinity to fat tissue being often completely embedded within a fatty globule. They are soft and have either a light brown or coffee color when they are fatty or dark, reddish brown color when they have richer blood supply. Their color also varies according to age being light pink in children while turning yellow to adults. Parathyroid glands may be intracapsular (being beneath the fibrous capsule of the thyroid) or extracapsular.

The superior parathyroid gland is usually located on the posteromedial aspect of the upper thyroid pole near the tracheoesophageal groove (Fig. 2.12). The superior

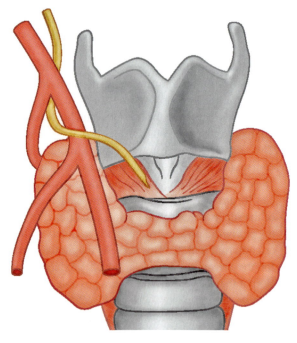

Fig. 2.11 External branch of the superior laryngeal nerve and superior thyroid artery. The nerve may be anterior, posterior, or between the arterial trunk branches

(the nerve remains cranial to the upper pole) and type b (the nerve comes below the upper thyroid pole)

2.7.5 Injury to the Superior Laryngeal Nerves

Injury to the superior laryngeal nerve is less easily recognized because it is associated with less severe

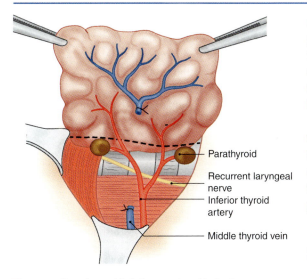

Fig. 2.12 Superior and inferior parathyroid glands

parathyroid glands arise from the dorsal part of the P IV. They follow the thyroid migration of the ultimobranchial bodies which is relatively short. Because of this short migration path, the superior parathyroid glands remain in a more or less more stable position (85% of cases) on the posterior aspect of the upper thyroid lobe situated in an area 2 cm in diameter about 1 cm above the crossing of the inferior thyroid artery and the recurrent laryngeal nerve. In 12–13% of cases, the glands are found on the posterior aspect of the upper thyroid lobe, but in more lateral positions and in 1% of cases they are found above the upper pole. In 1–4%, they are truly posterior found behind the pharynx or esophagus. The short migratory path also explains the unusual occurrence of congenital ectopic position. True superior intrathyroidal glands are extremely rare.

The inferior parathyroid glands are more widely distributed, although their normal position is found on the posterolateral aspect of the inferior thyroid pole (Fig. 2.12). Another common location for the inferior parathyroid glands is the area close or into the thyrothymic ligament or into the cervical part of the thymus. They arise from the dorsal part of the P III, the same pouch that gives the thymus. The embryonic descent of the thymus extends from the upper limit of the neck down to the pericardium, and this fact explains the high incidence of ectopias associated with the inferior parathyroid glands. High ectopias along the carotid sheath from the angle of the mandible to the lower pole of the thyroid are found in 1–2% of cases. Low ectopias are found in 3.9–5% of cases usually within the thymus at the posterior aspect of its capsule or in close proximity to the great mediastinal vessels. Therefore, inferior glands may be found in the fatty tissue of the anterior mediastinum or even at the carotid bifurcation. Intrathyroidal inferior parathyroid glands have been described in 3% of cases.

Supernumerary glands may also exist usually within the thymus or in relation to the thyrothymic ligament. Supernumerary parathyroid glands may develop from accessory parathyroid debris arising from fragmentation of the pharyngotracheal duct when the pharyngeal pouches separate from the pharynx.

2.8.1 Vascular Supply

In 80% of cases, there is a single artery that supplies the parathyroid glands being single in 65% of cases. Two distinct arterial branches are seen in 15% of cases. Both the superior and inferior glands derive their blood supply from the inferior thyroid artery. The superior parathyroid gland receives its arterial supply from the inferior thyroid artery in 80% of cases, in 15% from the superior thyroid artery, and in 5% from intercommunicating branches.

2.8.2 Relation of Parathyroid Gland to Recurrent Laryngeal Nerves

A predictable relation of the parathyroid glands to the recurrent laryngeal nerve has been described (Fig. 2.12). It involves the use of the recurrent nerve as an anatomic landmark where the superior parathyroid glands lie posterior and superior to the nerve, whereas the inferior parathyroid gland lies anterior to the nerve.

2.9 Lymph Nodes

The primary zone of lymphatic drainage is to the anterior compartment that is Delphian, tracheoesophageal, and superior mediastinal nodes. The nodes of the lateral neck (internal jugular, posterior triangle) constitute a zone of secondary drainage. The neck lymph nodes become of surgical interest only in the case of metastatic thyroid cancer. The description of the location of the lymph nodes in the neck is described in levels (Fig. 2.13):

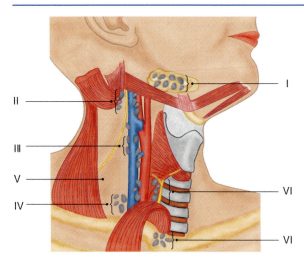

Fig. 2.13 Location of lymph nodes in the neck (see main text for more details)

Level I: submental and submandibular group
Level II: upper Jugular group
Level III: middle jugular group
Level IV: lower jugular group
Level V: posterior triangular group
Level VI: anterior compartment lymph nodes

More on the anatomy of the neck lymph nodes in Chap. 15.

Further Readings

Netter FH (1990) Atlas of human anatomy. CIBA-Geigy, Summit

Randolph GW (2003) Surgery of the thyroid and parathyroid glands. Elsevier, Philadelphia

Stewart WB, Rizzolo LJ (2007) Embryology and surgical anatomy of the thyroid and parathyroid glands. In: Oertli D, Udelsman R (eds) Surgery of the thyroid and parathyroid glands. Springer, Berlin

Thyroid Ultrasound

3

Irini S. Hadjisavva and Panayiotis A. Economides

3.1 Anatomy

The thyroid is a butterfly-shaped, vascular gland attached to the trachea and the larynx, situated at the anterior of the neck and inferior to the thyroid cartilage. It is composed of two oval-shaped lobes, the right and left, which are connected by the isthmus (Fig. 3.1). The right lobe is likely to be slightly bigger than the left. Even though the dimensions and shape of the thyroid may vary greatly among individuals, the mean lobe length is 40–60 mm, lobe thickness is less than 20 mm, and normal adult thyroid volume is 18.6±4.5 mL (±SD) (Hegedus et al. 1983; Solbiati et al. 2005). Thyroid volume is significantly associated with age and weight, and the difference in thyroid gland volume between males and females is explained by the difference in body weight. Thyroid volume is calculated by the ellipsoid formula: Volume=0.5×(length×depth×width).

In about 10–40% of normal patients, a third conical lobe – the pyramidal lobe – is present, even though most times it is not visible with ultrasound. The latter, which is a remnant of the fetal thyroglossal duct, branches off the isthmus and stretches left of the midline, anterior to the thyroid cartilage. The thyroid gland is covered by a fibrous sheath, the capsule, which has an echogenic U/S appearance. Generally, four parathyroid glands, even though more may be present, are situated posterior to the upper and lower thyroid lobes. The thyroid is vascularized by the inferior and superior

I.S. Hadjisavva, Ph.D. • P.A. Economides, M.D., Ph.D., FACE (✉)
Economides Nicosia Endocrinology Center,
9 Iona Nicolaou St., Engomi, Nicosia, 2406 Cyprus
e-mail: peconomi@cytanet.com.cy

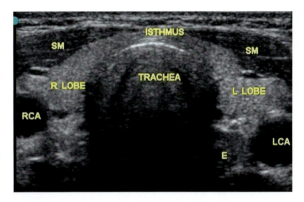

Fig. 3.1 Transverse image of a normal thyroid gland. *RCA*, *LCA* right and left carotid arteries, *E* esophagus, *SM* strap muscles

thyroid arteries and veins and the middle thyroid veins. Lymphatic vessels from the thyroid are extensive and drain into the pretracheal, paratracheal, and internal jugular chain nodes.

The gland is made up of several spherical groups of follicular cells that contain stored thyroid hormone in the form of colloid. Lying next to follicles are the parafollicular cells, which are responsible for the production of calcitonin. The thyroid parenchyma has a uniform medium to high echogenicity relative to the normally hypoechogenic surrounding muscle tissue. For this reason, any thyroid tissue heterogeneity or hypoechogenicity could imply pathology (Ruchała and Szczepanek 2010). The recurrent laryngeal nerve passes between the trachea, esophagus, and thyroid lobe, while the esophagus found posterior to the trachea and usually extending on the left – frequently mistaken for a thyroid nodule – has a hypoechoic rim due to its muscle composition and is clearly noted when the patient swallows (Ahuja 2000).

D. Linos and W.Y. Chung (eds.), *Minimally Invasive Thyroidectomy*,
DOI 10.1007/978-3-642-23696-9_3, © Springer-Verlag Berlin Heidelberg 2012

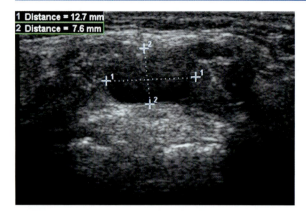

Fig. 3.2 Transverse image of an infrahyoid midline thyroglossal duct cyst

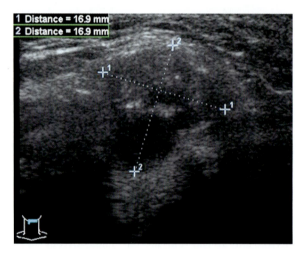

Fig. 3.3 Transverse image of thyroglossal duct papillary carcinoma

Incomplete degeneration of the thyroglossal duct leading to midline cystic lesions above the isthmus is often seen during neck scanning (Fig. 3.2). These lesions are mostly seen inferior to the hyoid bone and appear cystic although complex lesions are also detected. They are more easily noted when they become infected and enlarged. Ectopic thyroid tissue may be identified as a solid component, and although uncommon, thyroid carcinoma in the thyroglossal duct will need to be ruled out by FNA.

Other thyroid anomalies detected by thyroid and neck ultrasound imaging are complete absence of thyroid tissue (agenesis), absence of only one lobe (hemiagenesis), hypoplastic thyroid tissue, failed bifurcation of the gland, or presence of a hypertrophied pyramidal lobe (Baskin et al. 2008). Ectopic thyroid tissue may also be seen laterally, high in the midline neck (lingual, sublingual, or thyroglossal), retrosternal, or in the superior mediastinum. Although rare, these ectopic sites can harbor thyroid malignancy (Fig. 3.3) (Albayrak et al. 2011).

3.2 Ultrasound Technology

Ultrasound technology is based on longitudinal sound waves with frequency above the audible limit of humans that are produced by a probe or transducer consisting of piezoelectric crystals that change shape when voltage is applied to them. This converts electrical energy to ultrasound waves of frequencies anywhere between 2 and 18 MHz. In thyroid scanning, the linear array transducer is the one most commonly used, where the piezoelectric crystals are arranged linearly and produce a rectangular beam. Curved array transducers offer a large surface field of view and are commonly used for abdominal and pelvic applications.

Lower frequencies (5 MHz) are used to measure the size of the thyroid gland and assess deep lesions while higher frequencies (10–15 MHz) are used for high-resolution exams involving small nodules and lymph nodes (Guth et al. 2009). The higher the frequencies, the higher the resolution, whereas the lower the frequency, the deeper the penetration. High-frequency transducers can achieve resolution to less than 1 mm. Current ultrasound equipment utilize frequencies 5–15 MHz.

While in the body, ultrasound waves come across tissues with different densities, and part is reflected as an echo to the transducer, where they are converted to an electric signal and transformed by the scanner into an image. Substances with greater acoustic impedance will produce stronger echoes. Deeper tissues send back attenuated waves (due to loss of energy through the traveling medium) resulting in weaker echoes. If in the process the waves hit gases or solids, most of their energy is reflected, thus inhibiting the sonographer from getting an image of deeper tissues. More recent three-dimensional scanning involves sending sound waves in different angles/imaging planes so as to accurately construct an image, measure volume, and examine surface features (Holter 2010). Three-dimensional imaging is mostly used for obstetric/gynecologic and cardiac applications. There have not been many reports where three-dimensional thyroid ultrasound is used; however, evidence exists that such technique provides accurate measurement of thyroid volume (Lyshchik et al. 2004; Slapa et al. 2011). Three-dimensional thyroid imaging has been shown to provide precise, sonographic volumetric evaluation of morphology of thyroid nodules.

Doppler ultrasonography is based on the change in frequency of sound that increases when it is moving close to the transducer and decreases if it is moving away. Color flow Doppler imaging utilizes red or blue color according to whether blood flow is toward or away from the probe. Power mode Doppler imaging provides a highly sensitive color map that shows the power and amplitude of the Doppler signal instead of flow direction. B-flow imaging (BFI) is a non-Doppler technology that has been introduced to complement Doppler blood flow evaluation. B-flow technique uses a morphological approach with a higher spatial and temporal resolution than Doppler and with decreased number of artifacts. The BFI technique has been applied in the study of thyroid nodules where microcalcifications produced a twinkling sign (BFI-TS) that was highly suggestive of malignancy (Brunese et al. 2008).

Estimation of tissue stiffness by ultrasound (sonoelastography) is a novel dynamic technique based on the deformation of tissue after applying external force (Gietka-Czernel et al. 2010). It is increasingly used in evaluating thyroid, breast, and prostate tumors. Sonoelastography can be used as an adjunctive tool for the diagnosis of thyroid cancer especially in indeterminate nodules (Luo et al. 2011; Rago et al. 2010). Sonoelastography has also been evaluated in differentiating benign from malignant cervical lymph nodes with much promising results.

Ultrasound contrast agents have recently been used to improve the diagnostic yield of ultrasound. Microbubbles when injected intravenously enhance the echoes received from both the large and small blood vessels, therefore allowing the examination of the microvasculature of the thyroid parenchyma and nodules. Their use for differentiation of benign and malignant thyroid nodules is currently under investigation (Zhang et al. 2010; Xu 2009).

During ultrasound examination, the patient lies down with a small pillow under the shoulders, so the neck is hyperextended and the thyroid becomes accessible for imaging. Gel is applied in copious amounts on the skin, and a linear or curvilinear probe is pressed firmly back and forth against the neck in order to allow

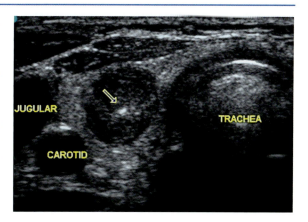

Fig. 3.4 U/S-guided FNA: echogenic needle tip (*arrow*) is seen within a right thyroid nodule (perpendicular approach)

for both longitudinal and transverse scanning. As sound waves pass through air poorly, it is important to make sure that air pockets between the transducer and the skin are eliminated. First, the thyroid gland is located and examined followed by inspection of the cervical lymph nodes along the carotid artery and jugular vein. The entire neck should be scanned.

Ultrasonography can provide accurate and reliable information on the presence of thyroid disease and aid in the monitoring of its progression. It can identify the position and size of solitary or multiple thyroid nodules and help in the determination of their characteristics such as echogenicity, composition, vascularization, and the presence of calcifications (Sheth 2010). Additionally, ultrasonography has been increasingly used for guidance during fine needle aspiration (FNA) of nodules and cysts (Fig. 3.4) (Kim et al. 2008). Ultrasound is also considered to be very sensitive in identifying and staging cervical lymph node metastasis from thyroid carcinoma. However, MRI may also be used in parallel, to examine areas where ultrasound examination is difficult such as retrotracheal and substernal locations (King et al. 2000). Use of ultrasound is also highly accurate for the detection of parathyroid tumors.

Overall, ultrasonography is an inexpensive procedure with high sensitivity and accuracy. However, limitations may arise in situations where the patient has a short neck, a large thyroid mass, or multiple nodules, or when the ultrasonographer lacks proficiency in thyroid ultrasound imaging. The main limitation of thyroid ultrasound imaging is that its results do not correlate well with histopathology, and it is therefore mandatory that the clinician uses the information in

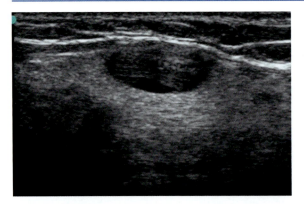

Fig. 3.5 Longitudinal image of a thyroid cystic lesion

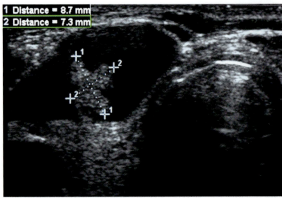

Fig. 3.6 Longitudinal image of a cystic lesion with solid elements

combination with clinical data (Hegedüs 2001). It is also very important that whoever performs the ultrasound examination either clinician or radiologist has the necessary clinical knowledge so as to be able to comprehend the findings and correctly interpret the results. More commonly, thyroid ultrasound is being performed by the endocrinologist – thyroidologist in the clinical practice-office.

3.3 Thyroid Pathologies

3.3.1 Thyroid Cysts

Thyroid cysts occur in less than 1% of thyroid lesions. Epithelial cysts usually contain serous transudate or colloid and are predominantly anechogenic. They are oval or round in shape (Fig. 3.5), have regular well-defined borders, and generally show no blood flow with Doppler examination. Complex thyroid cysts contain multiple septa with connective tissue and solid elements (Fig. 3.6). Doppler examination may show vascularity in the epithelial solid components. Comet tail artifact is a characteristic of dense colloid cysts (Fig. 3.7), and when present it strongly suggests a benign nodule (Ahuja et al. 1996). Cystic lesions are often the result of hemorrhage or degenerative change. Hemorrhagic cysts are divided into "young cysts" and "older cysts." "Young cysts" present with tiny echoes that are evenly scattered, while "older cysts" are usually anechogenic and may contain blood sediment (Ruchała and Szczepanek 2010).

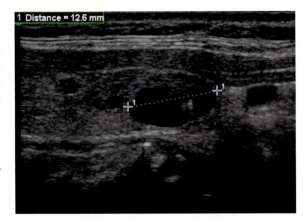

Fig. 3.7 Longitudinal image showing the comet tail sign in a colloid cystic nodule

3.3.2 Goiter

On U/S, the gland is either symmetrically or asymmetrically enlarged. In simple diffuse goiter, imaging will reveal homogeneous normal echogenicity, while in multinodular goiter the echogenicity is heterogeneous with multiple nodules (Fig. 3.8). However, even in simple diffuse goiter, some minimal heterogeneity with fibrotic or calcified areas may be noted. Ultrasound evaluation of a multinodular goiter is important as it can demonstrate the dominant or an enlarging nodule to be subjected for FNA. However, the prevalence of cancer in a nodule in a multinodular goiter is independent of the number of nodules present (Marqusee et al. 2000; Papini et al. 2002). As such, in a multinodular goiter, each nodule has its own cancer risk, and time

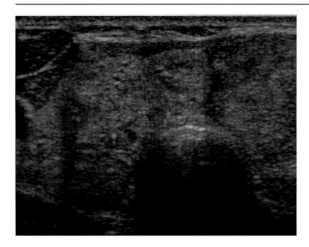

Fig. 3.8 Transverse image of a multinodular goiter with confluent nodules

should be spent by the sonographer to fully examine all nodules.

The most common type of nodule seen in a multinodular goiter is the colloid or hyperplastic (adenomatous) nodule. These nodules are usually rounded with well-defined margins. They are commonly isoechoic or hypoechoic and, less frequently, hyperechoic. Hyperplastic nodules that undergo degeneration have a cystic element often with septations. Calcifications may be seen either central or peripheral (eggshell). Comet tail sign is also noted secondary to the nodule's colloid composition. Halo may or may not be present, and the vascularity may range from completely avascular to peripheral and/or intranodular.

3.3.3 Thyroid Nodules and Characteristics

A thyroid nodule is a distinct ultrasonographically detected lesion within the thyroid gland, distinguished because it has a different echogenicity compared to the adjacent parenchyma. Palpable nodules are present in up to 7% of the population, but U/S examination can detect nodules in up to 68% of the population (Guth et al. 2009). Malignancy is more common in nodules found in patients younger than 20 or older than 60 years. Gender also plays a role, with men having a higher risk for malignancy. A previous history of neck irradiation or family history of thyroid cancer are also risk factors. Nodules that are hard and fixed on clinical examination and are associated with vocal cord paralysis or enlarged neck lymph nodes have a higher risk of malignancy.

Ultrasonography is extremely helpful in assessing cancer risk and should be performed in all patients with suspected thyroid nodules, as palpation alone is not accurate in at least a third of patients with solitary palpable nodules. It is important to note that even with ultrasound, 69% of benign nodules will have at least one suspicious finding of papillary thyroid cancer, and frequently papillary cancers will have non-suspicious features (Wienke et al. 2003; Yuan et al. 2006). It is therefore essential that ultrasonographic evaluation should be followed with fine needle aspiration (FNA) of the suspicious nodules. Important ultrasound features that are recorded are (1) solitary nodules or multinodularity; (2) size, as three orthogonal dimensions; (3) nodule composition; (4) echogenicity; (5) calcifications; (6) shapes and margins; and (7) vascularity.

3.3.3.1 Solitary Nodules Versus Multinodularity

Ultrasound may detect single or multiple nodules; however, oftentimes even in cases where a solitary nodule is discovered, closer and more detailed examination will reveal additional, small difficult-to-detect nodules. Malignant nodules can often coexist with benign ones, and in addition, papillary carcinoma is often multifocal. In multinodular goiter, ultrasound often shows multiple hypoechoic, isoechoic, and hyperechoic areas in combination with complex/cystic colloid lesions. In these cases, radionuclide imaging can also be used as it can help determine the areas to be biopsied. Multiple reports propose that the risk of malignancy in a thyroid with multiple nodules is comparable to the one with a solitary nodule. A solitary nodule had a similar likelihood of being malignant as a nodule that was one of several (18.8% vs. 17.3%) (Mihailescu and Schneider 2008).

U/S-guided FNA along with evaluation of nodule features will provide a good indication of benignity or suspicion of carcinoma. In the case where the patient presents with multiple nodules, one or more nodules may be selected for U/S-guided FNA. Prioritization of the significant nodules and subjecting those to FNA is a difficult clinical task and much dependent on the skills and experience of the ultrasonographer.

3.3.3.2 Size

The size of a nodule can be measured accurately by the scale on the ultrasound screen and is generally recorded in three orthogonal dimensions. Current high-resolution transducers can visualize nodules as small as 2 mm in diameter, making detection of miniscule thyroid and parathyroid tumors possible. The use of curved array transducers rather than linear array can provide accurate size measurements of large nodules. Determination of nodule size is essential in comparing changes over time. However, size alone is not considered a reliable means in predicting or excluding malignancy.

Both the European Thyroid Association and the American Thyroid Association have issued clinical practice guidelines suggesting that nodules larger than 1.0 cm and are nonfunctioning undergo further evaluation by FNA (Pacini et al. 2006). Nodules that are smaller than 1.0 cm but have suspicious ultrasound characteristics also require further investigation. These characteristics are hypoechogenicity, irregular margins, microcalcifications, intranodular vascularity, and regional lymphadenopathy. In malignancy, size is important, as smaller tumors tend to have more favorable prognosis (Hoang et al. 2007). Although nodules larger than 3–4 cm seem to have an increased risk of malignancy, benign nodules can also markedly enlarge.

3.3.3.3 Nodule Composition

A nodule can be solid, complex (mixed solid and cystic) (Fig. 3.9), or purely cystic. Additionally, nodules can be further subcategorized as predominantly solid or predominantly cystic. Most nodules are solid, while about a third appear to have some cystic component, and it is generally observed that the more the solid portion of the nodule, the greater the risk of malignancy (Lee et al. 2009). A cyst is a thin-walled, spherical structure without any internal solid elements allowing sound transmission with little reflection and subsequently posterior acoustic enhancement. Completely cystic nodules are rare, as high-resolution ultrasound will exhibit, upon close examination, small solid components or debris. Solid nodules pose a higher risk of malignancy, while complex nodules with a dominant fluid component, or purely cystic nodules, tend to be benign (Frates et al. 2005). These complex nodules most often represent benign lesions with cystic degeneration or hemorrhage. Although a predominantly cystic nodule is often benign, FNA should always be performed since rarely papillary thyroid carcinoma can present with cystic changes.

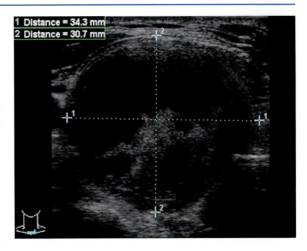

Fig. 3.9 Transverse image of a complex nodule

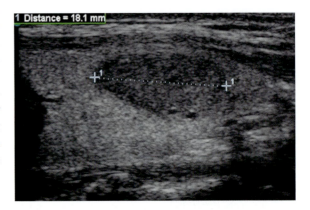

Fig. 3.10 Longitudinal image showing a hypoechoic nodule

3.3.3.4 Echogenicity

The echogenicity of the nodule is based on its ability to transmit or reflect the ultrasound wave. This is compared to the parenchymal echogenicity of the thyroid gland lobe. Another reference is the comparison to the surrounding neck muscles. Hypoechoic nodules have less echogenicity compared to the thyroid parenchyma (Fig. 3.10), whereas hyperechoic nodules are more echogenic (Fig. 3.11). Isoechoic nodules have the same ultrasound characteristics as normal thyroid tissue (Fig. 3.12). Malignant nodules most often appear solid and hypoechoic. However, a large number of benign nodules are also hypoechoic, so this feature has a low positive predictive value. A hypoechoic nodule is more likely to be benign as the substantial majority of nodules

3 Thyroid Ultrasound

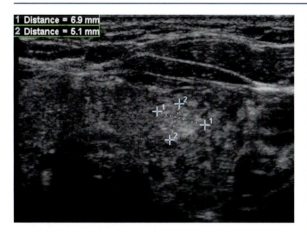

Fig. 3.11 Transverse image showing a small hyperechoic nodule in a patient with Hashimoto's thyroiditis

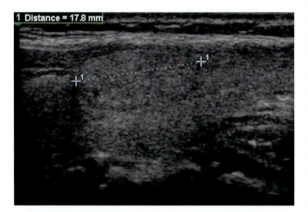

Fig. 3.12 Longitudinal image showing an isoechoic nodule with thin halo

are benign. On the other hand, a primarily hyperechoic nodule indicates benign nature, and FNA may not be needed unless other suspicious characteristics are present.

Isoechoic nodules are identified due to the presence of halo, a peripheral sonolucent rim of decreased echogenicity. A halo which can be thin or thick, complete or incomplete, and represents a capsule/pseudocapsule caused by compressed thyroid tissue, inflammatory changes, or peripheral vessels is often detected by color and power Doppler (Fig. 3.13). Although a thick, absent, or incomplete halo can be an indicator of malignancy, it cannot be considered as an accurate solitary predictive factor (Rago et al. 1998; Wong and Ahuja 2005). A smooth, thin, and complete halo is often seen in benign nodules.

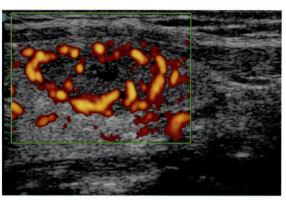

Fig. 3.13 Longitudinal image of a nodule with perinodular vascularity by power Doppler examination

3.3.3.5 Presence of Calcifications

Calcifications are reflective echogenic foci that cause ultrasound attenuation and appear as bright spots within or around a nodule or can be found alone in the thyroid parenchyma. With ultrasound, many nodules appear to have calcifications which can be classified into three groups: microcalcifications, coarse calcifications (macro), or peripheral calcifications (rim or eggshell). Clinically, the presence of calcifications in thyroid nodules raises suspicion for malignancy, but the type of calcifications and the location can provide more important information.

Microcalcifications are 1 mm or less round crystalline calcific deposits most often representing psammoma bodies. Depending on their size they may or may not cause acoustic shadowing. Among nodule characteristics identified with ultrasound, microcalcifications provide the strongest indication of malignancy with a high positive predictive value (Fig. 3.14) (Triggiani et al. 2008). They have been described in both differentiated and undifferentiated thyroid carcinoma, in benign follicular nodules as well as in autoimmune thyroiditis. The presence of microcalcifications without the presence of a definitive nodule also increases the risk of malignancy, and further evaluation should be undertaken.

Macrocalcifications represent dystrophic areas and tissue necrosis and can be found in both malignant and benign nodules. They are larger than 1 mm in size and are generally accompanied with acoustic shadowing (Fig. 3.15). Macrocalcifications can often coexist with microcalcifications in papillary carcinoma. Large, coarse calcifications are also prevalent in medullary carcinoma or metastatic cervical nodes from medullary carcinoma.

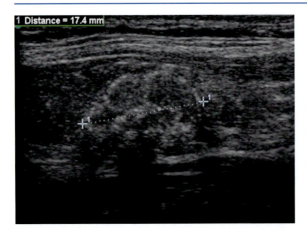

Fig. 3.14 Longitudinal image of papillary carcinoma with irregular margins and microcalcifications

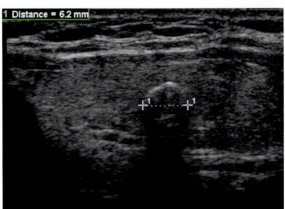

Fig. 3.16 Longitudinal image showing a small nodule with eggshell calcifications

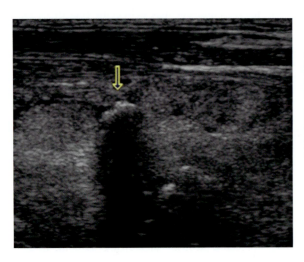

Fig. 3.15 Longitudinal image showing coarse calcifications (*arrow*) causing acoustic shadowing in a patient with Grave's disease

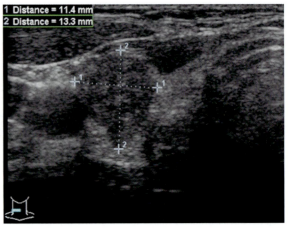

Fig. 3.17 Papillary carcinoma: transverse image showing a solid hypoechoic nodule with microlobulated margins and AT ratio >1

Peripheral calcifications surround the nodule like an eggshell (Fig. 3.16) and are thought to be a benign characteristic. Although such calcifications are commonly seen in benign multinodular goiters, there have been reports of malignancy as well (Yaturu and Rainer 2010). Associated penetration of the rim calcification should be particularly worrisome to the clinician as it can indicate aggressive behavior and invasion by the cancer (Park et al. 2009).

3.3.3.6 Shapes and Margins

Both the shape and margins of nodules are important characteristics to consider when evaluating thyroid nodules. On ultrasound, benign thyroid nodules are more likely to be smooth, well rounded, with regular, sharp, well-demarcated borders. Malignant nodules often appear ill-defined with irregular borders. The shape of a solid nodule is categorized as: ovoid to round, taller than wide (when the anteroposterior diameter is longer than its transverse: AT ratio >1) (Fig. 3.17), or irregular. There is high specificity and positive predictive value for malignancy when the nodule is taller than wide.

Nodule margins are categorized as smooth, spiculated/microlobulated, or ill-defined (Moon et al. 2011). A thyroid nodule is characterized as ill-defined when more than 50% of its border is not clearly marked. Ill-defined margins point to invasion of the surrounding thyroid and could signify an aggressive cancer. However, both ill-defined margins and microlobulations are often seen in benign nodules.

3.3.3.7 Vascularity

Both color flow imaging and power Doppler assess thyroid nodule vascularity with power Doppler being more sensitive in examining smaller lesions.

Color flow patterns are categorized as: (a) Type I: no blood flow, (b) Type II: perinodular flow, and (c) Type III: intranodular blood flow (perinodular vessels may or may not be present) (Ahuja 2000). Although nonspecific, thyroid cancers may have internal hypervascularity, whereas benign nodules may have peripheral vascularization. However, Type III vascularization can be found in both benign and malignant nodules (Cantisani et al. 2010). Completely avascular nodules are more likely to be benign. Color flow or power Doppler is also valuable in examining the solid component of complex nodules and determining the area to be subjected to FNA. Data obtained from color Doppler imaging should always be used in combination with other suspicious ultrasound features in a nodule.

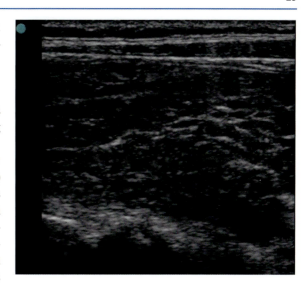

Fig. 3.18 Hashimoto's thyroiditis: longitudinal image showing an enlarged gland with heterogeneous echotexture and fibrous linear septations

3.3.4 Thyroiditis

3.3.4.1 Hashimoto's Thyroiditis (Chronic Autoimmune Lymphocytic Thyroiditis)

The thyroid appears enlarged and diffusely heterogeneous (Fig. 3.18) with several hypoechoic areas or inflammatory nodules. Multiple tiny cystic lesions may also be seen providing a "Swiss cheese" appearance (Fig. 3.19) (Yeh et al. 1996). The gland has a lobulated shape with an enlarged isthmus except in the case of the chronic form where the gland is small, atrophic, and diffusely fibrotic. Rarely, coarse calcifications may be noted in the echogenic septa or throughout the hypoechoic parenchyma. Regional cervical and paratracheal benign-appearing lymphadenopathy may be seen, mostly in the initial stages.

Vascularity is either normal or increased similar to Grave's disease. However, in the late stage, the vascularity can be normal, decreased, or absent. In a small number of patients, the gland parenchyma and vascularity may appear completely normal throughout the course of disease. The main difficulty in examining Hashimoto's thyroids is to differentiate between the

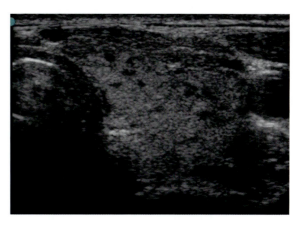

Fig. 3.19 Hashimoto's thyroiditis: transverse image of *left lobe* showing tiny (Swiss cheese appearance) hypoechoic nodules (micronodules)

inflammatory pseudonodules (Fig. 3.20) and the true nodules that can be either benign or malignant (papillary carcinoma or lymphoma) (Gul et al. 2010). Pseudonodules can be hyperechoic or hypoechoic, are poorly defined, and most often do not have sharp outline or a halo. In doubt or in the presence of calcifications, the physician should proceed to FNA in order to rule out malignancy (Anderson et al. 2010), while any associated marked cervical lymphadenopathy increases the suspicion for lymphoma.

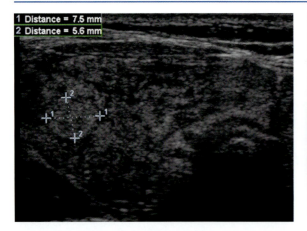

Fig. 3.20 Hashimoto's thyroiditis: transverse image showing hyperechoic areas and fibrosis (pseudonodules)

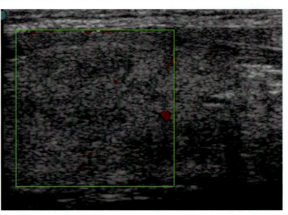

Fig. 3.21 Subacute thyroiditis: hypoechoic ill-defined areas with low vascularity

3.3.4.2 Silent (Painless) Thyroiditis (Subacute Lymphocytic Thyroiditis)

Ultrasonographic features are similar to that of chronic thyroiditis, with predominantly focal hypoechoic regions and hypoechogenicity (Miyakawa et al. 1992). The thyroid volume is slightly increased (but significantly lower than what is observed with Grave's). The gland's size and echotexture usually return to normal once the disease subsides. If it progresses to hypothyroidism, then the features of autoimmune chronic thyroiditis will prevail and become permanent.

3.3.4.3 Acute Thyroiditis

Ultrasonographic findings include focal or diffuse hypoechoic areas with ill-defined margins most often affecting one lobe. Progressively, cystic collections appear which then develop into abscesses extending to extrathyroid tissues. Rarely, the whole gland may be affected. The vascularity is decreased on Doppler examination because of tissue edema, and there is marked pain with transducer pressure. Ultrasound can help to monitor the abscess development, progression, and response to treatment.

3.3.4.4 De Quervain's Thyroiditis (Subacute Granulomatous Thyroiditis)

Subacute thyroiditis is an inflammatory disease often preceded by a viral infection, involving either one or both lobes. On ultrasound, the gland appears enlarged with focal or multiple hypoechoic nodules of unclear margins that are tender when pressed by the transducer (Omori et al. 2008). The extent of hypoechogenic areas in the thyroid is a possible marker for developing thyroid dysfunction (Nishihara et al. 2009). There are no calcifications seen, and the gland may be heterogeneous in texture with either normal or most often decreased vascularity (Fig. 3.21). Cervical lymphadenopathy may or may not be seen. As the disease/acute phase subsides, thyroid gland size decreases with normalization of the gland's parenchyma. Usually by 3–6 months, everything is back to normal, and at that point, the previously seen hypoechoic inflammatory lesions should be reexamined. If persistent, FNA should be performed.

3.3.4.5 Riedel's Thyroiditis

Riedel's thyroiditis is an extremely rare inflammatory disease of unknown cause leading to fibrosis of the gland and adjacent tissues and vessels. On ultrasound examination, the gland is enlarged and very hard to compress with the transducer. Its texture may vary to either inhomogeneous or homogeneously hypoechoic. Ultrasound examination is essential to determine the extent of extrathyroid involvement. Further imaging with CT or MRI may be needed.

3.3.4.6 Grave's Disease

Ultrasound reveals an enlarged thyroid gland often with a prominent pyramidal lobe, enlarged isthmus, and rounded lobes. At the initial stages of the disease, there are small, deeply hypoechoic areas (Fig. 3.22)

3 Thyroid Ultrasound

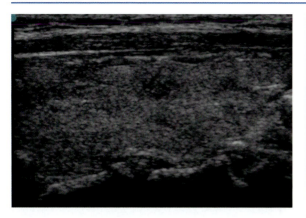

Fig. 3.22 Grave's disease: longitudinal image showing inhomogeneous parenchyma with hypoechoic areas

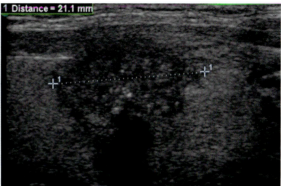

Fig. 3.24 Papillary carcinoma: transverse image showing a solid hypoechoic nodule with irregular margins and microcalcifications

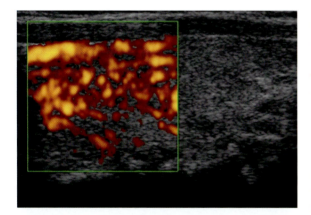

Fig. 3.23 Grave's disease: longitudinal image showing markedly increased vascularity ("thyroid inferno") by power Doppler examination

that will eventually progress to diffuse hypoechoic regions secondary to lymphocytic infiltration. In a small number of patients, the thyroid parenchyma may appear normal on ultrasound, while in patients with radioiodine-treated Grave's, the gland is small with diffuse linear hyperechoic areas of fibrosis.

Doppler examination most often shows markedly augmented symmetric thyroid vascularity, also characterized as "thyroid inferno" (Fig. 3.23) (Hari Kumar et al. 2009). Thyroid vascularity may correlate with the development of the disease, and treated Grave's patients show decreased arterial blood flow (Kumar et al. 2009). Thyroid inferno is much more commonly seen in Grave's as compared to Hashimoto's, where the gland's vascularity can be low or normal. In addition in Grave's, unlike in patients with Hashimoto's, the gland may appear normal during the time of remission.

3.4 Thyroid Carcinomas

3.4.1 Papillary Carcinoma

Although papillary carcinoma can present with various ultrasound characteristics, it most often appears as a solid and hypoechoic (70–90%) nodule secondary to the presence of minimal colloid. Calcifications may or may not be present (30%), but the presence of punctuate microcalcifications is a particularly identifiable characteristic of papillary carcinoma (Wong and Ahuja 2005; Jun et al. 2005). Coarse or peripheral calcifications can also be seen (Chan et al. 2003). On careful examination, one can find additional suspicious nodules as it is often multifocal. Nodule margins are irregular (Fig. 3.24) and ill-defined in most tumors, even though some nodules may be partially encapsulated and surrounded by halo. Chaotic, irregular hypervascularity may or may not be present. In more rare cases, it can present as an isoechoic or hyperechoic nodule or with complex composition.

Associated metastatic cervical lymphadenopathy is often present and should be carefully recorded so as to aid the surgeon for lymph node dissection (Moreno et al. 2011). Cervical lymph node examination should always follow a thyroid examination even if no thyroid nodule is identified, as there are rare cases of aggressive/metastatic thyroid microcarcinomas.

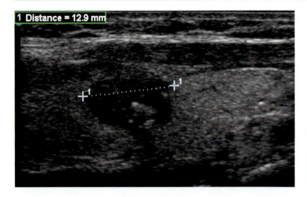

Fig. 3.25 Medullary carcinoma: longitudinal image showing a hypoechoic nodule with calcifications

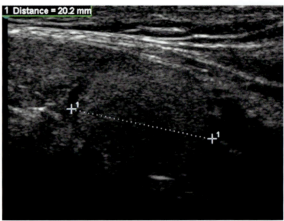

Fig. 3.26 Benign follicular lesion (adenoma): longitudinal image showing a solid homogeneous oval isoechoic nodule

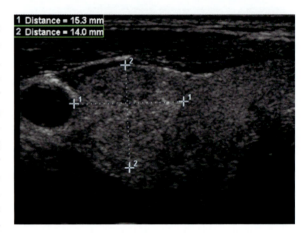

Fig. 3.27 Benign follicular lesion: transverse image showing a solid oval isoechoic nodule with some dot microcalcifications

3.4.2 Medullary Carcinoma

The ultrasound characteristics of medullary carcinoma are frequently similar to those seen in papillary carcinoma (Cai et al. 2010; Kim et al. 2009a; Lee et al. 2010b). Nodules are predominantly solid with marked hypoechogenicity (Fig. 3.25), and there is often an irregular halo or complete absence of halo. Calcifications are most often present and appear as dense echogenic foci due to amyloid depositions and subsequent calcifications (Wong and Ahuja 2005). In medullary cancer, there is a higher tendency for coarse calcifications with posterior shadowing. Nodules are irregularly shaped with either well-defined or spiculated, ill-defined margins. Color flow Doppler shows either chaotic intranodular vascularity or increased perinodular vascularization. In familial medullary carcinoma, the tumors are multifocal and bilateral. As in papillary carcinoma, there is often associated metastatic cervical lymphadenopathy.

3.4.3 Anaplastic Carcinoma

Anaplastic carcinoma presents as a diffuse enlarging irregular mass. These lesions are hypoechoic with ill-defined margins, calcifications, and large areas of necrosis (in 74% of the tumors) (Takashima et al. 1990). There is invasion of the gland capsule and infiltration of adjacent vascular structures and muscles.

3.4.4 Follicular Lesions

Follicular lesion implies either follicular adenoma or carcinoma, as it is not possible to distinguish between the two with either ultrasound imaging or FNA (Mihai et al. 2009). Follicular lesions appear predominantly oval, solid, and homogeneous (Figs. 3.26 and 3.27). They are either isoechoic, hyperechoic, or hypoechoic, whereas heterogeneous echotexture may raise suspicion for malignancy. Calcifications are rarely seen, and margins are well defined and regular. Follicular lesions often have hypoechoic halo secondary to perinodular vascularity. Intranodular hypervascularization is also common. Thyroid follicular lesions are often found enlarged and can present with cystic or hemorrhagic degenerating changes. Larger lesion size, absence of halo, hypoechoic appearance, and absence of cystic change may favor follicular carcinoma diagnosis (Sillery et al. 2010).

Hurthle cell lesions present similarly to follicular lesions. These nodules are commonly solid and can be either hypoechoic, isoechoic, or hyperechoic or can present with heterogeneous appearance. As in follicular lesions, they may have a halo that can be complete or incomplete. Calcifications are rarely encountered in these lesions, and vascularity can range from peripheral blood flow only with no internal vasculature to extensively vascularized nodules both peripherally and internally (Lee et al. 2010a).

3.4.5 Lymphoma

Malignant thyroid lymphoma can present as a solid focal mass or diffuse large lesion (Sakorafas et al. 2010). Lymphomas are mainly hypoechoic; however in some cases they may present with heterogeneous echogenicity and with areas of cystic necrosis. Ultrasound features of Hashimoto's thyroiditis are often present with inhomogeneity and fibrous strands. Lymphoma may spread beyond the thyroid in 50–60% of patients. On color Doppler imaging, lymphomas may appear either with low or increased disorganized vasculature. Enlarged and rounded, irregular cervical lymph nodes are often present.

3.5 Ultrasound Examination of Neck Lymph Nodes and Thyroid Carcinoma Follow-Up

There are about 300 lymph nodes in the normal neck, divided into seven different levels: level I: submental and submandibular; levels II, III, and IV: upper-mid-lower jugular; level V: posterior triangle; level VI: pretracheal and paratracheal; and level VII: anterior mediastinum and supraclavicular. Each lymph node has a cortical and a medullary region and is covered by a fibrous capsule. The main artery enters at the hilus and then branches into arterioles. With ultrasound, we examine the size, shape, echogenic hilum, level of echogenicity, presence of necrosis, extracapsular spread, and calcifications.

Normal lymph nodes are well defined and oval- or bean-shaped. They are hypoechoic or isoechoic compared to normal thyroid tissue and have an echodense central hilum (Fig. 3.28). Their vascular pattern can be categorized as (a) hilar, where blood flow is limited to the hilus; (b) peripheral, where blood flow is along the periphery and has branches that do not arise from the hilum; (c) mixed, where both hilar and peripheral flow

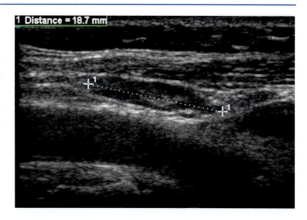

Fig. 3.28 Longitudinal image of a normal cervical lymph node with echogenic hilum

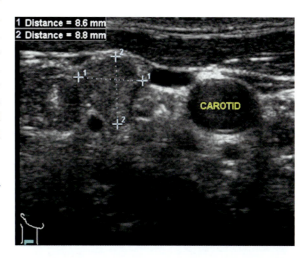

Fig. 3.29 Transverse image of a metastatic rounded lymph node in the right lateral neck (papillary carcinoma). Short/long axis ratio >0.5

is present; and (d) avascular, where no flow is detected. Reactive or inflammatory nodes are large, but they tend to maintain their oval shape. These nodes have increased hilar vascularity. In contrast, metastatic lymph nodes have a rounded shape (short/long axis ratio >0.5 in transverse view) (Fig. 3.29) with absence of the echogenic hilar line, contain calcifications (Fig. 3.30), may be fully or partially cystic, and have peripheral or chaotic vascularity (Landry et al. 2011; Kessler et al. 2003; Langer and Mandel 2008). Although ultrasonography is a good tool with high sensitivity for the detection of cervical metastases, it has low specificity since benign lymphadenopathies are very common occurrences.

Ultrasound-guided FNA is performed to evaluate suspicious lymph nodes. However, as lymph node

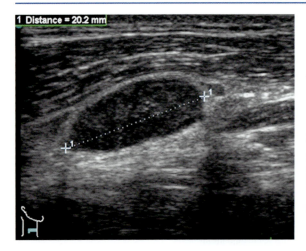

Fig. 3.30 Longitudinal image of metastatic papillary carcinoma lymph node with absent hilar line and microcalcifications

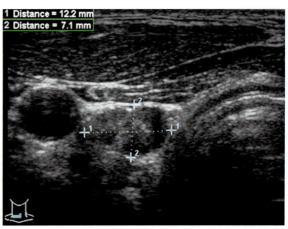

Fig. 3.32 Transverse image showing a right paratracheal metastatic lymph node with calcifications

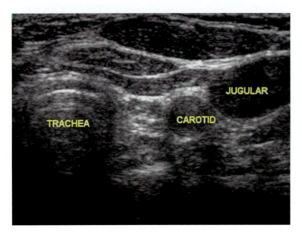

Fig. 3.31 Postoperative neck: transverse image of hyperechoic connective tissue at the left thyroid bed

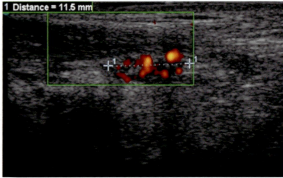

Fig. 3.33 Longitudinal image showing a metastatic highly vascular paratracheal lymph node (papillary carcinoma)

cytology is frequently negative (absence of malignant epithelial cells), thyroglobulin (Tg) measurement from the needle washout fluid should always be performed (Baskin 2004; Kim et al. 2009b; Cunha et al. 2007). The procedure involves washing the needle with saline solution and then measuring Tg levels. Although Tg washout measurement is more accurate compared to conventional cytology in confirming malignancy, the technique is highly dependent on the skills and experience of the ultrasonographer.

For thyroid carcinoma follow-up, in addition to lymph nodes, the ultrasonographer should pay particular attention in imaging the postoperative thyroid bed (Fig. 3.31). Any finding such as residual thyroid tissue, scar, fibrotic changes, or suture granulomas should be clearly marked (Kim et al. 2009c). Cystic lesions, solid hypoechoic/ irregular paratracheal lymph nodes (Fig. 3.32), areas with increased vascularity (Fig. 3.33), or calcifications should raise suspicion for thyroid cancer recurrence (Kamaya et al. 2011). Neck ultrasonography with lymph node mapping should always be performed preoperatively so as to guide the surgeon to perform appropriate cervical lymph node dissection (Hwang and Orloff 2011). Any disease should be clearly marked in an ultrasound neck diagram/map. This practice has been clearly proven to alter the surgical approach in patients undergoing thyroidectomy.

3.6 Ultrasound of the Parathyroids

Parathyroid glands have an oval or rounded shape and are between 2 and 7 mm in size. They are isoechoic and are extremely difficult to be visualized even with very-high-resolution ultrasound. Most people have four parathyroids, two at the upper poles of the thyroid and two at the lower poles with the two superior glands often having a smaller size compared to the two inferior. The superior parathyroids are found posterior to the mid-upper thyroid lobe, whereas the interior parathyroids are found near the inferior thyroid lobe. However, the location of the inferior glands can vary to intrathyroidal, upper mediastinum, retroesophageal, retrotracheal, or along the common carotid artery (undescended). Autopsy studies have demonstrated that a small percentage of people have three glands, five glands, six glands, or very rarely more glands.

Ultrasound is essential for the identification and localization of parathyroid adenomas (or carcinoma), parathyroid hyperplasia, or parathyroid cysts (Levy et al. 2011). For scanning, patient positioning is crucial where the neck has to be fully hyperextended especially for imaging low neck retrotracheal lesions. High-frequency ultrasound transducers are used for optimal imaging of superficial parathyroid lesions, whereas low-frequency transducers are used for examining deep retrosternal lesions. It is important that the thyroid gland is evaluated first before examining the parathyroids, and scanning should be performed both transversely and longitudinally throughout the neck (Gates et al. 2009; Halenka et al. 2008). Color and/or power Doppler examination must always be performed in addition to standard gray scale sonography.

Parathyroid adenomas are usually homogeneously hypoechoic (Fig. 3.34) compared to the thyroid secondary to high cellularity and decrease in adipose cells. Even though some adenomas may be isoechoic or with heterogeneous echotexture, most parathyroid lesions are solid, with well-defined margins. Rarely, a cystic component with septations may be seen. Parathyroid adenomas are mostly oval, but their shape can vary due to anatomical pressure, leading to a triangular, flat, bilobar, or elongated extended shape. A distinctive echogenic line can be seen between the adenoma and the thyroid lobe (compressed parathyroid capsule). Calcifications are rare, while a "vascular arc" pattern and diffuse hypervascularity within the adenoma are revealed by color flow imaging. Most adenomas characteristically have a feeding artery (polar) (Fig. 3.35), while avascular adenomas can also be seen (usually smaller lesions). Color and/or power Doppler helps differentiate parathyroid lesions from lymph nodes and thyroid nodules.

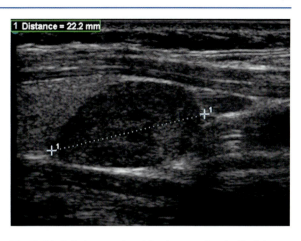

Fig. 3.34 Inferior parathyroid adenoma: longitudinal image showing an adenoma inferior to the right thyroid pole

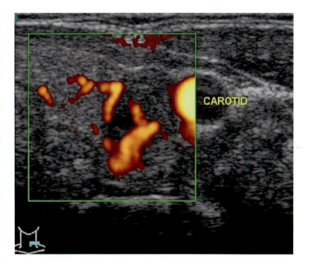

Fig. 3.35 Transverse image of a left superior parathyroid adenoma with polar artery

Although parathyroid hyperplasia lesions may be more rounded compared to adenomas, it is extremely difficult with U/S to differentiate between the two. Parathyroid carcinoma is uncommon, and it also cannot be differentiated by U/S from benign adenomas. Carcinomas are usually large and, although uncommon, can demonstrate invasion of nearby tissues. Their margins can be irregular, and calcifications can be seen. However, in most cases, parathyroid carcinomas look identical to benign adenomas.

When there is doubt, ultrasound-guided FNA of parathyroid lesions can be performed. It is now used more often to confirm the presence of a parathyroid tumor and to differentiate from other paratracheal or neck lesions. The technique is based on measuring parathyroid hormone (PTH) from the needle aspirate that is rinsed with normal saline (Kwak et al. 2009; Giusti et al. 2009). If the PTH level is high, then the presence of a parathyroid lesion is confirmed. It is highly specific compared to parathyroid cytology that most times provides inconclusive results. However, the majority of parathyroid lesions do not need to be subjected to FNA as the experienced ultrasonographer can easily localize and confirm them.

3.7 Thyroid Interventional Ultrasound

3.7.1 Percutaneous Ethanol Injections (PEI)

Ultrasound-guided percutaneous ethanol injection therapy of thyroid lesions has been used for the last two decades. It is an outpatient procedure where a thin (spinal) needle is used to inject sterile 95% ethanol percutaneously under U/S guidance. Alcohol is a sclerosing agent that draws water out of the cells, leading to denaturation of cellular proteins and direct coagulative necrosis. Subsequently, there is decrease in vascularity that will eventually lead to fibrosis. The amount of alcohol used depends on the type of lesion, and the procedure can be repeated multiple times (Brzac 2009). High-frequency transducers are used in order to obtain the highest resolution for needle guidance and control during the procedure.

PEI is most frequently used in thyroid cystic lesions where depending on the amount of ethanol injected, significant volume reduction or cyst disappearance can be achieved in lesions, causing local neck symptoms or for cosmetic issues (Sung et al. 2011; Kanotra et al. 2008). It is more difficult to treat toxic nodules as many treatment sessions may be required in order to normalize thyroid function, and this increases the risk of side effects. In poor surgical candidates, PEI can also be used to ablate parathyroid adenomas or hyperplastic parathyroid lesions as well as metastatic thyroid cancer neck lymph nodes. Side effects include burning sensation, severe neck pain, or transient vocal cord paralysis secondary to diffusion of ethanol into nearby tissues.

3.7.2 Percutaneous Laser Ablation (PLA)

Percutaneous laser ablation involves laser energy delivery through optical fibers positioned percutaneously into the thyroid nodule. This is done as an outpatient procedure under ultrasound real-time guidance, and the number of needles as well as their distribution depends on the size, shape, and position of the nodule. It is important that the needles are accurately placed in order to ensure successful laser irradiation and nodule shrinkage. Various sessions of PLA have shown to achieve nodule volume decreases of 50% or more (Valcavi et al. 2010). Complications include neck pain after the procedure, fever, hematoma, or skin burn. A major problem involved with the procedure is the difficulty to distinguish the boundaries of the laser-induced tissue damage, as ultrasonography findings do not correlate well with the area of thermal necrosis which results. Furthermore, there is a risk of damaging surrounding neck structures and so PLA should be performed in specialized centers only. PLA can be useful in treating benign large hypofunctioning nodules as an alternative option in patients who decline surgery or are poor surgical candidates.

3.7.3 Radiofrequency Ablation (RFA)

RFA is also a minimally invasive, relatively safe and effective technique with great potential for treating large thyroid nodules. It is performed in an outpatient setting and involves inserting large needle electrodes into the thyroid nodule under ultrasound guidance (Kharchenko et al. 2010). The radiofrequency electric fields pass ionic currents into the nodule causing local hyperthermia leading to cell death and coagulation necrosis.

Side effects included bleeding, neck swelling, and burning sensation in the neck. This technique has been proven effective in reducing nodule volume and treating hyperfunctioning thyroid nodules (Spiezia et al. 2009; Baek et al. 2010).

3.7.4 High-Intensity Focused Ultrasound (HIFU)

High-intensity focused ultrasound is another newly developed noninvasive technique that allows selective destruction of thyroid nodules without using needles or punctures. The procedure seems to be safe and is performed in an outpatient setting, where a converging beam of powerful acoustic waves is focused onto a given target causing thermal destruction of thyroid tissue by coagulation necrosis, hemorrhage, thrombosis, and fibrosis. Preliminary results from use of HIFU in treatment of thyroid nodules show the technique to be highly effective with minimal adverse events such as mild pain, skin burns, subcutaneous edema, or transient impaired vocal cord mobility. HIFU has also been evaluated for the treatment of primary hyperparathyroidism (Kovatcheva et al. 2010).

References

Ahuja AT (2000) The thyroid and parathyroids. In: Ahuja A, Evans R (eds) Practical head and neck ultrasound. Greenwich Medical Media Ltd, London

Ahuja A, Chick W, King W, Metreweli C (1996) Clinical significance of the comet-tail artifact in thyroid ultrasound. J Clin Ultrasound 24(3):129–133

Albayrak Y, Albayrak F, Kaya Z et al (2011) A case of papillary carcinoma in a thyroglossal cyst without a carcinoma in the thyroid gland. Diagn Cytopathol 39(1):38–41

Anderson L, Middleton WD, Teefey SA et al (2010) Hashimoto thyroiditis: part 2, sonographic analysis of benign and malignant nodules in patients with diffuse Hashimoto thyroiditis. AJR Am J Roentgenol 195(1):216–222

Baek JH, Kim YS, Lee D et al (2010) Benign predominantly solid thyroid nodules: prospective study of efficacy of sonographically guided radiofrequency ablation versus control condition. AJR Am J Roentgenol 194(4):1137–1142

Baskin HJ (2004) Detection of recurrent papillary thyroid carcinoma by thyroglobulin assessment in the needle washout after fine-needle aspiration of suspicious lymph nodes. Thyroid 14(11):959–963

Baskin HJ, Duick DS, Levine RA (2008) Thyroid ultrasound and ultrasound-guided FNA, 2nd edn. Springer Science and Business Media, New York

Brunese L, Romeo A, Iorio S et al (2008) A new marker for diagnosis of thyroid papillary cancer: B-flow twinkling sign. J Ultrasound Med 27(8):1187–1194

Brzac HT (2009) Ultrasonography-guided therapeutic procedures in the neck region. Acta Med Croatica 63(Suppl 3):21–27

Cai S, Liu H, Li WB et al (2010) Ultrasonographic features of medullary thyroid carcinoma and their diagnostic values. Chin Med J (Engl) 123(21):3074–3078

Cantisani V, Catania A, De Antoni E et al (2010) Is pattern III as evidenced by US color-Doppler useful in predicting thyroid nodule malignancy? Large-scale retrospective analysis. Clin Ter 161(2):e49–e52

Chan BK, Desser TS, McDougall IR et al (2003) Common and uncommon sonographic features of papillary thyroid carcinoma. J Ultrasound Med 22(10):1083–1090

Cunha N, Rodrigues F, Curado F et al (2007) Thyroglobulin detection in fine-needle aspirates of cervical lymph nodes: a technique for the diagnosis of metastatic differentiated thyroid cancer. Eur J Endocrinol 157:101–107

Frates MC, Benson CB, Charboneau JW et al (2005) Management of thyroid nodules detected at US: society of radiologists in ultrasound consensus conference statement. Radiology 237(3):794–800

Gates JD, Benavides LC, Shriver CD et al (2009) Preoperative thyroid ultrasound in all patients undergoing parathyroidectomy? J Surg Res 155(2):254–260

Gietka-Czernel M, Kochman M, Bujalska K et al (2010) Real-time ultrasound elastography – a new tool for diagnosing thyroid nodules. Endokrynol Pol 61(6):652–657

Giusti M, Dolcino M, Vera L et al (2009) Institutional experience of PTH evaluation on fine-needle washing after aspiration biopsy to locate hyperfunctioning parathyroid tissue. J Zhejiang Univ Sci B 10(5):323–330

Gul K, Dirikoc A, Kiyak G et al (2010) The association between thyroid carcinoma and Hashimoto's thyroiditis: the ultrasonographic and histopathologic characteristics of malignant nodules. Thyroid 20(8):873–878

Guth S, Theune U, Aberle J et al (2009) Very high prevalence of thyroid nodules detected by high frequency (13 MHz) ultrasound examination. Eur J Clin Invest 39(8):699–706

Halenka M, Frysak Z, Koranda P, Kucerova L (2008) Cystic parathyroid adenoma within a multinodular goiter: a rare cause of primary hyperparathyroidism. J Clin Ultrasound 36(4):243–246

Hari Kumar KV, Pasupuleti V, Jayaraman M et al (2009) Role of thyroid Doppler in differential diagnosis of thyrotoxicosis. Endocr Pract 15(1):6–9

Hegedüs L (2001) Thyroid ultrasound. Endocrinol Metab Clin North Am 30(2):339–360

Hegedus L, Perril H, Poulsen LR et al (1983) The determination of thyroid volume by ultrasound and its relationship to body weight, age and sex in normal subjects. J Clin Endocrinol Metab 56(2):260–263

Hoang JK, Lee WK, Lee M et al (2007) US features of thyroid malignancy: pearls and pitfalls. Radiographics 27:847–865

Holter MR (2010) Emerging technology in head and neck ultrasonography. Otolaryngol Clin North Am 43(6):1267–1274

Hwang HS, Orloff LA (2011) Efficacy of preoperative neck ultrasound in the detection of cervical lymph node metastasis from thyroid cancer. Laryngoscope 121(3):487–491

Jun P, Chow LC, Jeffrey RB (2005) The sonographic features of papillary thyroid carcinomas: pictorial essay. Ultrasound Q 21(1):39–45

Kamaya A, Gross M, Akatsu H, Jeffrey RB (2011) Recurrence in the thyroidectomy bed: sonographic findings. AJR Am J Roentgenol 196(1):66–70

Kanotra SP, Lateef M, Kirmani O (2008) Non-surgical management of benign thyroid cysts: use of ultrasound-guided ethanol ablation. Postgrad Med J 84(998):639–643

Kessler A, Rappaport Y, Blank A et al (2003) Cystic appearance of cervical lymph nodes is characteristic of metastatic papillary thyroid carcinoma. J Clin Ultrasound 31(1):21–25

Kharchenko VP, Kotlyarov PM, Mogutov MS et al (2010) Ultrasound diagnostics of thyroid disease. Springer, Berlin/Heidelberg

Kim MJ, Kim EK, Park SI et al (2008) US-guided fine-needle aspiration of thyroid nodules: indications, techniques, results. Radiographics 28(7):1869–1886

Kim SH, Kim BS, Jung SL et al (2009a) Ultrasonographic findings of medullary thyroid carcinoma: a comparison with papillary thyroid carcinoma. Korean J Radiol 10(2):101–105

Kim MJ, Kim EK, Kim BM et al (2009b) Thyroglobulin measurement in fine-needle aspirate washouts: the criteria for neck node dissection for patients with thyroid cancer. Clin Endocrinol (Oxf) 70(1):145–151

Kim JH, Lee JH, Shong YK et al (2009c) Ultrasound features of suture granulomas in the thyroid bed after thyroidectomy for papillary thyroid carcinoma with an emphasis on their differentiation from locally recurrent thyroid carcinomas. Ultrasound Med Biol 35(9):1452–1457

King AD, Ahuja AT, To EW (2000) Staging papillary carcinoma of the thyroid: magnetic resonance imaging vs ultrasound of the neck. Clin Radiol 55(3):222–226

Kovatcheva RD, Vlahov JD, Shinkov AD et al (2010) High-intensity focused ultrasound to treat primary hyperparathyroidism: a feasibility study in four patients. AJR Am J Roentgenol 195(4):830–835

Kumar KV, Vamsikrishna P, Verma A et al (2009) Utility of colour Doppler sonography in patients with Graves' disease. West Indian Med J 58(6):566–570

Kwak JY, Kim EK, Moon HJ et al (2009) Parathyroid incidentalomas detected on routine ultrasound-directed fine-needle aspiration biopsy in patients referred for thyroid nodules and the role of parathyroid hormone analysis in the samples. Thyroid 19(7):743–748

Landry CS, Grubbs EG, Busaidy NL et al (2011) Cystic lymph nodes in the lateral neck as indicators of metastatic papillary thyroid cancer. Endocr Pract 17(2):240–244

Langer JE, Mandel SJ (2008) Sonographic imaging of cervical lymph nodes in patients with thyroid cancer. Neuroimaging Clin N Am 18(3):479–489

Lee MJ, Kim EK, Kwak JY, Kim MJ (2009) Partially cystic thyroid nodules on ultrasound: probability of malignancy and sonographic differentiation. Thyroid 19(4):341–346

Lee SK, Rho BH, Woo SKJ (2010a) Hürthle cell neoplasm: correlation of gray-scale and power Doppler sonographic findings with gross pathology. J Clin Ultrasound 38(4):169–176

Lee S, Shin JH, Han BK, Ko EY (2010b) Medullary thyroid carcinoma: comparison with papillary thyroid carcinoma and application of current sonographic criteria. AJR Am J Roentgenol 194(4):1090–1094

Levy JM, Kandil E, Yau LC et al (2011) Can ultrasound be used as the primary screening modality for the localization of parathyroid disease prior to surgery for primary hyperparathyroidism? A review of 440 cases. ORL J Otorhinolaryngol Relat Spec 73(2):116–120

Luo S, Kim EH, Dighe M, Kim Y (2011) Thyroid nodule classification using ultrasound elastography via linear discriminant analysis. Ultrasonics 51(4):425–431

Lyshchik A, Drozd V, Reiners C (2004) Accuracy of three-dimensional ultrasound for thyroid volume measurement in children and adolescents. Thyroid 14(2):113–120

Marqusee E, Benson CB, Frates MC et al (2000) Usefulness of ultrasonography in the management of nodular thyroid disease. Ann Intern Med 133(9):696–700

Mihai R, Parker AJ, Roskell D, Sadler GP (2009) One in four patients with follicular thyroid cytology (THY3) has a thyroid carcinoma. Thyroid 19(1):33–37

Mihailescu DV, Schneider AB (2008) Size, number, and distribution of thyroid nodules and the risk of malignancy in radiation-exposed patients who underwent surgery. J Clin Endocrinol Metab 93(6):2188–2193

Miyakawa M, Tsushima T, Onoda N et al (1992) Thyroid ultrasonography related to clinical and laboratory findings in patients with silent thyroiditis. J Endocrinol Invest 15(4):289–295

Moon WJ, Baek JH, Jung SL et al (2011) Ultrasonography and the ultrasound-based management of thyroid nodules: consensus statement and recommendations. Korean J Radiol 12(1):1–14

Moreno MA, Agarwal G, de Luna R et al (2011) Preoperative lateral neck ultrasonography as a long-term outcome predictor in papillary thyroid cancer. Arch Otolaryngol Head Neck Surg 137(2):157–162

Nishihara E, Amino N, Ohye H et al (2009) Extent of hypoechogenic area in the thyroid is related with thyroid dysfunction after subacute thyroiditis. J Endocrinol Invest 32(1):33–36

Omori N, Omori K, Takano K (2008) Association of the ultrasonographic findings of subacute thyroiditis with thyroid pain and laboratory findings. Endocr J 55(3):583–588

Pacini F, Schlumberger M, Dralle H et al (2006) European consensus for the management of patients with differentiated thyroid carcinoma of the follicular epithelium. Eur J Endocrinol 154(6):787–803

Papini E, Guglielmi R, Bianchini A et al (2002) Risk of malignancy in nonpalpable thyroid nodules: predictive value of ultrasound and color-Doppler features. J Clin Endocrinol Metab 87(5):1941–1946

Park M, Shin JH, Han BK (2009) Sonography of thyroid nodules with peripheral calcifications. J Clin Ultrasound 37(6):324–328

Rago T, Vitti P, Chiovato L et al (1998) Role conventional ultrasonography and colour flow Doppler sonography in predicting malignancy in 'cold' thyroid nodules. Eur J Endocrinol 138:41–46

Rago T, Scutari M, Santini F et al (2010) Real-time elastosonography: useful tool for refining the presurgical diagnosis in thyroid nodules with indeterminate or nondiagnostic cytology. J Clin Endocrinol Metab 95(12):5274–5280

Ruchała M, Szczepanek E (2010) Thyroid ultrasound – a piece of cake? Endokrynol Pol 61(3):330–344

Sakorafas GH, Kokkoris P, Farley DR (2010) Primary thyroid lymphoma (correction of lympoma): diagnostic and therapeutic dilemmas. Surg Oncol 19(4):e124–e129

Sheth S (2010) Role of ultrasonography in thyroid disease. Otolaryngol Clin North Am 43(2):239–255

Sillery JC, Reading CC, Charboneau JW et al (2010) Thyroid follicular carcinoma: sonographic features of 50 cases. AJR Am J Roentgenol 194(1):44–54

Slapa RZ, Jakubowski WS, Slowinska-Srzednicka J, Szopinski KT (2011) Advantages and disadvantages of 3D ultrasound of thyroid nodules including thin slice volume rendering. Thyroid Res 4(1):1

Solbiati L, Charboneau JW, Osti V et al (2005) The thyroid gland. In: Rumack CM, Wilson SR, Charbonewu JW, Johnson JAM (eds) Diganostic ultrasound, 3rd edn. Elsevier/Mosby, Missouri

Spiezia S, Garberoglio R, Milone F et al (2009) Thyroid nodules and related symptoms are stably controlled two years after radiofrequency thermal ablation. Thyroid 19(3):219–225

Sung JY, Kim YS, Choi H et al (2011) Optimum first-line treatment technique for benign cystic thyroid nodules: ethanol ablation or radiofrequency ablation? AJR Am J Roentgenol 196(2):W210–W214

Takashima S, Morimoto S, Ikezoe J et al (1990) CT evaluation of anaplastic thyroid carcinoma. Am J Roentgenol 154:1079–1085

Triggiani V, Guastamacchia E, Licchelli B, Tafaro E (2008) Microcalcifications and psammoma bodies in thyroid tumors. Thyroid 18(9):1017–1018

Valcavi R, Riganti F, Bertani A et al (2010) Percutaneous laser ablation of cold benign thyroid nodules: a 3-year follow-up study in 122 patients. Thyroid 20(11):1253–1261

Wienke JR, Chong WK, Fielding JR et al (2003) Sonographic features of benign thyroid nodules: interobserver reliability and overlap with malignancy. J Ultrasound Med 22(10):1027–1031

Wong KT, Ahuja AT (2005) Ultrasound of thyroid cancer. Cancer Imaging 5(1):157–166

Xu HX (2009) Contrast-enhanced ultrasound: the evolving applications. World J Radiol 1(1):15–24

Yaturu S, Rainer L (2010) Thyroid nodule with eggshell calcification and oncocytic thyroid cancer. Med Sci Monit 16(3):CS25–CS28

Yeh HC, Futterweit W, Gilbert P (1996) Micronodulation: ultrasonographic sign of Hashimoto's thyroiditis. J Ultrasound Med 15:813–819

Yuan WH, Chiou HJ, Chou YH et al (2006) Gray-scale and color Doppler ultrasonographic manifestations of papillary thyroid carcinoma: analysis of 51 cases. Clin Imaging 30(6):394–401

Zhang B, Jiang YX, Liu JB et al (2010) Utility of contrast-enhanced ultrasound for evaluation of thyroid nodules. Thyroid 20(1):51–57

Fine-Needle Aspiration of Thyroid

Sofia Tseleni-Balafouta

4.1 Introduction

Thyroid enlargement, either diffuse or in the form of thyroid nodules (solitary or multiple), is a very frequent finding, mostly by normal thyroid function tests. The prevalence of the thyroid nodules is estimated about 4% in the population of the western countries with a much higher frequency after performance of ultrasonographic studies (Brander et al. 1991; Christensen et al. 1984). Since the thyroid cancer usually appears as a nodular lesion, it seems reasonable to develop safe tests for the detection of cancer among the by far most common benign hyperplastic nodules. The therapeutic approach for benign nodules can be conservative since the morbidity of the surgical complications would exceed the morbidity of cancer if all thyroid nodules would be removed surgically (Mazzaferri et al. 1988). In this context, the fine-needle aspiration of thyroid emerged as the most useful tool in recognizing thyroid cancer as well as the most accurate and cost-effective test, compared with all noninvasive tests and represents therefore the corner stone in most guidelines for the management of thyroid nodules (Gharib et al. 2010). After the introduction of this method, the number of malignancies among the surgical specimens of the thyroid increased dramatically, reflecting a more accurate selection of the suspicious nodules for surgery. However, it does not represent an independent diagnostic test since the cytological findings must be interpreted in relation to all clinical and imaging data prior to the final recommendation for the management. Insofar it is obvious that the cytopathologists involved must be aware of the clinical implications of their report and the clinicians must be familiar with the pathological substrate of the nodules as well as with the wording of the pathologists and the possibilities and limitations of the FNA (Buesseniers and Silver 2007).

4.2 The Diagnostic Approach by FNA of Thyroid

4.2.1 Indications and Aims of the Method

According to the mentioned guidelines for the management of the thyroid nodules, an indication for FNA are all thyroid nodules with a maximal diameter more than 1 cm and smaller nodules with suspicious findings on the ultrasound (Gharib et al. 2010). A lower limit for the maximal diameter does not exist; however, we had bad experience in terms of adequacy of the sample for nodules with a diameter smaller than 0.5 cm, probably due to technical difficulties in the sampling procedure in tiny lesions, even under US guidance.

The usual aims of the FNA are:
(a) To recognize an aggressive thyroid tumor and to recognize or at least to suspect a clinically relevant low-grade tumor among all nodular enlargements of thyroid
(b) To confirm the benign diagnosis of a nodule justifying the clinicians for a conservative approach avoiding an unnecessary surgery

---

S. Tseleni-Balafouta
First Department of Pathology,
Medical School – University of Athens,
M. Asias 75, Athens 11527, Greece
e-mail: stseleni@med.uoa.gr

(c) To classify or to suspect some tumor types demanding a special therapeutic approach (like medullary CA, lymphoma, anaplastic CA, or metastatic CA from a primary site other than the thyroid)
(d) To confirm the clinical diagnosis of a diffuse goiter like Hashimoto's disease or subacute thyroiditis de Quervain
(e) To clarify eventual postoperative enlargements in the thyroid region, differentiating mainly between residual or recurrent disease versus granulomas or lymph node enlargements
(f) To explore various neck enlargements outside the thyroid gland, mainly cystic lesions of the neck, and differentiating between ectopic thyroid cysts, thyroglossal duct cysts, branchial cleft cysts, and cystic degenerated lymph node metastases of thyroid papillary CA
(g) To confirm the presence of lymph node metastases

The aims of the FNA cannot be:
(a) The detection of a microscopic focus of papillary CA
(b) The final classification of follicular neoplasias as adenomas or carcinomas
(c) The determination of the extent of the thyroid tumors
(d) The exclusion of lymph node metastases
(e) The safe recognition of a parathyroidal lesion

4.2.2 Contraindications

There are not any established contraindications for performing the method since it is generally safe and simple. A severe hemorrhagic diathesis should be taken under consideration, although the needle chosen can be very thin, minimizing the risk of bleeding. The use of anticoagulative drugs does not represent a contraindication for the method; however, their administration should be discontinued prior to the aspiration.

4.3 The FNA Procedure

4.3.1 The General Concept

The concept of the method is based on the entering of a thin needle in a lesion in order to disrupt the tissue, to gain small pieces of it, to expel them on a slide and to make smears at the site ("direct smears") or to rinse the needle in a solution (either a balanced salt solution or a preservative), and then to centrifuge the solution and to prepare smears from the sediment ("indirect smears"). Any cyst fluid obtained by aspiration also undergoes centrifugation (eventually with admixture of a fixative) and preparation of indirect smears from the sediment.

Simple as it may seem, the whole procedure frequently leads to unsatisfactory samples, caused mainly by inexperience in entering the nodule, sampling it, or preparing the smears. It is obvious that the FNA diagnostic approach of thyroid nodules is a teamwork, demanding special skills in performing the sampling, evaluating the smears, and correlating the findings with the clinical data.

4.3.2 Who Should Perform the FNA?

Much debate has been made in the past about this question. The only honest answer would be "whoever has the experience to detect a nodule either by palpation or by ultrasound and the training to sample adequate material." The biopsy may be performed either by clinicians (mostly endocrinologists or endocrine surgeons), by radiologists (under US guidance), or by skilled cytopathologists. Many workers on this field suggest that there are significant advantages to the aspiration being performed by a skilled cytopathologist: a better quality of the smears prepared at the site, an immediate evaluation of the quality and of the adequacy of the material, and the personal assessment of the clinical findings, including the "feeling" of the aspirated lesion (Fig. 4.1). If the aspirator is experienced enough, he can get some information already at the time of the FNA procedure. Besides the clinical finding, he acquires a "feeling" of the lesion during the procedure of the biopsy. Soft vascular nodules produce, for example, a feeling of the needle entering and stroking, which is very different from that produced by viscuous colloid nodules or by calcified lesions. The aspiration of a cyst can also be very informative in terms of the amount, the color, and the consistency of the fluid. A cytopathologist performing the biopsy can take advantage of all this initial information when evaluating the smears under the microscope (Hall et al. 1989).

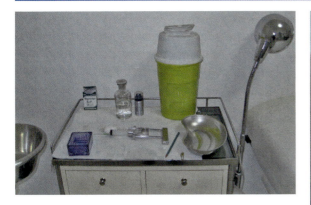

Fig. 4.1 The basic equipment for FNA includes alcohol pads, a 10- or 20-mL syringe (eventually attached to a syringe holder) with a fine needle (preferable a 22-g needle) and glass slides. The slides have to be clearly labeled with a pencil immediately after smearing

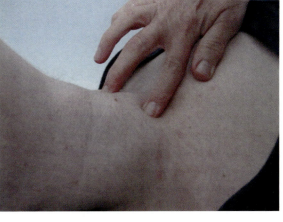

Fig. 4.2 The nodule has to be palpated between the second and third finger with the patient in supine position in order to find the best place for the aspiration

4.3.3 Planning of the Procedure: Choice of the Guidance

For planning the whole procedure, a physical examination of the patient in correlation to the findings of the ultrasonography is good in place. All nodules having an indication for FNA have to be determined, and it must be decided whether a palpation-guided FNA is reliable enough, otherwise the use of an ultrasonographical guidance will be necessary. The palpation should be skillful enough to ensure that the material can be aspirated from the appropriate area without a direct visualization by ultrasonography. The reliability of the palpatory finding depends on the physician's experience but also on the nodule's size, localization, consistency, and on the patient's neck structure. Skilled persons can be able to reliably palpate and aspirate nodules as small as 5 mm located on the isthmus. Nodules of hard consistency are easily palpable even in smaller size and are more frequently observed in neoplasms, fibrosed, or calcified nodules, as well as in largely cystic degenerated ones. Nodules located at the posterior surfaces of the lobes are difficult to palpate and so are nodules of the inferior parts of the lobes, extending to the mediastinum. The latter may be palpated during swallowing, due to the moving toward the trachea; however, they are extremely difficult to immobilize for the sampling. Furthermore, the adequacy of the material gained by an FNA under palpation is mostly questionable since the lower parts are possibly missed to the control. Obese patients or those with well-developed neck muscles, mainly males, are bad targets for palpation. Multinodular goiters represent a further limitation for the palpation-guided FNA, especially in cases of coexistent nodules, some of which have a benign, whereas others a suspicious ultrasound. In those cases, the most suspicious foci should be targeted via the ultrasound and so should solid areas in largely cystic nodules. Easy access to an ultrasonic equipment would be an advantage. In any case, the final decision about the possibility to aspirate under palpation is taken with the patient supine in an examination couch in a slight hyperextension of the neck, using a small pillow under his shoulders (Fig. 4.2). The degree of the neck extension varies, and the patient is asked to swallow during the search for the best place for the aspiration, with the neck muscles relaxed and the thyroid nodule palpable. A clear palpation finding is crucial in obtaining an adequate sample, but also in avoiding aspiration in the extrathyroidal tissues, which can cause discomfort and neck hematomas. We must point out the importance of taking time in evaluating the palpation finding, in keeping the patient under control, and in the planning of the whole procedure.

Clearly palpable solitary nodules of a thyroid lobe are ideal targets for FNA under palpation. This approach has the advantage of being simple, having a lower cost, since it does not require a US equipment, and being very quick, minimizing the patient's discomfort, as well as the bleeding in the nodule. It is therefore strongly recommended for nodules with rich vascularity, as well as for anxious patients or those with blood coagulation disturbances, mostly caused by anticoagulant medication. The ideal setting for the thyroid biopsy would be an aspiration clinic, allowing a multidisciplinary team approach and creating optimal conditions to obtain representative samples.

4.3.4 Fine-Needle Aspiration of the Thyroid: How Fine Should the Needle Be?

By definition, needles 19–27 g are fine needles suitable for FNA in various organs. The thyroid is an organ with rich vascularity and 21 g seems to be the largest needle recommended. Most aspirators of thyroid nodules prefer needles 21–25 g. According to our experience and to the experience of others (Droese 1995), a 22-g needle (external diameter, 0.6 mm) seems to be the most suitable one for an initial aspiration since it is large enough to aspirate thick colloid or slightly fibrotic lesions without extensive bleeding as a side effect. Even larger needles (21 g) are preferable for evacuating cystic nodules, especially those containing a viscous colloid, as well as for aspirating nodules with extensive fibrosis, mostly on the ground of Hashimoto's thyroiditis. The needle length recommended lies between 20 and 32 mm.

We normally use a 20-mL syringe attached to the needle to perform the suction of the tissue. Others prefer a 10-mL syringe, and some aspirators advocate an "aspiration without aspiration," obtaining the tissue sample without any suction, just with a needle moving toward and back in the tissue. We had bad experience with this technique in thyroid nodules, especially in fibrosing lesions or cysts with thick colloid.

4.3.5 Procedure of the FNA Under Palpation

4.3.5.1 Informing the Patient
Before the biopsy, the patient should be clearly informed about the need for the biopsy and its key role in the management of the thyroid nodules. The diagnostic limitations of the procedure should be mentioned, including the possibility of obtaining inadequate material with a need of rebiopsy as well as of getting an inconclusive or even more a false-negative or false-positive diagnosis. The patient should also be clearly informed about eventual rare complications and asked to sign an informed consent, accepting the possibility of some complications, namely, bleeding, infection, or a vasovagal episode. However, to minimize the patient's anxiousness and to gain his collaboration, the steps of the procedure should be briefly described and its simplicity and painlessness should be pointed out. An extensive informing can be especially helpful in reducing the patient's anxiety. The patients taking anticoagulatives should have discontinued the administration after consultation of their physician.

4.3.5.2 How Necessary Is Local Anesthesia?
We do not advocate the application of a local anesthetic since we consider it superfluous. The biopsy is not painful and generally well tolerated by the patient. Furthermore, we avoid an eventual allergic reaction, the obscuring of the palpated nodule by a lump created by the injection as well as an eventual admixture of the anesthetic fluid to the sample compromising the quality of the smears. An anesthetic ointment can be applied 30 min prior to biopsy in very anxious patients or children. However, we have best experience with talking to the patients during the whole procedure to give them a feeling of safety, especially if more passes are needed.

4.3.5.3 The Aspiration Technique
A right-handed aspirator should always stay on the right side of the patient independent of the nodule's location. After skin disinfection, the aspirator should ask the patient to swallow in order to feel the nodule move following the swallowing and in order to ensure the finding of palpation and then immobilize the nodule between the index and middle finger. Then he should ask the patient not to swallow, insert the needle attached to the syringe into the nodule with the right hand (Fig. 4.3), and apply a gentle suction by reaching a negative pressure in the syringe retracting the piston of the syringe back rapidly (5–12 mL). This action can be facilitated with the use of a mechanical device (Fig. 4.1), enabling the aspirator to perform the suction with the inserting hand, keeping the nodule fixed with the other hand. However, by this approach, the feeling of being in the nodule is more difficult, and the calculation of the depth of the lesion gets confounded, mainly in deeper located

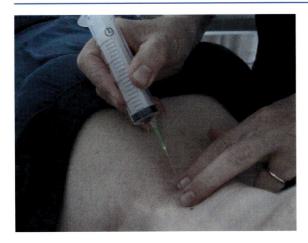

Fig. 4.3 The needle enters the immobilized nodule. The selection of the place for every pass is crucial for the adequacy of the sample

small nodules. Alternatively, the aspirator performs the suction quickly with the left hand and maintains it with the right hand in order to fix the nodule again with the left hand. The fixation of the nodule during sampling is crucial, being possible in the palpation-guided FNA, whereas getting lost in the US-guided FNA. The amount of suction to be performed depends widely on the consistency of the nodule and should be applied gradually in order to minimize bleeding in a highly vascularized substrate. The next, most critical step is to obtain the tissue sample moving the needle two to three times quickly back and forth in slightly different directions in the sense of a "needle stroke," dislodging small pieces of tissue. Without any doubt, suction seems to be helpful, but by far not the major factor of tissue disruption, and should not be extremely aggressive in order to avoid unpleasant bleeding. Crucial for the adequacy seem to be multiple "strokes" of the needle dislodging tissue fragments, which are then forced into the bore of the needle (Boerner and Asa 2010).

During this procedure, the aspirator should be aware to keep the needle in the nodule and stop the aspiration immediately when the aspirated material appears in the hub of the needle in order to avoid contamination of the sample with large amounts of blood (hemodilution). Ideally, the aspiration is stopped just before the material appears in the needle hub at all.

The epithelial tissue components, which are of main interest, are regularly easily dislodged from their stromal surroundings. Cellular epithelial lesions, such as hyperplastic nodules, adenomas, and carcinomas, offer usually adequate samples. Much more difficult is to obtain adequate material from fibrosing or calcified lesions, as well as from highly vascularized lesions (like hyperfunctioning nodules) due to hemodilution.

If fluid is obtained during the suction, the aspirator should continue until the fluid stops filling the syringe because either the cyst or a part of a multilocular lesion has been evacuated. Needle strokes are not recommended during the cyst evacuation. If a rest nodule is palpable, the aspiration is immediately repeated, either evacuating another cystic component or aspirating a solid component with "needle strokes." At the end of the aspiration and before the exit of the needle, the suction has to be terminated by releasing the piston of the syringe in order to equalize the negative pressure, otherwise the atmospheric pressure would push the material obtained into the syringe and it would get lost.

4.3.5.4 The Number of Passes

The number of passes needed depends primarily on the size of the nodule since heterogeneity in the nodule is possible, and FNA might miss a relevant area, like all small-sized biopsies. Generally, each pass performed with a slight movement to different directions into the tissue covers an area of approximately 1–1.5 cm. Any nodule of greater size should need more passes respectively. For example, a nodule of a maximal diameter of 3.0 cm should be biopsied two to three times, with the passes keeping a distance of at most 1 cm in order to avoid missing a suspicious area larger than 1 cm. Some aspirators perform routinely several passes; however, we do not recommend an unlimited number of passes since repeated biopsies exhibit inadequate, bloody smears to a significant percentage, due to an immediate post-FNA intranodular bleeding. We assessed indeed the sample obtained by the first pass to be the most representative one since FNA-caused intranodular bleeding obviously compromises the subsequent passes. In case of a nondiagnostic FNA result, we recommend waiting for an intranodular ultrasonographically detected hematoma to be absorbed before repeating the biopsy, otherwise the risk of having again a bloody, nondiagnostic smear is significant.

4.3.5.5 Post-FNA Patient Care

After the exit of the needle, a direct pressure via a dry swab should be applied on the site of the biopsy to produce hemostasis, preferably by the patient himself, if he is cooperative enough, since he is able to assess the degree of the pressure he can tolerate. In case of a noncooperative patient, some assistance would be very helpful. Most of the times, 3–5 min of pressure is sufficient; however, the time needed can be longer, depending on the number of passes, the vascularization of the nodule, the presence of a hematoma, and the patient's status of blood coagulation. Then, the patient can be released to go home.

4.3.5.6 Frequent Mistakes Concerning the Aspiration Procedure

- If an accurate fixation of the nodule is not achieved, it may move during the aspiration and render it difficult to obtain an adequate tissue sample.
- Performing the aspiration by suction alone without "strokes" in the nodule rarely achieves an adequate sampling.
- Continuing the aspiration after the sample has appeared in the hub of the needle causes hemodiluted smears and blood clots unsuitable for evaluation.
- If the negative pressure is not equalized prior to the exit of the needle from the nodule, the aspirated tissue will intrude in the syringe and get lost for the direct smearing.

4.3.5.7 US-Guided FNA

In principle, the whole procedure is the same, keeping the advantage of direct visualization with main disadvantage the higher cost and the longer duration of the procedure. The latter may cause discomfort of the patient, as well as increased bleeding, resulting frequently in suboptimal smears. Admixtures of the contact medium (gel) to the tissue expelled should be avoided, otherwise the smears exhibit precipitated material, and the cell morphology can be obscured.

4.3.6 Complications: Side Effects of the Biopsy

Intranodular hematomas can occur after FNA of nodules especially if the post-FNA pressure was not correctly targeted, or not of sufficient duration, or if the coagulation status of the patient was not correctly considered. Most intranodular hematomas may cause acute local pain, sudden enlargement of the lesion, and discomfort in swallowing; however, they are as a rule rapidly absorbed. The patients should be advised to locally apply ice and to avoid aspirin as an analgetic drug. In rare cases, an evacuation of the hematoma is indicated for the relief of the symptoms.

Extensive aspiration in the extrathyroidal tissues may lead to painful neck hematomas.

Infection has been reported to be another possible complication; however, in a series of nearly 300,000 FNA over a period of over 27 years, we never recorded an infection, even on the grounds of a post-FNA hematoma.

Some lesions seem to have an increased risk for hemorrhage. Mainly, the oncocytic lesions frequently cause extensive bleeding, and the tissue undergoes a post-FNA to hemorrhagic necrosis. This may be very confusing for the subsequent histology since the pathological substrate cannot be recognized in the histological sections, and an evaluation of the invasiveness of the lesion may be inaccurate due to the fibrous organization of the hematoma (Saxen et al. 1978). We suggest that the post-FNA changes leading to false histological diagnoses are an important "side effect" of this diagnostic approach (Tseleni S, 1986).

The most alerting complication we faced were sudden vasovagal episodes probably due to a stimulation of the vagal nerve. However, most of them lasted for only a short time, and the patient recovered in a supine position without any further treatment. Rare cases demanded the administration of atropine sulfate intramuscularly.

Penetration of the trachea may occur predominantly in nodules located at the isthmus. The experienced aspirator recognizes a loss of the vacuum in the syringe due to the air aspirated from the tracheal lumen as well as a sudden cough episode of the patient. Rarely, a blood admixture in the sputum can be noticed by the patient, which lacks any clinical significance. The smears prepared from such an aspiration of the trachea should however be extra labeled since the admixture of tracheal epithelial cells or mucous can be misleading and compromising the diagnostic accuracy.

4.4 Processing of the Sample

There are several alternatives for the processing of the sample prior to the microscopic evaluation, and the way of achieving the better results is a matter of debate (Keebler 1991; Crystal et al. 1993). The best way of processing depends largely on the experience of the cytopathologist in interpreting the prepared samples by the various methods. It is obvious that the cytopathologist involved in the FNA should give exact advice to the aspirator about the handling of the aspirate, according to his favorite methods. Generally, direct smears of the sample give the greatest amount of information since many epithelial structures remain intact, and many stomal elements are present and well interpretable. Nevertheless, the preparation of direct smears of good quality demands special skill and practice in handling, and in case of inexperience in smearing, indirect smears and liquid-based preparations can be of advantage (ThinPrep and SurePath are FDA-approved liquid-based techniques).

4.4.1 Gain of the Aspirate: Preparing the Smears

4.4.1.1 Expelling the Sample

After its exit from the lesion, the needle must be disconnected from the syringe and the syringe be filled with air (10–20 mL), then reconnected and the material remaining in the needle hub should be quickly expelled onto one or more slides, depending on its amount and consistency, in order to make direct smears. If the aspirator is not experienced in preparing smears, he should prefer to expel the sample rinsing thoroughly the syringe and the needle in a liquid medium (either saline or fixative) and send it to the laboratory for centrifugation and preparation of indirect smears from the sediment or directly for liquid-based cytology preparations according to the cytopathologist's preferences (Kocjan 2006).

If a fluid is obtained, the content of the syringe can proceed to liquid-based cytology, or it can be centrifuged at 1,500 rpm (400×g) for 5 min, and smears can be made from the sediment. However, we have good experience disconnecting the needle from the syringe and expelling just the content of the needle on a slide using another syringe. Such preparations frequently exhibit some cellular aggregates, probably captured in the needle, and they provide in a good percentage adequate smears. On the contrary, smears made from sediments are frequently acellular or just inadequate, mainly if the fluid contains blood, coagulating with the cellular elements and leading to clots, unsuitable for the microscopic evaluation. The smears prepared from the content of the needle in the way we described should also be labeled separately from those made from the sediment of the fluid.

Eventual residual tissue in the bore of the needle after direct smears can be collected by rinsing it with a fluid, either a balanced salt solution or a fixative, depending largely on the way the rinse will be used. Then, it can be further processed as described for the fluids obtained with the aspiration. It seems reasonable to use the rinse for thin-layer preparations or for the production of cell blocks, embedding the sediment in a paraffin mold to prepare paraffin sections, mainly suitable for immunohistochemical applications (Zito et al. 1995).

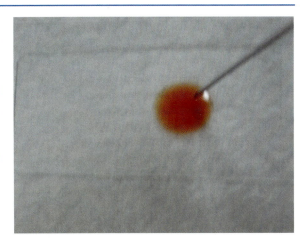

Fig. 4.4 A drop of the aspirated material is released on a slide with the needle being on the slide surface

4.4.1.2 Preparing Direct Smears

To make direct smears, the expelled tissue must be placed at a distance of 0.5–1 cm from the frosted end of the slide in order to facilitate the smearing. During expelling, one should keep in mind to put the needle tip on the glass slide, in order to avoid tissue distribution in the form of tiny droplets, technically unsuitable for any further preparation. Generally, a good drop of tissue, frequently containing some amount of colloid, is enough for a direct smear (Figs. 4.4 and 4.5). The amount of material needed for a proper smearing as well as the smearing process itself are a matter of experience and have to be demonstrated on site.

Best smearing of the material is achieved by the use of another glass slide in a way "like the take off of a plane," estimating simultaneously the degree of the pressure needed to put on the smearing glass for an optimal thickness of the smear (Figs. 4.6 and 4.7). We always smear just once; the whole procedure including aspirating, expelling, and smearing should be completed quickly for the following reasons: to minimize bleeding and thereby any annoying hemodilution and to avoid any coagulation of a tissue sample with blood

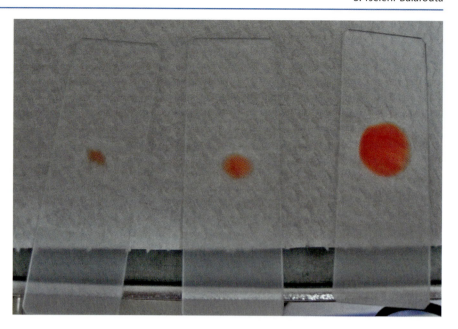

Fig. 4.5 The drop can be of variable size in the range shown in the figure

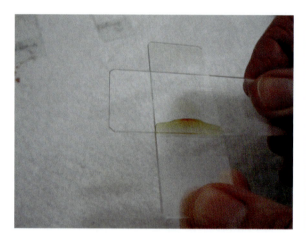

Fig. 4.6 The best smearing is performed with another glass slide like a "take off" of a plane

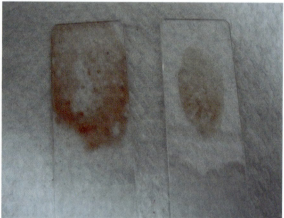

Fig. 4.7 Best smeared is the sample with the rounded edge

admixture. Properly smeared slides exhibit a rounded edge (Fig. 4.8). The labeling of the slides has to be performed immediately after smearing in order to avoid any mislabeling. Proper labeling is crucial, especially if the smears are sent to a cytopathologist not implicated in the biopsy. The localization of the aspirated nodules must be recorded (preferably on a brief sketch) and labeled separately. In case of inadequate material when aspirating a multinodular goiter, the repeat biopsy concerns just the nodule with inadequacy. Moreover, we recommend to label separately every pass even in the same nodule since it may be of importance for the cytopathologist to assess the heterogeneity of the tissue. Special conditions should also be indicated, for example, smears probably containing diagnostically irrelevant tissues such as tracheal elements or extrathyroidal soft tissues.

4.4.2 Fixating and Staining the Smears

Direct smears can be either air-dried or wet-fixed. Air-dried smears containing some fluid should be dried

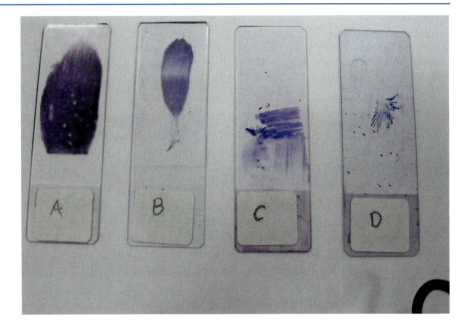

Fig. 4.8 MGG-stained smears: (**a**) and (**b**) are well-prepared smears with a rounded edge; (**c**) and (**d**) are improperly smeared

quickly, eventually using gently a hair dryer in order to avoid "wet artifacts," whereas wet fixation should be applied immediately by spraying the smears with a fixative or putting them in a fixative solution, like 96 alcohol. Immediate processing protects from "drying artifacts" of the wet-fixated smears.

After the initial type of fixation, the smears can be stained differentially (Boon 1992). Air-dried smears undergo a Romanowsky-type stain, like May-Gruenwald-Giemsa (MGG), Diff Quick, or Hemacolor (the latter both are rapid stains suitable for an immediate evaluation of adequacy, missing however the high quality of MGG-stained smears). Wet-fixed smears are best stained with the Papanicolaou technique, modified according to the formula used from the laboratory of the involved cytopathologist. Some pathologists prefer the hematoxylin and eosin stain, best correlating with the histological sections. To compare the stains, the air-dried MGG-stained smears have an excellent contrast and are of advantage in evaluating the background elements (colloid, lymphoid populations, necrosis) and the cell cytoplasm (e.g., visualization of the azurophilic granules in medullary carcinoma); they, however, miss the nuclear details. Wet fixation offers a nuclear transparency and more information about chromatin and nucleoli. It is obvious that both stains are complementary and it would be of advantage to perform both of them, if several smears are available. Often, however, only a few smears can be obtained from the aspirated nodule, in which case they should be processed according to the cytopathologist's preferences. We have the best experience with air-dried, MGG-stained smears, and most of the diagnoses can be made with those preparations. Even in the gross evaluation of the slides, the amount of colloid is obvious (Fig. 4.9). We should mention that air-dried smears are very popular among the European cytopathologists and are best represented by the majority of the figures in the textbooks. Also, most of the established criteria for FNA smears in the literature are based on air-dried smears since FNA of thyroid has been established primarily by Swedish pathologists evaluating mainly air-dried, MGG-stained smears.

4.4.3 Additional Techniques

Additional techniques are rarely needed in the routine diagnostic if the cytopathologist is experienced enough. They should be avoided since they are time- and cost-consuming. However, in rare cases, some ancillary techniques may be useful and add substantially to the diagnostic accuracy, namely, some immunohistochemical and recently some molecular applications.

4.4.3.1 Immunohistochemical Applications

The immunohistochemistry has been assessed by most pathologists as an art rather than a science, and its

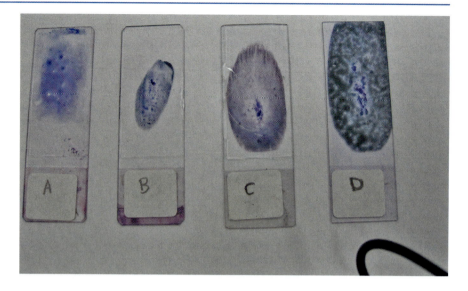

Fig. 4.9 MGG-stained smears exhibit an excellent contrast in gross evaluation: (**a**) and (**b**) represent smears from a colloid-rich nodule, (**c**) and (**d**) contain tissue particles in the center of blood ("cellular smears")

interpretation demands standardization in the laboratory and experience in the evaluation. Immunocytochemistry exhibits more difficulties and less possibilities than the immunohistochemistry and should be used with caution. The most suitable preparations for the immunocytochemical applications are the cellblock preparations (samples collected from sediments of centrifuged fluids or rinses of the needle embedded in paraffin blocks providing paraffin serial sections).

FNA of thyroid rarely needs an immunocytochemical support in the routine diagnostic. It might be helpful to detect a nonclassical medullary carcinoma by the immunocytochemical detection of calcitonin and neuroendocrine markers in the cells, also to suggest the parathyroidal origin of a nodule expressing parathormone and chromogranin or to confirm the primary nature of a nontypical thyroid neoplasm by the detection of thyroglobulin. The clonality of a lymphoid population can also be checked by the immunocytochemistry, if several smears are available, by suspicion of a thyroidal lymphoma (Henrique et al. 1999). However, most problems, namely, the indeterminate diagnoses, cannot be resolved through immunocytochemistry.

4.4.3.2 Molecular Applications

Several molecular studies are in principle possible in FNA material, and commercially available kits have been developed for some of them; however, they increase the cost without offering a reliable tool in the diagnostic challenges of thyroid nodules. For example, the detection of the specific B Raf V600 mutation confirms the diagnosis of a papillary carcinoma, its absence, however, does not exclude a papillary carcinoma since the sensitivity of the method is insufficient (lower than 50%, varying in the various studies). Furthermore, no magic markers are by now available for the classification of the follicular lesions, responsible for most indeterminate smears, and none of the suggested molecular signatures have been established in the routine diagnostic.

4.5 The Cytological Evaluation

Evaluating FNA smears resembles to the construction of a puzzle. The dispersed pieces must be put together in a reasonable way to get an integrate picture. Like a puzzle constructor, the cytopathologist must have an exact knowledge of the possible histologic pictures ("the wanted final pictures") and some degree of fantasy to reproduce the picture of the dislodged and smeared tissue. Sometimes, the pieces are insufficient (or unsuitable) for the reconstruction ("nondiagnostic material"), or a reproduction of different pictures by the same pieces is possible ("indeterminate smears"). Furthermore, the sample may be composed of various pieces, some of them corresponding to different pictures than the majority of the pieces ("focally suspicious material"). The main "pieces of the puzzle" are recorded in the cytological report. Since the FNA diagnostic is a teamwork, we consider the knowledge of the basic cytological terms to be important for the development of a common language for the communication between the clinicians and the cytopathologists.

4.5.1 The Wording of the Cytopathologist

The cytopathologists describe various microscopic features of the samples, having a varying degree of significance and a different impact on the diagnostic accuracy (Delibasis et al. 2009). The cooperating clinicians should ideally be familiar with the cytological language in order to facilitate the scientific communication. The sample features assessed microscopically cover a broad range of elements with a varying degree of specificity and diagnostic relevance.

4.5.1.1 Nonspecific Elements
(a) Amorphous background: Colloid, amyloid, stromal fragments, and psammoma bodies.
(b) Cellular elements: Blood (present in most aspirates, especially in the well-vascularized lesions), inflammatory infiltrates (mostly lymphocytic, sometimes polymorphonuclear granulocytes in acute inflammation, mainly on a cystic substrate or on a necrotic background of a high-grade malignancy or histiocytic epithelioid, pointing to a granulomatous inflammation), phagocytes (pigmented macrophages indicative of cystic degeneration), and multinucleated giant cells (numerous and huge in subacute thyroiditis and sparse in thyroiditis Hashimoto and in the papillary carcinoma). Cells of nonthyroidal origin are also nonspecific (like fat cells or striated muscle cells). Nonspecific cells cannot support a diagnosis; however, they can be enhancing a suspicion. The coexistence of multinucleated giant cells with microcalcifications in the ultrasound needs an intensive exploration to exclude a papillary CA, or the presence of regenerating muscle cells in a papillary CA is indicative of invasion of the muscles by the tumor cells.

4.5.1.2 Cellular Elements Relevant for the Diagnosis
Most diagnoses are based on the interpretation of epithelial cells, namely:
(a) *Follicular cells*: In benign lesions mostly arranged in monolayered sheets and dissociated, exhibiting oval, uniform nuclei and friable cytoplasm with indistinct cell borders. The follicular cells may exhibit a functional atypia with anisokaryosis and hyperchromatic nuclei, sometimes observed on the ground of nodular hyperplasia or even more in Hashimoto's thyroiditis.
(b) *Oxyphilic cells (oncocytes)*: The follicular cells may undergo an oxyphilic (oncocytic) metaplasia. Metaplastic oxyphilic cells exhibit a rather good cohesiveness and abundant, granular cytoplasm with distinct cell borders and an intense oxyphilic staining. They may exhibit various degrees of atypia. They frequently cause inconclusive diagnoses with no clear distinction between oncocytic metaplasia, a Huerthle cell neoplasm, and the oncocytic type of papillary carcinoma.
(c) *C cells*: They may be included in samples from thyroid aspiration; however, they are hardly identifiable since they are pale cells with round nuclei and generally similar morphology to the follicular cells.
(d) *Parathyroidal* chief or oxyphilic cells: Aspirated by mistake; also cannot be safely distinguished from thyroidal follicular cells.
(e) *Squamous cells*: May also be included, either due to metaplastic foci in a Hashimoto's thyroiditis or to the squamous epithelium of a neck cyst (thyroglossal duct or branchial cleft cyst).
(f) *Tumor cells*: Most tumor cells in the thyroid exhibit some degree of epithelial differentiation, reflecting the development of malignancies of mainly epithelial differentiation. Mesenchymal tumors are extremely rare. Malignant lymphomas are the second most common malignancies.

The epithelial tumor cells can strongly mimic the follicular cells (well-differentiated phenotype, sometimes difficult to recognize as neoplastic cells) or they can be absolutely abnormal, exhibiting high-grade features (huge, hyperchromatic nuclei, nuclear pleomorphism and anisokaryosis, prominent nucleoli, abnormal mitoses). Various intermediate phenotypes are possible. The classification of the tumors on cytological grounds depends on the specificity of the phenotypic appearance.

4.5.2 Basic Patterns in Thyroid Smears

The assessment of the above-mentioned elements according to their amount and arrangement on the smears leads to the reconstruction of the basic

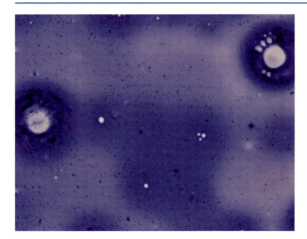

Fig. 4.10 Benign "colloid" nodule: abundant diffuse colloid with sparse dissociated follicular cells. MGG stain

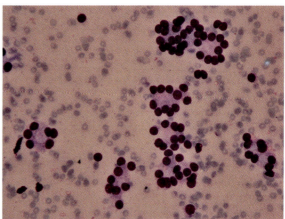

Fig. 4.11 "Microfollicular pattern": follicular cells arranged in small-sized follicular formations around an empty center, moderate anisokaryosis (indeterminate smear). MGG stain

histological patterns most likely to underlie as the pathological substrate of a nodule as follows:

(a) Macrofollicular pattern (colloid predominance)

It represents the prototype of a benign pattern with rare exceptions (like the macrofollicular variant of papillary CA). The smears exhibit abundant diffuse colloid and uniform follicular cells, dissociated, in monolayered sheets and in three-dimensional microfollicles with some basement membrane material (Fig. 4.10). An admixture of pigmented macrophages ("phagocytes") is a common finding, due to areas of a microcystic degeneration.

(b) Microfollicular pattern (cellular, "gray zone" pattern)

The smears are cellular with little or no colloid at all and abundant follicular cells, arranged mainly in circular formations around an empty center or around a thick particle of colloid (Fig. 4.11). Anisokaryosis and some degree of nuclear atypia are common findings in this pattern. Histologically, they correspond either to an "adenomatous" hyperplastic nodule or to a follicular neoplasia (adenoma or carcinoma). Most of the times, the diagnosis differentiates between hyperplasia and neoplasia; however, there are cellular smears borderline on cytological grounds between hyperplasia and neoplasia, best designated as "follicular lesion." In that sense, this pattern represents the large group of indeterminate smears since the main diagnostic clue is the evaluation of the nodule's capsule, not possible in the smears.

(c) Pattern of cystic degeneration

It is characterized particularly by the presence of abundant pigmented phagocytes (Fig. 4.12). From the statistical point of view, most of the cystic nodules

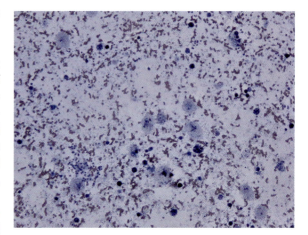

Fig. 4.12 Pattern of cystic degeneration, characterized by the presence of abundant, pigmented phagocytes. Coexistence of colloid and sparse follicular cells. MGG stain

represent benign hyperplastic nodules; however, cystic degenerated neoplasms may occur (in particular papillary carcinomas and oncocytic neoplasms). Insofar, the presence of abundant thick colloid and of many phagocytes in absence of any epithelial cells is just indicative of a benign degenerating nodule, but a neoplastic condition cannot be excluded. The presence of coexistent epithelial cells, specific for the substrate, are necessary for a safe diagnosis, otherwise the adequacy of the smear is questionable.

(d) Inflammatory pattern

It concerns mainly smears of autoimmune thyroiditis Hashimoto, consisting largely of lymphocytic elements of variable type (Fig. 4.13). Groups

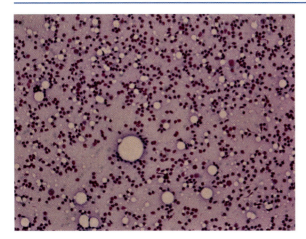

Fig. 4.13 "Inflammatory pattern" from a lymphocytic thyroiditis. A mixed lymphocytic population with cells of variable nuclear size with scanty cytoplasm (they concern mainly mature lymphocytes, follicular center cells, and plasma cells). MGG stain

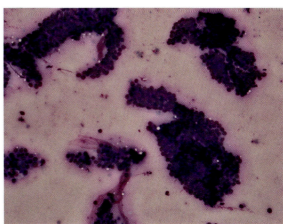

Fig. 4.14 Papillary CA: cellular papillary pattern. MGG stain

of epithelial cells, follicular or oncocytic, are admixed, and they ensure the sampling of thyroid gland and not of a lymph node. The coexistence of histiocytic elements and many multinucleated giant cells is indicative of a granulomatous thyroiditis (focal palpation thyroiditis or diffuse subacute thyroiditis de Quervain). Acute inflammatory patterns (polymorphonuclear granulocytes) are very rare in thyroid nodules, and in such cases, the possibility of an inflamed thyroglossal duct cyst should be taken under consideration. Sparse lymphocytic infiltrates are a frequent finding in benign hyperplastic nodules. In a follow-up series of such benign nodules, we correlated the presence of lymphocytes in the smears with a higher risk for increasing of the size of the nodule (Tseleni-Balafouta et al. 1991).

(e) Neoplastic pattern

The smears lack colloid and are largely cellular and monomorphous, with different cell phenotypes and various patterns of cell arrangement, according to the various histological types. Many architectural patterns may coexist in most thyroid tumors:

Papillary pattern: Elongated and spheroidal papillary formations, monolayered sheets, good cell cohesiveness, and nuclear overlapping, a pattern typical for the papillary CA (Figs. 4.14 and 4.15).

Microfollicular pattern: As described above, with varying degree of cellularity and nuclear anisokaryosis and atypia, mainly observed in the follicular tumors but also in the papillary CA, partly or even exclusively (in the follicular variant of papillary CA).

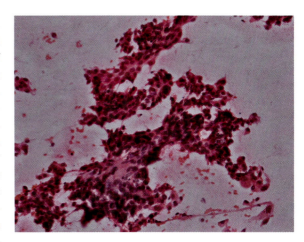

Fig. 4.15 Papillary CA: papillary structures with nuclear crowding. HE stain

Solid pattern: Solid cell arrangement, observed in the poorly differentiated follicular cell CA, in the medullary CA, and in the oncocytic and squamous cell tumors (Figs. 4.16, 4.17, 4.18, 4.19, and 4.20).

Diffuse pattern: Dissociated neoplastic cells (poor cell cohesion), mainly seen in the high-grade carcinomas (anaplastic CA), in the medullary CA, in the lymphomas, and in the rare mesenchymal tumors (Figs. 4.21 and 4.22).

4.5.3 The Nondiagnostic Smear

All smears lacking specific cellular elements, well preserved and prepared, sufficient for a diagnosis, should

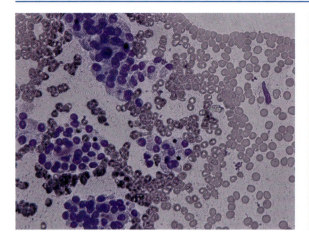

Fig. 4.16 Poorly differentiated CA ("insular" type). Solid sheets of small cells with nuclear crowding. MGG stain

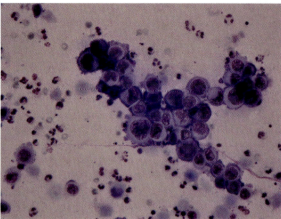

Fig. 4.18 Squamoid carcinoma on the ground of a papillary CA with high-grade cellular features and neutrophils in the background (due to necroses). MGG stain

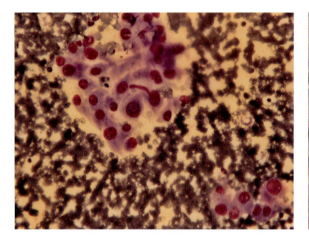

Fig. 4.17 Papillary CA with poorly differentiated areas: solid sheets of oxyphilic polygonal cells, intranuclear pseudoinclusions (cytoplasmic protrusions, exhibiting the same color with the cytoplasm and a peripheral condensation of chromatin). MGG stain

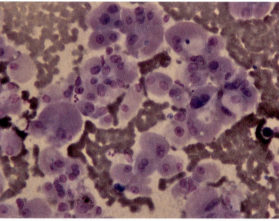

Fig. 4.19 Solid neoplastic pattern: sheets of an oncocytic neoplasm with a poor cell cohesion, abundant oxyphilic cytoplasm (violet in MGG stain), prominent nucleoli. (Huerthle cell neoplasm not possible to classify as an adenoma or a carcinoma since the invasiveness of the lesion cannot be assessed on cytological grounds)

be characterized as nondiagnostic. The clinician should manage the patient on the basis of all others findings, asking for a rebiopsy, in an interval estimated according to the clinical needs (Chow et al. 2001; Hamburger and Hussein 1988). Most nondiagnostic smears concern bloody smears (consisting exclusively of blood or exhibiting admixtures of cells entrapped in the blood clots and therefore unsuitable for evaluation) or smears with cystic fluid and phagocytes only (from cystic degenerated nodules). However, sometimes the smears are nondiagnostic due to a bad preparation (like too thick smearing or artifacts in fixation and staining). The standardization of the preparation has a significant impact on the diagnostic accuracy, and all smears prepared according to the cytopathologist's preferences make it easy for him to reach his maximal diagnostic potential. The amount of cells needed for the diagnosis varies greatly. Just one papillary sheet with the typical nuclei with definite intranuclear inclusions can lead to the diagnosis of a papillary carcinoma, whereas abun-

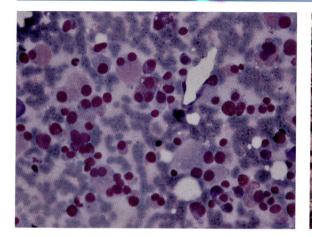

Fig. 4.20 Medullary carcinoma: plasmocytoid cells dissociated and in clusters, with eccentric nuclei, anisokaryosis, azurophilic discrete cytoplasmic granulation, and multinucleated tumor cells. MGG stain

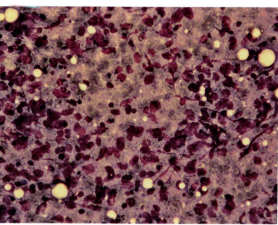

Fig. 4.22 Diffuse pattern in a malignant non-Hodgkin lymphoma (high grade). Necrotic background and atypical lymphoid cells. MGG stain

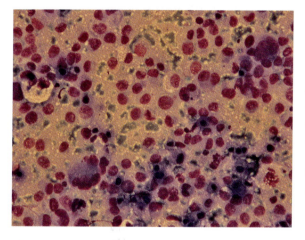

Fig. 4.21 Anaplastic carcinoma. Necrotic background, poor cell cohesion with mainly dissociated cells, marked nuclear polymorphism and atypia, tumor giant cells, and atypical mitoses. MGG stain

dant sheets of follicular cells can under certain circumstances be inconclusive. A nondiagnostic smear is not necessarily a benign smear, only because no malignant cells have been found. On the contrary, the percentage of a neoplastic lesion seems to underlie nearly to half of the nondiagnostic smears (Buesseniers and Silver 2007). The clinicians should accept the limitation of a nondiagnostic smear and avoid to force the cytopathologist to exceed his potential, otherwise a false diagnosis might result in a corresponding mismanagement.

4.5.4 Information Needed by the Cytopathologist for the Evaluation of the FNA Smears

Besides correct sampling and preparing of the smears, the microscopic evaluation by the cytopathologist demands some minimal clinical data for the correct interpretation of the cytological patterns. Insofar, each smear sent to the cytopathologist for evaluation should be accompanied by the following useful information:

(a) Age and sex of the patient with a special remark in case of a pregnancy. Smears from young people and especially of pregnant women can be very cellular and this should be taken under consideration to avoid false-positive diagnoses.

(b) Any relevant information from medical history pointing toward an increased risk of malignancy. These include familial medical history and disturbances of other endocrine organs (like MEN syndromes, familial medullary CA, or hyperparathyroidism). For example, having in mind the actual possibility of a medullary CA facilitates enormously the recognition of this tumor or a cellular smear in the presence of a well-known hyperparathyroidism raises the need for the differential diagnosis from a parathyroidal lesion.

(c) The functional status of the thyroid referring to an eventual antithyroidal drug administration since functional atypia and huge nuclei observed in antithyroidal treatment may lead to an overdiagnosis of malignancy. In the case of a clinical hyperthyroidism, the scintigraphical imaging of a nodule can clarify if it consists of a hyperfunctioning tissue.

(d) The most important information concerns the findings of the ultrasonography. They should include the number, the localization, the size, the shape, the borders, and the echogenicity of the nodules, with special remarks to the presence of microcalcifications and the type of the vascularization.

4.6 The Diagnostic Possibilities of FNA in Thyroid Nodules

The diagnostic accuracy of fine-needle aspiration after excluding the nondiagnostic samples and in experienced hands is generally greater than 95%, with the sensitivity ranging between 65% and 98% (mean value 77.7%) and the specificity between 72% and 100% (mean value 85.4%) (Droese 1995; Gharib and Goellner 1993; Hamburger and Hamburger 1986; Jayaram et al. 1999; Ko et al. 2003; Revetto et al. 2000). All statistical assessments of FNA accuracy are based on correlations to the histological reports of resected thyroids since the histological diagnosis has been considered as a gold standard. However, the histology is not absolutely reliable, given the high interobserver variability even among thyroid specialists (Saxen et al. 1978). Moreover, sometimes the diagnosis of a papillary carcinoma, based mainly on cytological grounds, is easier to diagnose in well-prepared smears than in histological sections, especially if a post-FNA necrosis or fibrosis confuses the histological evaluation. Noteworthy would also be that false-negative rates are probably mostly overestimated since clinically suspicious nodules are higher represented among the surgical specimens.

4.6.1 The Limitations of the Method

The main limitations of the diagnostic approach of the thyroid nodules with FNA are the inadequate and the indeterminate smears (Gharib 1994; Gharib et al. 1993).

(a) *Inadequate smears*: It is very difficult to define the adequacy of the sample since it depends of several factors, including various technical issues concerning the aspiration technique and the processing of the material, but also different clinical issues and the correlation between the sample and the clinical data. Some previously proposed quantitative criteria cannot be strictly followed since a smear adequate for a small indolent nodule might be insufficient for a large suspicious one. Insofar, none of the suggested criteria has been established in the routine diagnostic. We estimate the matter of evaluating the adequacy to be the most challenging issue of this diagnostic approach, being responsible for most false diagnoses and demanding an experienced cytopathologist, familiar with the cytological pictures but also with the clinical implications. We propose the following general definition of adequacy: "Adequate is a properly processed smear containing well preserved, sufficient and specific elements for a diagnosis compatible with the clinical and sonographical findings." We always point out the comparison of the cytology with the clinical findings as an additional factor in checking the reliability of the sample.

(b) *Indeterminate smears*: This group includes two different categories of lesions: first, all samples containing cellular elements with a not clearly characterized phenotype or containing benign-looking cells in coexistence with suspicious for malignancy cells ("suspicious"), and secondly all highly cellular samples of follicular cells without any definite signs of malignancy ("follicular lesion, gray zone"). In the former subgroup, we found a malignant focus in about 65% whereas in the latter, about 21% neoplastic lesions among the surgically removed thyroids (unpublished data).

4.6.2 The Degree of Accuracy Varies Among the Various Lesions

The diagnostic reliability of FNA in thyroid nodules depends mainly on the experience of the aspirator and the cytopathologist but also on the lesion under investigation (Baloch and Livolsi 2004). Some pathological substrates provide specific cytological pictures, whereas others may be confusing (Lowhagen and Sprenger 1974; Nguyen et al. 1991; Orell and Philips 1997).

Among *benign nodules*, hyperplastic nodules with typical patterns can be accurately diagnosed. Areas with oxyphilic metaplasia, functional atypia, or hypercellularity may lead to overdiagnoses. Hashimoto's thyroidi-

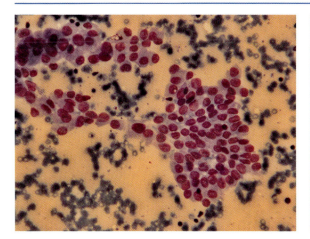

Fig. 4.23 Papillary carcinoma. Typical papillary pattern, disoriented nuclei with crowding. MGG stain

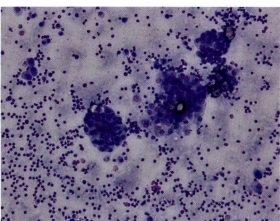

Fig. 4.25 Diffuse sclerosing variant of papillary CA. Abundant lymphocytes in the background and polygonal squamoid cells and concentric psammoma bodies. MGG stain

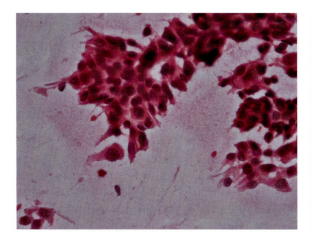

Fig. 4.24 Papillary CA. Polygonal cells with a thick nuclear membrane with irregularities. The nuclei are more transparent in wet fixation. HE stain

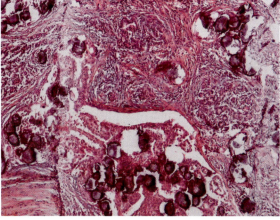

Fig. 4.26 The histological picture of Fig. 4.22. Lymphocytic infiltrates, psammoma bodies and squamoid cells. Paraffin section, hematoxylin, and eosin stain

tis can be confirmed cytologically; however, the smears are frequently challenging toward over- as well as underdiagnoses (Guarda and Baskin 1987). The follicular cells in Hashimoto's thyroiditis, including the oncocytic ones, may exhibit severe atypia, sometimes overdiagnosed as neoplasia (Ravinsky and Safneck 1988). On the contrary, dense lymphocytic infiltrates may obscure the presence of atypical neoplastic cells. The fibrous type of thyroiditis can be extremely difficult to sample. Thyroiditis de Quervain is often painful during aspiration, and the smears are frequently poor. If the aspiration has been performed in the regression phase, the typical multinucleated giant cells may be missed, and the confirmation of the diagnosis is not possible.

Among the tumors, the highest accuracy can be expected by adequate sampling for the papillary carcinoma since this type of tumor is the most common one and since the diagnosis can be accurately made by established cytological patterns and nuclear morphology (correct diagnoses over 90%) (Figs. 4.23 and 4.24). Even some variants of papillary carcinoma with characteristic phenotypes can be recognized with safety, like the aggressive diffuse sclerosing variant (Figs. 4.25 and 4.26). The anaplastic carcinoma is also mostly correctly diagnosed due to the obviously malignant phenotypes; however, paucicellular, inadequate smears are not a rarity, as a consequence of extensive necroses. The medullary carcinoma can reach a high diagnostic accuracy especially in air-dried smears (75–80%); however, the interpreting cytopathologist must be familiar with the different phenotypes of the tumor. The preoperative recognition of a medullary carcinoma can be challenging and, at the same time, of significant importance since it influences the planning of the treatment. Insofar, we would strongly recommend the estimation of calcitonin levels in all smears suspicious for neoplasia, without any further specification. A frequent diagnostic challenge concerns some types of poorly differentiated carcinomas, especially the insular type, leading to monomorphous smears of cells without significant atypia (Nguyen and Akin 2001; Pietribiasi et al. 1990).

The follicular-patterned cellular lesions including hyperplastic nodules and follicular neoplasias (adenomas and carcinomas), exhibiting a conventional follicular cell differentiation or an oncocytic differentiation ("Huerthle cell lesions"), form the large cytologically indeterminate group as mentioned above (Baloch et al. 2002) Goellner et al. 1987. There are the main differences in reporting and the greatest interobserver variability. The more experienced the cytopathologist, the fewer the indeterminate diagnoses. This "gray zone" can be, by increasing experience of the cytopathologist, substantially shortened; however, it can never disappear on morphological grounds (Kini et al. 1985; Raber et al. 2000). Some "indeterminate" smears can, for example, actually represent thick-smeared samples, misleading to an overdiagnosis of a cellular lesion (Fig. 4.27). An oncocytic papillary carcinoma can be misinterpreted as an oxyphilic nodule if the typical nuclear features are underestimated. Nevertheless, even the most experienced cytopathologists cannot afford a definite diagnosis in evaluating a real microfollicular cellular pattern since the potential of invasiveness cannot be assessed on cytological grounds. In that sense, this "borderline" group is a real limitation of the method. In surgically resected specimens, this group exhibited malignancy in about 30–35% (Buesseniers and Silver 2007). We would like to point out the significance of correlating this cytological diagnosis to all other findings prior to making the decision for the management. We suggest the maximal diameter of the lesion to be the most critical parameter since large cellular lesions are more likely to be invasive malignancies than the smaller ones. Furthermore, the differentiation of a parathyroidal lesion from an "adenomatoid" thyroid nodule can be extremely difficult, especially if a parathyroidal adenoma has been aspirated by mistake

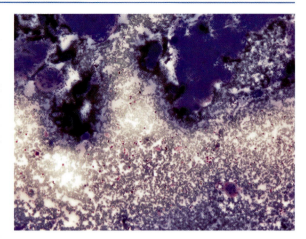

Fig. 4.27 "Pseudocellular" thick preparation of an adenomatous nodule. Most of the areas are too thick for evaluation; however, benign three-dimensional microfollicles with metachromatic basement membrane material are visible. MGG stain

(as a thyroid nodule). Based on the lack of colloid and the high cellularity, most of these cases are overdiagnosed as thyroidal neoplasias, leading to an unnecessary thyroidectomy (Tseleni-Balafouta et al. 2007). Therefore, we suggest to include the possibility of a parathyroidal adenoma in the differential diagnosis of the cellular indeterminate smears. The medullary carcinoma may also sometimes lack the typical cell phenotype and exhibit a rather follicular to solid pattern, mimicking a follicular lesion. Insofar, we find as reasonable the exclusion of the latter two possibilities by comparing the parathormone and calcitonin blood values in all "cellular," indeterminate smears.

Malignant lymphomas are relatively accurately diagnosed (78%), especially if they are of high-grade malignancy. Since the morphology is not sufficient for the classification of the lymphomas, by suspicion of a lymphoma, extra passes would be needed to get additional material for flow cytometry or immunocytochemical detection of the immunophenotype of the lymphoid cells (Dong et al. 2001; Henrique et al. 1999; Matsuzuka et al. 1993).

4.6.3 How Accurate Is FNA in Exploring the Neck Lymph Nodes in the Presence of a Thyroid CA?

A positive finding of a metastasis is principally a safe diagnosis, whereas a negative smear does not exclude the presence of a metastasis since it might be missed by sampling. Cervical lymph node metastases frequently undergo extensive cystic degeneration, resulting in acellular smears. Cystic foci in lymph nodes remain highly suspicious, even by negative FNA results. The measurement of thyroglobulin in the cystic fluid would be another interesting option to confirm a suspicion if the amount of cancer cells is not sufficient for the diagnosis.

4.6.4 How Useful Can FNA Be in the Postoperative Follow-Up?

FNA is an ideal tool in elucidating an enlargement in the anatomic site of the thyroid or in the vicinity after the removal of the gland. It can accurately differentiate between a foreign body granuloma, a lymph node enlargement, and a thyroid residual tissue, as well as others unrelated to the operation lesions. Especially in the case of a thyroid carcinoma, it is very helpful in detecting a local recurrence or a lymph node metastasis.

4.7 The Communication Between the Clinicians and the Cytopathologists

A good working cytopathologist-clinician interaction represents the final step, highly significant in this diagnostic approach, very crucial for the best decision-making. The microscopic report should serve as a guide for the clinicians to manage the nodules, insofar it should reflect the possibilities and limitations of the diagnosis in each case. Many reporting systems have tried to standardize the information of the smears, creating classifications helpful for the management.

4.7.1 Reporting of the FNA Findings

Over the last years, several proposals for the cytological reporting appeared reflecting the wide use of the method and the increasing experience in the communication. The presence of different formats is rather confusing especially for clinicians inexperienced in the cytological evaluation (Wang 2006). The Papanicolaou Society of Cytopathology worked out a reporting system widely used by the cytopathologists (Papanicolaou Society of Cytopathology Task Force on Standards of Practice 1996). We consider the recently issued Bethesda System for Reporting Thyroid Cytopathology (BSRTC) (Baloch et al. 2008), based on an NCI-sponsored conference (2007), to be the most suitable for communicating the findings from the smears to the clinicians. It is a 6-tiered system with the following general format:

I. Nondiagnostic or unsatisfactory
II. Benign
III. Atypia of undetermined significance or follicular lesion of undetermined significance
IV. Follicular neoplasm or suspicious for a follicular neoplasm
V. Suspicious for malignancy
VI. Malignant

Each group includes different possible diagnoses. The estimated risk of malignancy is increasing from 0% to 3% in group II (benign) to 97–99% in group VI (malignant) (Baloch et al. 2008).

4.7.2 Our Suggestions for the Reporting

The clinicians are frequently asking the cytopathologists about the safety of their cytological report and the risk of a false-negative or a false-positive diagnosis. In order to include in the reporting system some issues usually discussed in personal communication, we suggest the following modifications:

Since the "benign" smears may interfere at the one end with the "nondiagnostic" and at the other end with the "indeterminate" ones and no quantitative criteria can help to eliminate this problem, we suggest a sub-classifying of this group as follows:

Benign smears
(a) *Of uncertain adequacy*

We can move here the "nondiagnostic" smears consisting of abundant colloid without any or with few follicular cells and the smears with lymphocytes on a ground of Hashimoto's disease as well as "cyst fluid only" smears (with many phagocytes). We can also include some cases with incon-cordance of the cytology and US findings, like cases with cystic lesions in US and just lymphocytes in cytology, indicating that the needle might have missed the lesion. In that class, we also could include the cases with sparse cells in the presence of large nodule's size since we think the US findings should be kept in mind by the pathologists, as well as by endocrinologists (according to our proposal for the definition of the adequacy).

(b) *With low risk of false negative* (obviously benign, permitting the clinicians to feel safe):

Includes cases with abundant material, exhibiting abundant diffuse colloid, and many follicular cells dissociated, in monolayered sheets and in three-dimensional follicles. Phagocytes may be present (colloid, macrofollicular pattern, eventually with areas of cystic degeneration).

(c) *With high risk of false negative*

Concerns all cases with a cellular, "adenomatoid" pattern (borderline to the indeterminate), the cases with oxyphilic metaplasia, and the cases with focal atypia in Hashimoto's thyroiditis.

Using this classification and alerting the clinicians for the benign group c, we were able to minimize over the last decade the mismanagement of thyroid cancer based on false-negative diagnoses.

Most cases of the benign group (a) can be alternatively classified as "nondiagnostic." In that case this group could also be subclassified as follows:

Nondiagnostic

(a) Without any specific elements (blood, fibrous fragments)
(b) Favors benign (colloid cysts, cystic fluid only)
(c) With evidence of suspicion (evidence of atypical cells, however, with a poor quality of the smear in terms of smearing, fixation or staining, or suspicious background elements such as multinucleated giant cells or psammomas) or evidence of inadequacy of the sampling (as previously analyzed)

It is obvious that FNA of the c group should be repeated immediately, in contrast to the group b. Even for the nondiagnostic smears, it might be helpful for the clinicians to know how urgent is the need to repeat the FNA since some nodules are small with an indolent sonographic appearance and since some patients principally refuse to repeat the whole procedure.

4.7.3 Reading "Between the Lines" of the FNA Report ("How Accurate Is It?")

Beyond any reporting system whenever used, the personal communication in the frame of a teamwork is the best way to maximize the benefit of the FNA diagnosis. Some general conclusions are possible, regarding the reliability of the cytological diagnosis. First of all, the clinicians should read the cytological report carefully in order to personally estimate the degree of the sample's adequacy, especially if the cytopathologist is not aware of the clinical findings. Even in the case of a satisfying adequacy, the degree of reliability varies among the various cytological diagnoses as follows:

1. *Benign diagnoses*
(a) "Colloid nodules"

Colloid-rich nodules containing typical follicular cells and eventual phagocytes may generally with safety be treated and followed up as indolent hyperplastic nodules.

(b) "Adenomatoid nodules"

Cellular nodules with scanty colloid ("adenomatoid nodules") are less safely diagnosed as benign since a well-differentiated neoplasm may be able to mimic an adenomatoid nodule. In that sense, adenomatoid hyperplastic nodules – more than the colloid ones – should be evaluated in correlation to the clinical and sonographical findings and should have a shorter interval for follow-up.

(c) Smears with oncocytic (oxyphilic) metaplasia

Metaplastic oxyphilic cells are very frequent in Hashimoto's thyroiditis, but they can be focally observed in nodular hyperplasia. Insofar, sheets of oncocytic cells may be present in benign smears, and they should not alert the clinicians, unless exclusively represented, dissociated, and with some degree of atypia. Yet, we would like to mention that some inexperienced cytopathologists underestimate oxyphilic neoplastic cells (mainly of papillary carcinoma) as metaplastic cells. Generally, smears of atypical or oncocytic nodules in a Hashimoto's thyroiditis can be very challenging, and it is recommended that they should be evaluated by very experienced cytopathologists.

(d) Smears with lymphocytic infiltrates

Smears exhibiting a dense lymphocytic infiltrate may be highly confusing, either toward false-positive or false-negative diagnoses. Atypical epithelial cells with lymphocytic thyroiditis in the absence of biochemical or sonographical evidence of Hashimoto's thyroiditis must be considered as possible neoplasia with peritumoral lymphocytic thyroiditis (Tseleni-Balafouta et al. 1989). We advice the clinicians to correlate the FNA diagnosis of lymphocytic-rich smears to the ultrasonographic and the clinical findings and to keep the follow-up intervals short, in the case of a decision for a conservative approach.

2. *Malignant diagnoses*

The more specific the tumor classification, the more unlikely to have a false-positive diagnosis. Smears with "some evidence of suspicion" not further classified are likely to be overdiagnosed due to functional atypia.

The diagnostic accuracy and specificity varies greatly among the various histological types of the tumors. The most accurate diagnoses can be made in representative samples of papillary carcinoma, especially of the conventional type and of the aggressive tumor variants. Some difficulties are observed in the follicular variant, mainly of the macrofollicular type due to the lack of papillary structures and to the admixture of abundant colloid, obscuring the neoplastic cells. Extensive cystic degeneration of lymph node metastases of papillary CA is a common finding. The aspirates of such nodes are frequently inadequate lacking the neoplastic cells. Therefore, colloid and phagocytes in lymph node samples are highly suspicious for a metastatic focus of papillary CA, even in the absence of neoplastic cells.

The suspicion of a follicular neoplasm based mainly of the high cellularity of the smears is frequently a matter of debate among the cytopathologists, with a significant interobserver variability. Such findings should be correlated to the clinical data since high cellularity can be observed in benign nodules of young individuals, on the ground of thyroiditis, or in pregnant women. Nevertheless, the follicular variant of a papillary CA may be misdiagnosed as follicular neoplasia. A second opinion from an expert can sometimes result in a more definite diagnosis.

The medullary carcinoma can most of the times be detected by an experienced cytopathologist, preferably in air-dried direct smears. However, this tumor can exhibit a diversity of morphologies, and it can be easily underdiagnosed – not at least due to a lack of awareness on the ground of the relative rarity of the tumor. On suspicion, the diagnosis can be confirmed by immunocytochemistry (or just by comparing the blood calcitonin levels).

Anaplastic carcinomas can be most of the times easily diagnosed since they exhibit high-grade atypia and polymorphism. Frequently, the diagnosis has been made clinically by the rapid progression of this extremely aggressive tumor and needs just a confirmation. One limitation is the eventual inadequacy of the sample due to the extensive necroses, as well as the difficulty to recognize the epithelial nature of the tumor as well as to confirm the thyroid gland as the primary site of origin.

The diagnosis of a poorly differentiated carcinoma can be easily missed, especially in the insular type, exhibiting smears of high cellularity, however with only mild to moderate nuclear atypia. Furthermore, poorly differentiated CA frequently cannot be delineated from differentiated carcinoma since both tumor components may coexist. A component from an anaplastic carcinoma may also be underdiagnosed.

It is obvious that, given the heterogeneity of phenotypes in the thyroid tumors, FNA can serve as an initial tool for the classification of thyroid nodules and the selection for surgery since the final diagnosis has to be made on histological grounds.

References

Baloch ZW, Livolsi VA (2004) Fine needle aspiration of thyroid nodules: past, present and future. Endocr Pract 10: 234–241

Baloch ZW, Fleisher S, Livolsi VA et al (2002) Diagnosis of "follicular neoplasm": a gray zone in thyroid fine-needle aspiration cytology. Diagn Cytopathol 26:41–44

Baloch ZW, Livolsi VA, Asa SL et al (2008) Diagnostic terminology and morphologic criteria for cytologic diagnosis of thyroid lesions: a synopsis of the National Cancer Institute thyroid fine needle aspiration state of the science conference. Diagn Cytopathol 36:425–437

Boerner SL, Asa SL (2010) Biopsy interpretation of thyroid. Lippincott, Williams and Wilkins, Philadelphia, pp 13–37

Boon M (1992) Routine cytologic staining procedures. In: Weid GL, Bibbo M, Keebler CM et al (eds) Tutorials of cytology. International Academy of Cytology, Chicago

Brander A, Viikinkoski P, Nickels J et al (1991) Thyroid gland: US screening in a random adult population. Radiology 181: 683–687

Buesseniers AE, Silver SA (2007) Fine needle aspiration cytology of the thyroid. In: Oertli D, Udelsman R (eds) Surgery of the thyroid and parathyroid glands. Springer, Berlin/Heidelberg, pp 61–80

Chow LS, Gharib H, Goellner JR et al (2001) Nondiagnostic thyroid fine needle aspiration cytology: management dilemmas. Thyroid 11:1147–1151

Christensen SB, Ericson UB, Janzon L et al (1984) The prevalence of thyroid disorders in a middle-aged female population with special reference to the solitary thyroid nodule. Acta Chir Scand 150:13–19

Crystal BS, Wang HH, Ducatman BS (1993) Comparison of different preparation techniques for fine needle aspiration specimens. A semiquantitative and statistical analysis. Acta Cytol 37:24–28

Delibasis KK, Asvestas PA, Matsopoulos GK, Zoulias E, Tseleni-Balafouta S (2009) Computer-aided diagnosis of thyroid malignancy using an artificial immune system classification algorithm. IEEE Trans Inf Technol Biomed 13(5):680–686

Dong HY, Harris NL, Preffer FI, Pitman MB (2001) Fine needle aspiration biopsy in the diagnosis and classification of primary and recurrent lymphoma: a retrospective analysis of the utility of cytomorphology and flow cytometry. Mod Pathol 14:472–481

Droese M (1995) Aspiration cytology of the thyroid. Schattauer, Stuttgart/New York, pp 3–25

Gharib H (1994) Fine needle aspiration biopsy of thyroid nodules: advantages, limitations and effect. Mayo Clin Proc 69:44–49

Gharib H, Goellner JR (1993) Fine needle aspiration biopsy of the thyroid: an appraisal. Ann Intern Med 118:282–289

Gharib H, Goellner JR, Johnson DA (1993) Fine needle aspiration cytology of the thyroid: a 12-year experience with 11000 biopsies. Clin Lab Med 13:699–709

Gharib H, Papini E, Paschke R, Duick DS, Valcavi R, Hegedüs L, Vitti P, AACE/AME/ETA Task Force on Thyroid Nodules (2010) American Association of Clinical Endocrinologists, Associazione Medici Endocrinologi, and European Thyroid Association medical guidelines for clinical practice for the diagnosis and management of thyroid nodules: executive summary of recommendations. J Endocrinol Invest 33(5 Suppl):51–56

Goellner JR, Gharib H, Grant CS et al (1987) Fine needle aspiration of thyroid, 1980 to 1986. Acta Cytol 31:587–590

Guarda LA, Baskin HJ (1987) Inflammatory and lymphoid lesions of the thyroid gland: cytomorphology by fine needle aspiration. Am J Clin Pathol 87:14–22

Hall TL, Layfield LG, Philippe A, Rosenthal DL (1989) Sources of diagnostic error in fine needle aspiration of the thyroid. Cancer 63:718–725

Hamburger JI, Hamburger SW (1986) Fine needle biopsy of thyroid nodules: avoiding the pitfalls. N Y State J Med 86:241–249

Hamburger JI, Hussein M (1988) Semiquantitative criteria for fine needle aspiration diagnosis: reduced false negative diagnosis. Diagn Cytopathol 4:14–17

Henrique RM, Sousa ME, Godinho MI et al (1999) Immunophenotyping by flow cytometry of fine needle aspirates in the diagnosis of lymphoproliferative disorders: a retrospective study. J Clin Lab Anal 13:224–228

Jayaram G, Razak A, Chan SK et al (1999) Fine needle aspiration of the thyroid: a review of experience in 1854 cases. Malays J Pathol 21:17–27

Keebler CM (1991) Cytopreparatory techniques. In: Bibbo M (ed) Comprehensive cytopathology. Saunders, Philadelphia

Kini SR, Miller JM, Hamburger JI et al (1985) Cytopathology of follicular lesions of the thyroid gland. Diagn Cytopathol 1: 123–132

Ko HM, JhuIK YSH et al (2003) Clinicopathologic analysis of fine needle aspiration cytology of the thyroid. Acta Cytol 47:727–732

Kocjan G (2006) FNAC technique and slide preparation. In: Fine needle aspiration cytology. Springer, Berlin/Heidelberg, pp 7–33

Lowhagen T, Sprenger E (1974) Cytologic presentation of thyroid tumors in aspiration biopsy smear: a review of 60 cases. Acta Cytol 18:192–197

Matsuzuka F, Miyauchi A, Katayama S, Narabayashi I, Ikeda H, Kuma K, Sugawara M (1993) Clinical aspects of primary thyroid lymphoma: diagnosis and treatment based on our experience of 119 cases. Thyroid 3:93–99

Mazzaferri FL, de los Santos ET, Rofagha Keyhani S et al (1988) Solitary thyroid nodule: diagnosis and management. Med Clin North Am 72:1177–1211

Nguyen GK, Akin MR (2001) Cytopathology of insular carcinoma of the thyroid. Diagn Cytopathol 25:325–330

Nguyen GK, Ginsberg J, Crockford PM (1991) Fine needle aspiration biopsy cytology of the thyroid. Its value and limitations in the diagnosis and management of the solitary thyroid nodules. Pathol Annu 26:63

Orell SR, Philips J (1997) The thyroid: fine needle biopsy and cytological diagnosis of thyroid lesions. Karger, Basel/London/New York, pp 8–29

Papanicolaou Society of Cytopathology Task Force on Standards of Practice (1996) Guidelines of the Papanicolaou society of cytopathology for the examination of fine-needle aspiration specimen from thyroid nodules. Diagn Cytopathol 15:84–89

Pietribiasi F, Sapino A, Papotti M et al (1990) Cytologic features of poorly differentiated "insular" carcinoma of the thyroid, as revealed by fine needle aspiration biopsy. Am J Clin Pathol 94:687–692

Raber W, Kasserer K, Niederle B et al (2000) Risk factors of malignancy of thyroid nodules initially identified as follicular neoplasia by fine needle aspiration: results of a prospective study of one hundred twenty patients. Thyroid 10: 109–112

Ravinsky E, Safneck JR (1988) Differentiation of Hashimoto's thyroiditis from thyroid neoplasms in fine needle aspirates. Acta Cytol 32:854–861

Revetto C, Colombo L, Dottorini ME (2000) Usefulness of fine needle aspiration in the diagnosis of thyroid carcinoma: a retrospective study in 37,895 patients. Cancer 90:357–363

Saxen E, Franssila K, Bjarnason O, Norman T, Ringertz N (1978) Observer variation in histologic classification of thyroid cancer. Acta Pathol Microbiol Scand A 86:483–486

Tseleni S (1986) Fine needle aspiration of thyroid: confusion v. subsequent histology. J Clin Pathol 39(6):697–698

Tseleni-Balafouta S, Kyroudi-Voulgari A, Paizi-Biza P, Papacharalampous NX (1989) Lymphocytic thyroiditis in fine-needle aspirates: differential diagnostic aspects. Diagn Cytopathol 5(4):362–365

Tseleni-Balafouta S, Katsouyanni K, Kitsopanides J, Koutras DA (1991) The outcome of benign thyroid nodules correlates with the findings of fine needle biopsy. Thyroidology 3(2):75–78

Tseleni-Balafouta S, Gakiopoulou H, Kavantzas N, Agrogiannis G, Givalos N, Patsouris E (2007) Parathyroid proliferations: a source of diagnostic pitfalls in FNA of thyroid. Cancer 111(2):130–136

Wang HH (2006) Reporting thyroid fine needle aspiration: literature review and proposal. Diagn Cytopathol 34:67–76

Zito FA, Gadaleta CD, Salvatore C et al (1995) A modified cell block technique for fine needle aspiration cytology. Acta Cytol 39:93–99

Thyroid Pathology

5

Zubair W. Baloch and Virginia A. LiVolsi

5.1 Normal Thyroid

The gross and microscopic features of the normal thyroid are:
- A bilobed gland, connected by an isthmus.
- It is enveloped by a thin capsule which contains sizable venous channels.
- The weight of normal thyroid in the United States ranges from 10 to 20 g.
- The functional unit of the thyroid is known as "follicle" which averages about 20 μm in diameter (Dozois and Beahrs 1977; Akimova and Zotikov 1969; Mansberger and Wei 1993; Miller 2003).
- An aggregate of 20–40 follicles bound together by a thin sheath of connective tissue gives rise to a thyroid lobule (Mansberger and Wei 1993; Zampi et al. 1994).
- *The thyroid follicles* are lined by a single layer of low cuboidal follicular epithelium. The follicular lumen contains colloid, partly composed of thyroglobulin.
  - The nucleus of the follicular cell is round to ovoid in shape with evenly distributed nuclear chromatin; it is usually centrally placed with a not so readily identifiable nucleolus (Kondalenko et al. 1970).
- *The C cells* are seen next to the follicular cells and within the basal lamina that surrounds each follicle of the normal gland.
  - Usually concentrated in the central portions of the middle and upper thirds of the thyroid lobes (Mansberger and Wei 1993).
  - Typically increase in number in thyroids of infants as compared to adult glands (Sugiyama 1971; Kovalenko 1999).
  - Develop from the C cells which arise from the neural crest and migrate with the ultimobranchial body into the thyroid.
  - Microscopically, they are polygonal- to spindle-shaped and contain numerous membrane-bound cytoplasmic granules harboring calcitonin. A small number of C cells (or cells similar to them) contain somatostatin (Gibson et al. 1980; Wolfe et al. 1975; Baschieri et al. 1989; Dhillon et al. 1982).
  - Hyperplasia of C-cell aggregates can occur in some adults without any known endocrinologic abnormality (O'Toole et al. 1985).
  - The C-cell hyperplasia is defined as consisting of more than 40 C cells/cm^2 and the presence of at least three low-power microscopic fields containing more than 50 C cells (Guyetant et al. 1997).
  - The small solid cell nests, considered to be of ultimobranchial origin (Guyetant et al. 1997), have the same spatial distribution in the thyroid lobes as the C cells (Harach 1986, 1988).
  - Thyroid follicles which are lined by follicular cells and epidermoid cells (and sometimes C cells) and contain both colloid and mucoid material. These are known as "mixed follicles" (most likely originating from the ultimobranchial body rests) (Harach 1987).
- *The oncocytic cells* (oxyphil, Askanazy cells, Hürthle cells) represent metaplastic follicular cells.

- They are usually larger than follicular cells and have granular eosinophilic cytoplasm and round nucleus with prominent nucleolus (Baloch and LiVolsi 1999a).
- By electron microscopy, the cytoplasm is filled with enlarged mitochondria.
- Commonly seen in long-standing Graves' disease, autoimmune thyroiditis, thyroids affected by radiation, follicular-derived neoplasms, and some adenomatoid goiter (Baloch and LiVolsi 1999a; Weiss et al. 1984; Mikhailov et al. 1980).
• Small collections of lymphocytes and rare dendritic cells (antigen-presenting cells) can be seen in normal thyroid gland parenchyma. These are usually limited to the interstitial tissue (Mitchell et al. 1984).

5.2 Developmental Variations

5.2.1 The Thyroglossal Tract

• It extends in the midline from the foramen cecum at the base of the tongue to the isthmus of the normal gland (Katz and Hachigian 1988).
• It is usually attached to and may extend through the center of the hyoid bone and is intimately related to the surrounding skeletal muscle.
• By light microscopy, it consists of connective tissue, the thyroglossal duct, lymphoid tissue, and thyroid follicles.
• The thyroglossal duct is typically lined by ciliated pseudostratified epithelium.
• In case of trauma or infection, the epithelium may undergo transitional or squamous metaplasia or maybe totally be replaced by fibrous tissue.
• Fluid accumulation in the duct can lead to development of thyroglossal cyst (Topf et al. 1988; Mansberger and Wei 1993; Allard 1982).
• In rare instances, portions of thyroglossal duct are embedded within the thyroid gland proper and can give rise to an intrathyroidal cyst (Katz and Hachigian 1988).

5.2.2 The Ectopic Thyroid and Other Developmental Variations

• Thyroid maldescent can result in the presence of *lingual thyroid* located in the back of the tongue; as this tissue grows, it could become a surgical emergency in young children. In some patients, this may be the only thyroid that is present. Its removal, therefore, could result in profound acute hypothyroidism. Any type of diffuse thyroid disease can involve lingual thyroid and the thyroid tissue along the thyroglossal tract (Allard 1982; Baughman 1972; Heshmati et al. 1997).
• Due to its close association with the development of other tissues, thyroid tissue may be seen in association with the esophagus, larynx, trachea, jugular carotid lymph nodes, soft tissues of the neck, and even in association with the heart and great vessels (Kaplan et al. 1978; Kantelip et al. 1986).
• Developmental considerations also explain the finding of normal thyroid tissue in the cervical fat or muscle (Carpenter and Emery 1976). Fat, cartilage, or muscle may occasionally be found within the thyroid capsule (Finkle and Goldman 1973; Gardner 1956). These minor developmental variations must be remembered lest they be confused with infiltrative neoplastic growth.
• Parathyroid glands, thymic tissue, small collections of cartilage, and glands lined by ciliated cells may be seen in normal thyroids, likely related to defective development of the branchial pouches (Apel et al. 1994; Carpenter and Emery 1976; Harach et al. 1993).

5.2.3 Benign Thyroid Inclusions

• Thyroid follicles in lateral cervical lymph nodes should be considered metastatic carcinoma (papillary carcinoma) (Baloch and LiVolsi 2002a; LiVolsi 1990; Gerard-Marchant 1964).
• Normal thyroid tissue lying only within the capsule of a central midline node may represent an embryologic remnant/normal thyroid inclusion and not metastatic cancer (Roth 1965; Meyer and Steinberg 1969).

5.3 Diffuse Processes and Enlargements of Thyroid

5.3.1 The Thyroiditides

Although occasionally presenting as nodules or asymmetric enlargement of the gland, thyroiditis commonly involves the gland diffusely.

5.3.1.1 Acute Thyroiditis

- It is rare and is almost always due to infection, however may be encountered in the thyroid shortly following radiation exposure (Imai et al. 2002; Lambert et al. 1980).
- A variety of organisms cause thyroiditis including bacteria, fungi, and viruses (Leesen et al. 2001).
- It is most commonly encountered in malnourished children, elderly debilitated adults, immunocompromised individuals, or in otherwise healthy patients following trauma to the neck (Golshan et al. 1997; Imai et al. 2002).
- Most patients present with painful enlargement of the gland.
- By light microscopic examination, the diagnostic features include acute inflammation and microabscess formation. Microorganisms may be seen.

5.3.1.2 Granulomatous Thyroiditis

- It is usually a self-limiting disease which is also referred to as nonsuppurative thyroiditis or de Quervain's disease, is a rare entity that usually presents in women, and has been associated with HLA Bw35 (Hnilica and Nyulassy 1985).
- The microscopic picture is dependent upon the stage of the disease.
  - Early in the disease, there is loss of the follicular epithelium and colloid depletion.
  - The inflammatory response composed initially of polymorphonuclear leukocytes and even microabscesses progresses until lymphocytes, plasma cells, and histiocytes become the major inflammatory cells.
  - Histiocytes and giant cells replace the follicular epithelium.
  - A central fibrotic reaction is seen in late stages (Harach and Williams 1990).
  - Recovery is associated with regeneration of follicles from the viable edges of the involved areas (Meachim and Young 1963).

5.3.1.3 Palpation Thyroiditis

Palpation thyroiditis is found in 85–95% of surgically resected thyroids and most likely represents the thyroid's response to minor trauma associated with physical examination (Carney et al. 1975; Harach 1993).

5.3.1.4 Chronic Lymphocytic Thyroiditis

Mizukami et al. divided their patients with lymphocytic infiltration of the thyroid gland into four groups:

1. Chronic thyroiditis, oxyphilic: This group contains patients with classic Hashimoto's disease histology.
2. Chronic thyroiditis, mixed: This group shows less of an infiltrate than group 1 with minimal fibrosis. Patients demonstrate either eu-, hyper-, or hypothyroidism.
3. Chronic thyroiditis, hyperplastic: This group shows glandular hyperplasia associated with only a small lymphocytic reaction. Most patients are hyperthyroid.
4. Chronic thyroiditis, focal: This group shows only a focal lymphocytic reaction, and most patients are euthyroid.

5.3.1.5 Autoimmune Thyroiditis

- Common synonyms for autoimmune thyroiditis include Hashimoto's thyroiditis, lymphocytic thyroiditis, and struma lymphomatosa (Mizukami et al. 1982).
- It is most common in women and displays a variety of clinical and pathologic changes which include: hypothyroidism, rarely hyperthyroidism, large goiter, atrophic gland, and scattered clusters of infiltrating lymphocytes evolving to extensive chronic inflammation and scarring with almost complete loss of follicular epithelium (Mizukami et al. 1982; Hayashi et al. 1985).
- The thyroiditis may be found in the same families in which idiopathic hypothyroidism and Graves' disease are common. It may follow typical Graves' disease (Tomer et al. 2003).
- The hyperthyroid variant of autoimmune thyroiditis is closely related to Graves' disease and may be indistinguishable on the basis of gross and microscopic features, suggesting that this variant may indeed be Graves' disease (Fatourechi et al. 1971).
- In Hashimoto's thyroiditis:
  - The thyroid gland is firm and symmetrically enlarged weighing from 25 to 250 g (Mizukami et al. 1982). It has a tan yellow appearance attributed to the abundant lymphoid tissue.
  - By light microscopy (Fig. 5.1a, b):
    The thyroid follicles are small and atrophic.
    Colloid appears dense or may be absent.
    Follicular cells are metaplastic and include oncocytic (Hürthle cell), clear cell, and squamous (epidermoid) types.
    In the interstitium and in atrophic follicles, a lymphoplasmacytic infiltration with well-developed lymphoid germinal centers is found.

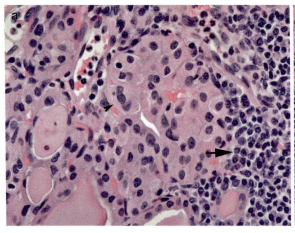

Fig. 5.1 (**a**) Chronic lymphocytic thyroiditis (Hashimoto's thyroiditis) demonstrating oncocytic metaplasia of follicular cells/Hürthle cell metaplasia (*arrowhead*) and infiltration by lymphocytes (*arrow*). (**b**) The lymphocytic infiltration can be extensive leading to lymphoid follicle formation (*center of the micrograph*)

Interlobular fibrosis can be seen in varying amounts (Mizukami et al. 1982; LiVolsi 1990).

The lymphocytic infiltrate is composed of both T and B cells in an almost 1:1 ratio, which differs from the peripheral blood, which shows T-cell predominance (Aozasa et al. 1989; Iwatani et al. 1983, 1993).

Patients with Hashimoto's thyroiditis are at increased risk of neoplasia with the most common malignancy being malignant lymphoma, B-cell type (Kossev and Livolsi 1999; Lam et al. 1999). In addition, a rare malignant tumor known as sclerosing mucoepidermoid carcinoma with eosinophilia has been recognized in patients with Hashimoto's disease (Baloch et al. 2000b).

5.3.1.6 Fibrosing Variant of Hashimoto's Thyroiditis

- This comprises approximately 10–13% of all cases of Hashimoto's disease.
- On microscopic examination, the thyroid architecture is abolished by severe follicular atrophy, dense keloid-like fibrosis, and prominent squamous/epidermoid metaplasia (most likely representing hyperplasia of the ultimobranchial body rests) of the follicular epithelium (Katz and Vickery 1974; Papi et al. 2003b).

5.3.1.7 Painless/Silent Thyroiditis

- This is an autoimmune disease, which causes painless enlargement of thyroid gland along with brief hyperthyroidism followed by hypothyroidism.
- It can be encountered in postpartum period and is also termed as postpartum thyroiditis (LiVolsi 1993; Weetman et al. 1990; Papi et al. 2003a).
- The histology shows disruption of follicular architecture and lymphocytic infiltration. Stromal fibrous and oxyphilic changes are rare (LiVolsi 1993).

5.3.1.8 Focal Nonspecific Thyroiditis

- Focal lymphocytic infiltration of the thyroid is found more frequently at autopsy and in surgical specimens.
- It has been suggested that iodide (iodine) in diet may combine with a protein, act as an antigen, and evoke an immune response localized to the thyroid gland (Vollenweider et al. 1982).
- It is characterized by focal lymphocytic aggregates and occasional germinal center formation. Follicular atrophy and oncocytic metaplasia are encountered rarely in these cases (Mizukami et al. 1988b).

5.3.1.9 Amiodarone-Induced Injury with Thyrotoxicosis

Administration of amiodarone may cause thyrotoxicosis, primarily due to the large quantity of iodine in the drug (Bogazzi et al. 2001; Roti and Uberti 2001).

5.3.1.10 Riedel's Disease (aka Riedel's Thyroiditis)

- This is a rare multisystem disorder with female predominance that involves the thyroid as well as other structures in the neck or even systemic structures,

sclerosing mediastinitis, retroperitoneal fibrosis, pseudotumor of the orbit, and sclerosis of the biliary tract (sclerosing cholangitis) (Arnott and Greaves 1965; Bartholomew et al. 1963; Davies and Furness 1984; Rao et al. 1973).
- Most patients are euthyroid, although hypothyroidism and hyperthyroidism have been reported (Schwaegerle et al. 1988; Katsikas et al. 1976).
- The gross descriptions of the thyroid range from stony hard to woody fixed ("ligneous thyroiditis").
- The microscopic examination shows:
  - The involved gland is destroyed and replaced by keloid-like fibrous tissue, associated with lymphocytes and plasma cells (Schwaegerle et al. 1988; Papi et al. 2002).
  - The fibrous tissue extends into muscle, nerves, and fat and entraps blood vessels. There is an associated vasculitis (predominantly a phlebitis) with frequent thrombosis (Meij and Hausman 1978).
  - In about 25% of cases, the parathyroid glands are also encased (Papi et al. 2002; Casoli and Tumiati 1999).
- Recently, it has been suggested that Riedel's disease belongs to the spectrum of IgG4-related systemic disease as they share the histopathologic features, and both have similar pattern of multiple organ involvement. Recognition of this link between Riedel's thyroiditis and IgG4-related systemic disease has implication for diagnosis, treatment, and prognosis (Dahlgren et al. 2010).

5.3.1.11 Combined Riedel's Disease and Hashimoto's Thyroiditis

In rare instances, the thyroid gland can show features of both Riedel's disease and Hashimoto's thyroiditis (Baloch et al. 2000a).

5.3.2 Graves' Disease/Diffuse Toxic Goiter

- It is characterized by diffuse enlargement of the thyroid up to several times the normal size.
- On gross examination, the cut surfaces are fleshy and lack normal translucence because of loss of colloid.
- The microscopic picture may vary due to treatment.
- *If the patient is untreated*, or treated briefly, the microscopic appearance shows (Fig 5.2):
  - Cellular hypertrophy and hyperplasia (LiVolsi 1990; LiVolsi 1994).

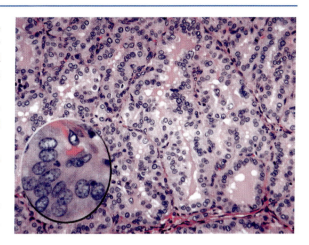

Fig. 5.2 Graves' disease showing cellular hypertrophy and hyperplasia with minimal colloid production. The high power (*inset*) demonstrating nuclear chromatin clearing which can be mistaken for papillary thyroid carcinoma

  - The follicular cells are tall columnar and are arranged into papillary formations that extend into the lumina of the follicles.
  - Blood vessels are congested.
  - Lymphoid infiltrates are seen between the follicles confined to interstitium.
- *In patients who receive antithyroid medication* before surgery, the glands can:
  - Appear almost normal except for numerous large follicles filled with colloid. A few papillae may remain.
  - The vascular congestion is notably decreased, especially if there has been preoperative administration of iodide (LiVolsi 1990).
  - If the patient has only been treated for symptoms, i.e., with beta-blockers, the histology of the gland resembles that of the untreated state (Kawai et al. 1993; Hirota et al. 1986).
- *In some patients*, the lymphocytic infiltration is very prominent and resembles the gland affected by chronic lymphocytic thyroiditis (LiVolsi 1990).

5.3.3 Dyshormonogenetic Goiter

- This pathology is seen in cases of inborn error of thyroid metabolism.
- The increase in TSH due to insufficient thyroid hormone leads to a larger, more active thyroid.

- Microscopically, enlargement of follicular cells and virtual absence of colloid are seen (Cassano 1971; Rosenthal et al. 1990).
- Most often, the follicular cells will demonstrate nuclear enlargement and pleomorphism. The hyperplastic nodules along with nuclear changes can be mistaken for carcinoma (Ghossein et al. 1997). Cancer can occur in a dyshormonogenetic goiter, but it is very rare (Ghossein et al. 1997; Vickery 1981).

5.3.4 Iatrogenic and Related Hyperplasias

- *Chronic ingestion of excess iodide*, for whatever reason, can lead to diffuse hyperplasia. In these cases, nodules with papillary formations may be numerous. Infiltration of lymphocytes may also occur (Roti and Uberti 2001).
- *A minority (approximately 3%) of patient taking lithium salts* for a prolonged period develop goiter or hypothyroidism or both (Strauss and Trujillo 1986).
- *Bromide ingestion may lead to hypothyroidism*; this leads to follicular cell hyperplasia, papillary architecture, and loss of colloid (Mizukami et al. 1988a).

5.3.5 Miscellaneous Disorders Causing Thyroid Enlargement

5.3.5.1 Radiation Fibrosis
- Radiation exposure can lead to an array of pathologic changes in thyroid gland. These are often related to dose in cases of external radiation. When radioiodine is administered, hypothyroidism is common, and the incidence increases with time (Constine et al. 1984).
- Pathologic changes in the thyroid following external radiation include foci of follicular hyperplasia (88%), lymphocytic infiltration (67%), oncocytic metaplasia (42%), fibrosis (25%), and adenomatous nodule formation (51%) (Komorowski and Hanson 1977).
- After a period of months in some and years in other cases after radiation, the thyroid gland becomes grossly shrunken that histologically shows fibrosis, follicular atrophy, oncocytic and squamous metaplasia, lymphocytic infiltration, and nuclear abnormalities. Vascular changes are prominent and include intimal thickening and sclerosis of arterial walls with a circumferential inflammatory cell infiltrate (Komorowski and Hanson 1977).

5.3.5.2 Amyloidosis
- Amyloid is found in the thyroid in the stroma of medullary thyroid carcinoma (Kennedy et al. 1972), amyloid goiter, and systemic amyloidosis (D'Antonio et al. 2000; Goldsmith et al. 2000).

5.3.5.3 Fibrosis due to Collagen Vascular Disease
- Approximately, 14–24% of patients with scleroderma experience thyroid dysfunction owing to interfollicular fibrosis (Marasini et al. 2005).

5.3.5.4 Pigments in the Thyroid
- *Pigmentation of the thyroid may be caused by iron (hemosiderin) deposition* due to bleeding within thyroid nodules or may be found in disorders of iron metabolism such as hemochromatosis. In the former, the pigment is found in macrophages, whereas in the latter, it is present in cytoplasm of the follicular epithelium (Alexander et al. 1985).
- Chronic administration of minocycline (or occasionally, other tetracycline antibiotics) can lead to deposition of minocycline-associated pigment in follicular cells that produces coal-black coloration to the thyroid (Alexander et al. 1985; Gordon et al. 1984). Thyroid function is rarely altered in these cases.

5.4 Nodular Processes/Enlargements of Thyroid

This category consists of thyroid lesions that present as solitary or multiple nodules: benign nodular goiter, toxic nodules, and benign and malignant neoplasms. The nodular thyroid lesions are of most interest to surgeons and patients since the major differential diagnosis is cancer.

5.4.1 Nontoxic Goiter

- Worldwide, the most common cause of nontoxic goiter is deficient output of thyroid hormone due to

inadequate amount of iodine in the diet causing iodine-deficiency goiter (endemic goiter) (Gaitan et al. 1991; Braverman 2001).
- Other causes of nontoxic goiter include inborn errors of thyroid metabolism (dyshormonogenetic goiter) (Ghossein et al. 1997; Rosenthal et al. 1990), dietary goitrogens, and goitrogenic drugs and chemicals (Bala et al. 1996; Fenwick and Griffiths 1981; Gabrilove et al. 1952; Amdisen et al. 1968).
- The pathologic changes of simple nontoxic goiter include one or more of the following: (1) follicular cell hyperplasia, (2) colloid accumulation/colloid goiter, and (3) nodularity/nodular goiter (Maloof et al. 1975; Bataskis et al. 1963; Struder et al. 1987):
    - *Follicular cell hyperplasia* represents the response of the thyroid follicular cells to TSH, to other growth factors, or to circulating stimulatory antibodies (Struder et al. 1987; LiVolsi 1990; Murray 1998). A hyperplastic gland is diffusely enlarged and not nodular (Murray 1998; LiVolsi 1990). Thyroid follicles are collapsed and contain only scanty colloid. The follicular cells are enlarged and columnar in shape with nuclear enlargement, hyperchromasia, and even pleomorphism. Because of follicular collapse and epithelial hyperplasia and hypertrophy, papillary formation can occur (Ramelli et al. 1982). The extremes of hyperplastic stage combined with papillary architecture and nuclear pleomorphism can be confused with carcinoma (Fig. 5.3). The recognition of the benign nature of this process is possible because of its (Ramelli et al. 1982) diffuse nature, unlike carcinoma, in which the tumors grow as often encapsulated nodular proliferation of abnormal cells in a background of nonneoplastic parenchyma.
    - *The colloid accumulation/colloid goiter phase* represents involution of the hyperplastic thyroid follicles and reaccumulation of colloid. The gland is diffusely enlarged, soft, and has a glistening cut surface because of the excess of stored colloid. The epithelium lining the follicles is low cuboidal or flattened and resembles that of the normal thyroid gland. In addition to large follicles (macrofollicles) filled with colloid, the thyroid may still retain patches of follicular hyperplasia (Fialho and de Oliveira 1971; Greer et al. 1967) (Fig. 5.4).
    - *The nodular stage/nodular goiter* is seen in patients with long-standing thyroid disorders

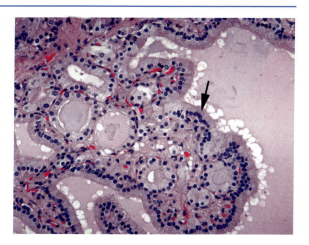

Fig. 5.3 Papillary hyperplasia in case of nodular goiter. Notice the cells (*arrow*) lining the papillary structures show round nuclei with evenly distributed nuclear chromatin

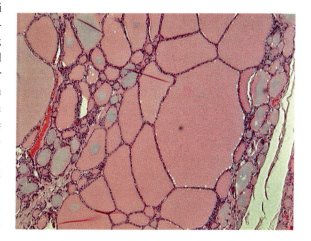

Fig. 5.4 Nodular goiter demonstrating large follicles (macrofollicles) filled with colloid

associated with deficiency of circulating thyroid hormone. It is essentially a process that involves the entire gland, but the nodularity may be asymmetric, and individual nodules within the same gland may vary greatly in size. The nodular goiters result from over distention of some involuted follicles intermixed with zones of persistent epithelial hyperplasia. The new follicles form nodules and may be heterogeneous in their appearance, in their capacity for growth and function, and in their responsiveness to TSH. The vascular network is altered through the elongation and distortion of vessels leading to hemorrhage, necrosis, inflammation, and fibrosis.

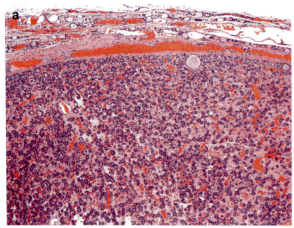 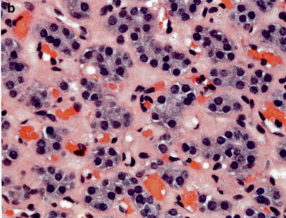

Fig. 5.5 (**a**, **b**): Follicular adenoma. (**a**) Follicular adenoma showing thin capsule and compression of the surrounding thyroid parenchyma. (**b**) The high power demonstrating a monotonous population of follicular cells arranged in microfollicles with minimal colloid

These localized degenerative and reparative changes give rise to nodules that are poorly circumscribed and others that are well demarcated and resemble true adenomas (adenomatous goiter) (Nair 1951; Hirosawa et al. 1983). Growth of goiters therefore may be related to focally excess stimulation by TSH, stimulation by growth factors, focally abnormal iodide concentration, growth-promoting thyroid antibodies, and poorly understood intrathyroidal factors (Braverman 2001). Several studies have shown that about 70% of dominant nodules in nodular goiter are indeed clonal proliferations.

5.4.2 Neoplasms

Thyroid neoplasms demonstrate a variety of morphologic patterns, which complicate their pathological interpretation (LiVolsi and Feind 1976). All neoplasms that arise either from follicular or C cells may have some functional capacities. They may respond to TSH and may even produce excessive amounts of thyroid hormones or, if medullary carcinoma, release abnormal quantities of calcitonin and/or other hormones (LiVolsi 1990). Localization of thyroid transcription factor (TTF-1) and thyroglobulin or calcitonin by immunohistochemistry aids in the classification of unusual thyroidal tumors and in providing definite identification of metastatic thyroid carcinomas (Baloch and LiVolsi 2002a).

5.4.2.1 Benign Neoplasms

Adenomas and Adenomatous Nodules

- A follicular adenoma or solitary adenomatous or adenomatoid nodule is defined as a benign encapsulated mass of follicles, usually showing a uniform morphology throughout the nodule (Baloch and LiVolsi 2002a; Rosai et al. 1992).
- Encapsulated nodules with papillary hyperplasia (some of which are functional) should not be classified as papillary adenomas (Mai et al. 2001), but as papillary hyperplastic nodules (LiVolsi 1996).
- Though adenomas are defined as solitary neoplasm in otherwise normal thyroid, they can occur in a background of multinodular thyroid gland. Therefore, many pathologists prefer the terminology of adenomatoid or adenomatous nodule. The features that distinguish histologically between adenoma and adenomatous nodules included encapsulation, uniformity of pattern within the adenoma which appears distinct, and compression of the surrounding gland by the adenoma and its capsule (LiVolsi and Baloch 2004) (Fig. 5.5).
- Some nodules share characteristics of adenomatous nodules and adenomas, such as partial encapsulation. Pathologists use a variety of terms for these, but the rebric "benign follicular nodule" has been suggested (Rosai and LiVolsi personal communication).
- On the basis of growth pattern, adenomas can be further classified as macrofollicular, microfollicular, fetal, embryonal, and trabecular (Rosai et al. 1992).

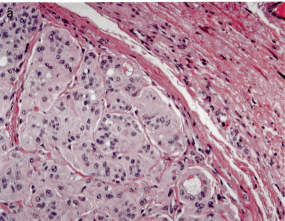 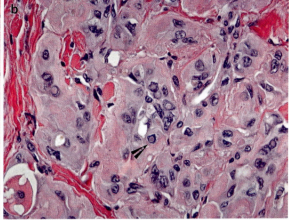

Fig. 5.6 (**a, b**): Hyalinizing trabecular neoplasm. (**a**) Hyalinizing trabecular neoplasm demonstrating tumor cells growing in nests in a background of dense hyaline stroma. (**b**) The high power demonstrating nuclear features similar to papillary thyroid carcinoma. The *arrowhead* points to a well-formed intranuclear inclusion

- Relatively common changes found in adenomas include hemorrhage, edema, fibrosis, and calcification, especially in the central portions of the tumor (Rosai et al. 1992). Nowadays, it is not uncommon to see post-fine-needle aspiration biopsy changes in follicular adenomas which include necrosis, increased mitotic activity, and cellular atypia in the area of the needle tract (LiVolsi and Merino 1994).

Hyalinizing Trabecular Neoplasm of the Thyroid

- This is a distinct-patterned follicular-derived lesion of the thyroid (Carney et al. 1987).
- By light microscopic examination, these adenomas grow in nests that are surrounded by dense hyaline stroma (Fig. 5.6a, b).
- The nuclear features of the follicular cells are similar to those seen in papillary carcinoma (LiVolsi 2000). By immunohistochemistry, the cells of hyalinizing trabecular adenoma stain positive for thyroglobulin and cytokeratin19 and negative for calcitonin, although the presence of other neuroendocrine markers has been described (Fonseca et al. 1997).
- Some authors have proposed that these adenomas actually represent an encapsulated variant of papillary carcinoma. This is due to similar nuclear cytology, immunoprofile, and RET oncogene rearrangements in both tumors (Papotti et al. 2000). However, a benign behavior has so far been described in all cases of hyalinizing trabecular neoplasm, and none of these tumors have been shown to harbor BRAF mutations (Nakamura et al. 2005).

Atypical Follicular Adenoma

- This term is applied to those follicular tumors that show features of aggressive behavior such as spontaneous necrosis and infarction, numerous mitoses, or unusual cellularity but do not show invasive characteristics.
- The overwhelming majority of the atypical adenomas follow a benign clinical course (Hazard and Kenyon 1954; Fukunaga et al. 1992; Lang et al. 1977).

5.4.2.2 Malignant Neoplasms

- The well-differentiated carcinomas of follicular epithelial origin make up the majority of malignant neoplasms of the thyroid; up to 80% of these are papillary carcinomas (Rosai et al. 1992).
- The nonneoplastic diseases of the thyroid do not seem to be the precursors of malignant diseases, with the exception that autoimmune thyroiditis can give rise to malignant lymphoma (Baloch and LiVolsi 2002a).
- Anaplastic carcinomas often arise in goiterous thyroids, in close association with well-differentiated carcinoma or rarely a benign neoplasm. Such findings have led to suggestions that the benign tumor or low-grade carcinoma can "transform" into the anaplastic carcinoma (Carcangiu et al. 1985c). This theory has been corroborated by molecular studies (Nikiforova et al. 2003).

Papillary Thyroid Carcinoma

- This is the most common malignant tumor of the gland in countries having iodine-sufficient or iodine-excess diets and comprises about 80% of thyroid malignancies in the United States (LiVolsi 1992; Mazzaferri and Young 1981). Papillary Thyroid Carcinoma (PTC) can occur at any age and rarely has been diagnosed as a congenital tumor (Mills and Allen 1986). Most tumors are diagnosed in patients in the third and fifth decades. Women are affected more than men in ratios of 2:1 to 4:1 (Schottenfeld and Gershman 1977).
- It clinically behaves in an indolent fashion and carries an excellent prognosis (>90% at 20 years) (Mazzaferri and Young 1981).
- The preferred mode of spread in the tumor is lymphatics leading to regional lymph node metastases (Mazzaferri and Young 1981). Venous invasion rarely occurs, and metastases outside the neck are unusual (5–7% of cases) (Furlan et al. 2004).

Etiologic Factors

- *Iodide*: The addition of iodine to the diet in endemic goiter areas in Europe has been associated with a decreased incidence of follicular cancer and an increase in papillary carcinoma (Williams et al. 1977; Harach et al. 2002).
- *External radiation*: External radiation probably plays a role in the development of papillary cancer (Petrova et al. 1996; Ron et al. 1987). The average time from radiation exposure to tumor development can be variable; however, it is classically been reported as 20 years (Ron et al. 1987; Cetta et al. 1997). Following most reported nuclear accidents, the increased incidence of PTC is seen predominantly in young children. Most of which show aggressive features including extracapsular extension and vascular invasion; however, mortality is extremely low (Cetta et al. 1997; Pacini et al. 1999).
- *Autoimmune disease*: It has been reported that up to one-third of papillary cancers arise in the setting of chronic thyroiditis. It has been suggested that both PTC and chronic lymphocytic thyroiditis are common conditions, the possibility of coincidental coexistence is more likely than an etiologic relationship (Tamimi 2002; Nikiforova et al. 2002). However, loss of heterozygosity for various tumor suppressor genes has been demonstrated in the cytologically atypical areas/nodules in chronic lymphocytic thyroiditis suggesting a link between chronic lymphocytic thyroiditis and PTC (Hunt et al. 2003a).
- *Hormonal and reproductive factors*: Since PTC papillary is more common in women than in men, the role of various hormonal factors in the development of papillary carcinoma has been suggested (La Vecchia et al. 1999).
- *Genetic syndromes*: PTC can occur in patients with familial adenomatous polyposis coli (FAP), Cowden's syndrome, nonpolyposis colon cancer syndrome (HNPCC), Peutz-Jeghers' syndrome, and ataxia talengectasia (Cetta et al. 2000; Harach et al. 1999; Haggitt and Reid 1986).
- *Thyroid/parathyroid adenomas*: Occasionally, PTC can be seen in goiterous nodules or adenomas. It is believed that this is likely to be a random event of location and does not indicate a casual relationship. Several authors have described the association of papillary carcinoma and parathyroid adenoma and/or hyperplasia (Meshikhes et al. 2004; Dralle and Altenahr 1979). Both types of lesions are associated with a history of low-dose external radiation to the neck.

Pathology

- *Gross pathology*
  - The lesions can be situated anywhere within the thyroid gland. The clinical papillary carcinomas are >1.0 cm in size, and tumors measuring ≤1.0 cm are classified as microcarcinoma. The lesions are usually firm and white in color, and tumoral calcification is a common feature. The tumor may resemble a scar due to extensive sclerosis. Cystic change can also be seen in PTC, this may be seen involving part or majority of the tumor mass (Rosai et al. 1992; LiVolsi 1990; Carcangiu et al. 1985a).

- *Microscopic pathology*
  - The classic variant of PTC displays papillae containing a central fibrovascular core lined by one or occasionally several layers of cells with crowded/overlapping oval nuclei (Fig. 5.7).
  - The pathologic diagnosis of PTC is based upon its nuclear features (major diagnostic feature) regardless of the growth pattern. The nuclei of PTC have been described as clear, ground glass, empty, or Orphan Annie eyed. They are larger and more oval than normal follicular nuclei and contain hypodense/clear chromatin. Intranuclear inclusions of cytoplasm are often found. Another

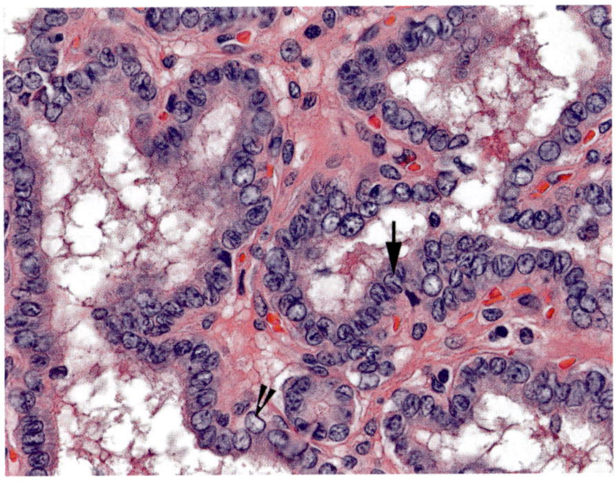

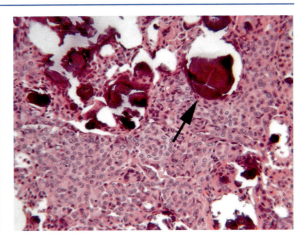

Fig. 5.7 Papillary thyroid carcinoma – classic variant demonstrating tumor cells surrounding a well-developed fibrovascular cores with nuclear features diagnostic of papillary thyroid carcinoma, nuclear chromatin clearing aka "Orphan Annie nuclei" (*arrowhead*), and intranuclear grooves (*arrow*)

Fig. 5.8 Lamellated round to oval calcified structures "psammoma bodies" (*arrow*) that represent the "ghosts" of dead papillae are seen in a case of diffuse sclerosis variant of papillary thyroid carcinoma

characteristic of the papillary cancer nucleus is the nuclear groove/crease (Carcangiu et al. 1985a; Baloch and LiVolsi 2002a; LiVolsi 1992). Nuclear grooves can also be seen in benign lesions of the thyroid such as Hashimoto's disease, adenomatous hyperplasia, and diffuse hyperplasia, as well as in follicular adenomas (particularly hyalinizing trabecular neoplasm) (Francis et al. 1995). Therefore, the mere presence of nuclear grooves especially in cytologic preparation should not lead to unequivocal diagnosis of PTC.

- Psammoma bodies are lamellated round to oval calcified structures that represent the "ghosts" of dead papillae (Fig. 5.8). These are seen usually within the cores of papillae or in the tumor stroma of PTC (Carcangiu et al. 1985a; Rosai et al. 1992); however, they can also be seen in intrathyroidal lymphatics representing intraglandular spread. Rarely, psammoma bodies are found in benign conditions of the thyroid gland (Riazmontazer and Bedayat 1991; Hunt and Barnes 2003). The finding of psammoma bodies in a cervical lymph node is a strong indicator of a PTC in the thyroid (Hosoya et al. 1983).
- Cyst formation may occur in primary tumor as well as in lymph node metastases. The cystic degeneration can be extensive making it difficult to distinguish from a branchial cleft cyst (Ruiz-Velasco et al. 1978; de los Santos et al. 1990;

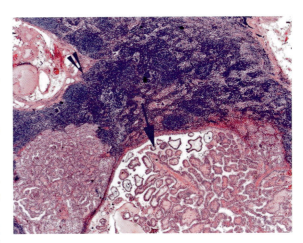

Fig. 5.9 A cervical lymph node showing metastases form papillary thyroid carcinoma (*arrow*). Notice the residual lymphoid tissue (*arrowhead*)

LiVolsi 1990). In such cases, an aliquot of the cystic fluid can be submitted for thyroglobulin analysis to confirm the diagnosis of metastatic PTC (Baloch et al. 2008).
- Papillary carcinoma early in its development invades the glandular lymphatics (LiVolsi 1990), which accounts for high incidence of regional node metastases (Fig. 5.9).
- Papillary carcinoma can also present as multifocal tumors within the same gland (Carcangiu et al. 1985a). It has been shown that papillary carcinomas are clonal proliferations. Recent

RET/PTC and LOH studies have shown that multifocal papillary microcarcinomas can be separate primaries instead of intraglandular spread from one tumor source (Fusco et al. 2002; Hunt et al. 2003b).
- Venous invasion can be identified in up to 7% of papillary cancers (Petkov et al. 1995).
- Regional lymph node metastases are extremely common (50% of more) at initial presentation of usual papillary cancer (Mazzaferri and Young 1981). The histology of the nodal metastases in papillary cancer may appear papillary, mixed, or follicular. This feature does not adversely affect long-term prognosis (Carcangiu et al. 1985a; LiVolsi 1992).
- Tumor grading is of no use in this tumor since over 95% of these lesions are grade 1 (Akslen and LiVolsi 2000b). Recently, Tallini has recommended that adverse histological features such as numerous mitotic figures, abnormal mitoses, and tumor necrosis in a tumor that demonstrates a papillary growth pattern should warrant a diagnosis of a high-grade or poorly differentiated papillary carcinoma; studies testing this hypothesis remain to be published (Akslen and LiVolsi 2000a, b; Tallini 2011).
- In some tumors, either in the primary site or in recurrences, transformation to poorly differentiated carcinoma can occur. This change is characterized by solid growth of tumor, mitotic activity, and cytologic atypia can be found. Such lesions have a much more guarded prognosis (Akslen and LiVolsi 2000a). Anaplastic transformation in a papillary cancer can occur, although it is uncommon (Carcangiu et al. 1985c).
- Distant metastases of papillary carcinoma to lungs, bones, and brain occur in 5–7% of cases (Tachikawa et al. 2001).
- *Immunohistochemistry*
  - PTC expresses thyroglobulin, TTF1, and not calcitonin (Baloch and LiVolsi 2002a). From an extensive list of these immunohistochemical markers, the ones that have shown some promise include cytokeratin19, HBME1, and galectin-3 (Prasad et al. 2005; Casey et al. 2003; Cheung et al. 2001; Eimoto et al. 1987; van Hoeven et al. 1998; Baloch et al. 1999a). However, none of these have proven to be specific since all can be expressed in some benign lesions of thyroid.

Molecular Pathology of Papillary Carcinoma
- Rearrangements of RET gene, known as RET/PTC, have been identified in papillary carcinoma of thyroid (Grieco et al. 1990; Santoro et al. 1990). The RET proto-oncogene is normally expressed in cells of neural crest origin and is located on chromosome 10q11.2 and cell membrane receptor tyrosine kinase (Grieco et al. 1990; Santoro et al. 1994). In normal thyroid wild type, RET is only expressed in C cells and not follicular cells. RET/PTC seen in papillary carcinomas occurs due to fusion of tyrosine kinase domain of RET to the 5′ portion of the various genes. To date, more than ten novel types of rearrangements have been described in papillary carcinoma. RET/PTC 1 and 3 are the most common forms that occur in sporadic papillary carcinoma. The prevalence of RET/PTC in papillary carcinoma varies significantly among various geographic regions; in the United States, it ranges from 11% to 43% (Nikiforov 2002). In sporadic tumors, RET/PTC1 is the most common form of rearrangement (60–70%) followed by RET/PTC3 (20–30%) (Nikiforov 2002; Fusco et al. 1995). The other rare forms of RET/PTC rearrangements have been mainly found in radiation-induced papillary carcinomas. Several studies have shown a strong association between radiation-induced papillary carcinoma and expression of RET/PTC; RET/PTC3 was found to be the most common form of rearrangement followed by RET/PTC1 (Nikiforov et al. 1997; Bounacer et al. 1997).The expression of RET/PTC is not exclusive to malignant thyroid tumors; it can also occur in some benign lesions. These include hyalinizing trabecular neoplasm Hashimoto's thyroiditis (Wirtschafter et al. 1997; Sheils et al. 2002) and hyperplastic nodules and follicular adenoma (Elisei et al. 2001).
- It is now well known that the Raf/MEK/ERK pathway is a significant contributor to the malignant phenotype associated with deregulated Ras signaling (Cohen et al. 2003; Nikiforova et al. 2003). BRAF-activating mutations in thyroid cancer are most commonly the BRAF V600E mutation and have been found in 29–69% of papillary thyroid cancers, 13% of poorly differentiated cancers, and 10% of anaplastic cancers (Nikiforova et al. 2003; Soares et al. 2004; Puxeddu et al. 2004; Begum et al. 2004). Interestingly, presence of BRAF V600E correlates with variants of PTC. More recent studies consisting

of large cohorts of patients have shown a strong correlation of BRAF mutation with nonfavorable clinicopathological features (Namba et al. 2003; Xing 2005). BRAF mutations are independent of RET/PTC translocations and RAS mutations. Molecular analysis of FNA samples for BRAF and RAS mutations and RET/PTC translocations have been shown to be of value in the preoperative diagnosis of papillary thyroid carcinoma in cases diagnosed as indeterminate or suspicious for malignancy (Xing et al. 2004; Nikiforov et al. 2009).

Prognostic Factors
- These include older age at diagnosis, male sex, large tumor size, and extrathyroidal growth (Mazzaferri and Young 1981; Mazzaferri 1987). Histopathologic variables associated with a more guarded prognosis include less-differentiated or solid areas, vascular invasion, and aneuploid cell population (Akslen and LiVolsi 2000b). Some authors have found that prognostic factors vary among males and females. In men, age and presence of gross lymph node metastases were important, while in females, age, presence of gross lymph node metastases, tumor size, and the number of structures adhered to the gland were important (Mazzaferri 1987, 1999).

Subtypes of Papillary Carcinoma
- Papillary Microcarcinoma (Occult Papillary Carcinoma)
  – Papillary microcarcinoma (PMC) is defined as tumor measuring 1 cm or less; however, some experts have also defined as tumors measuring up to 1.5 cm as microcarcinomas (DeLellis et al. 2004; Rodriguez et al. 1997). The term "occult" should not be used by pathologists as a diagnostic designation; it may be employed by clinicians for small lesions not easily identified by physical or radiological examination.
  – These lesions are quite common as incidental findings at autopsy or in thyroidectomy for benign disease or in completion thyroidectomies in patients with a history of carcinoma involving the opposite thyroid lobe (Hay et al. 1992). Therefore, it is important to recognize that the incidentally found microcarcinoma confined within the thyroid is probably of no clinical importance and should not be overtreated.
  – Lymph node metastases from papillary microcarcinoma can occur; metastases from lesions less than 0.5 cm have been reported (Hay et al. 1992; Rodriguez et al. 1997). Distant metastases, although very rare, are also documented (Braga et al. 2002).
  – Histologically, the tumors may be either completely follicular-patterned or show papillary architecture as well. Sclerosis may be prominent; the lesions can be encapsulated or infiltrate the surrounding thyroid (LiVolsi 1990) (Fig. 5.10).
  – A familial form of papillary microcarcinoma has been recognized; these tumors are characterized by multifocality with increase tendency toward vascular and lymphatic invasion, distant metastasis, and even death (Fernandez-Real and Ricart 1999; Lupoli et al. 1999).

- Follicular Variant of Papillary Cancer
  – This variant of PTC shows follicular growth pattern and diagnostic nuclear features of papillary carcinoma (Lindsay 1960; Chen and Rosai 1977) (Fig. 5.11).
  – Grossly and histologically, the tumor may appear encapsulated (Baloch et al. 1999b). The prognosis of the follicular variant is apparently similar to usual papillary cancer although there may be a greater risk for vascular invasion; regional nodal metastases are less common than in classic papillary cancer (Baloch et al. 2002; Tielens et al. 1994).
  – Three distinct types of follicular variant include the infiltrative type, the diffuse follicular variant,

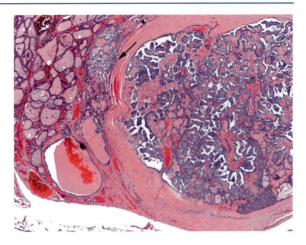

Fig. 5.10 Encapsulated papillary thyroid microcarcinoma with papillary growth pattern. Notice the tumor infiltration into normal thyroid (*arrow*)

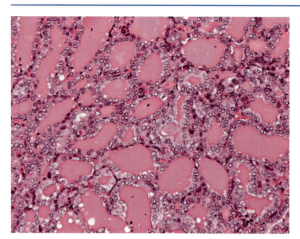

Fig. 5.11 Follicular variant of papillary thyroid carcinoma characterized by follicular growth pattern and tumor cells with nuclear cytology of papillary thyroid carcinoma

and the encapsulated follicular variant. In the infiltrative type, the tumor which is a solitary mass or nodule is unencapsulated and invades the surrounding thyroid gland. Lymphatic invasion, nodal metastases, and extraglandular extension are common (almost as common as classical papillary carcinoma) (LiVolsi. 1990). In the diffuse follicular variant, the gland is diffusely replaced by tumor (Baloch and Livolsi 2002b). Lymph node and distant metastases are common in these patients. The prognosis appears to be poor in these patients, although only a handful of cases have been described (Mizukami et al. 1995; Ivanova et al. 2002).

 – The encapsulated follicular variant is characterized by the presence of a capsule around the lesion (Liu et al. 2006). Encapsulated FVPTC are associated with an excellent prognosis (Baloch and Livolsi 2002b). In some cases, the diagnosis of this particular variant of papillary carcinoma can be difficult due to presence of multifocal rather than diffuse distribution of nuclear features of papillary thyroid carcinoma. Because of this peculiar morphologic presentation, these tumors can be misdiagnosed as adenomatoid nodule or follicular adenoma (Baloch and Livolsi 2002b; LiVolsi and Baloch 2004). Some authors have suggested that these tumors be classified as "tumors of undetermined malignant potential" due to excellent prognosis (Williams et al. 2000); however, others have shown that some cases belonging in this category can lead to distant metastasis (Baloch et al. 2002).
 – Rarely, FVPTC can be composed almost entirely of distended, colloid-filled large tumors; such tumors are termed as *macrofollicular variant* of papillary carcinoma.
 – It has been shown that FVPC does share some morphologic and clinical features with follicular carcinoma. This has been further corroborated by gene expression profiling studies and comparative genomic hybridization analysis; RAS gene mutations, an abnormality seen in follicular adenoma and carcinoma, is exclusively seen in FVPTC and not in classical PTC (Giordano et al. 2005; Wreesmann et al. 2004) in the papillary carcinoma group; similarly, RET gene translocations and BRAF mutations which are common in classic PTC are rare in cases of FVPC (Wreesmann et al. 2004; Giordano et al. 2005; Zhu et al. 2003). Therefore, in view of morphologic features, clinical behavior and molecular analysis encapsulated FVPC most likely is a hybrid of papillary carcinoma and follicular adenoma or carcinoma. Thus, a well-sampled tumor without any capsular and vascular invasion will behave more as a follicular adenoma, and the ones with capsular and vascular invasion, as follicular carcinoma (Baloch et al. 2010).

• Tall Cell Variant
 – The tall cell variant of PTC is an aggressive variant of papillary carcinoma which tends to occur in elderly patients. These tumors are usually large (>6 cm), extend extrathyroidally, and show mitotic activity and vascular invasion more often than usual papillary cancer.
 – The tall cell variant of PTC consists of tumor cells three times as tall as they are wide and shows eosinophilic cytoplasm (Johnson et al. 1988; Sobrinho-Simoes et al. 1989) (Fig. 5.12).
 – Dedifferentiation to squamous cell carcinoma has been described in tall cell variant of PTC (Bronner and LiVolsi 1991{Gopal 2011 #2906}).

• Columnar Cell Variant
 – The columnar cell variant is a rare form of papillary carcinoma (Sobrinho-Simoes et al. 1988). The tumor is characterized microscopically by papillary growth. Tall columnar cells line the

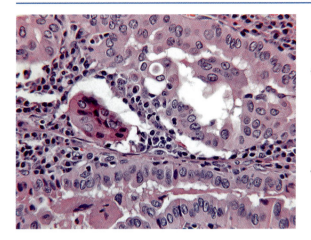

Fig. 5.12 Tall cell variant of papillary thyroid carcinoma demonstrating tumor cells three times as tall as they are wide with eosinophilic cytoplasm and diagnostic nuclei of papillary thyroid carcinoma

papillae. The nuclear features are usually not those of typical papillary carcinomas.
- Extrathyroidal extension is common as are distant metastases (Sobrinho-Simoes et al. 1988; Chan 1990; Wenig et al. 1998). Studies of such tumors that are partly encapsulated and gland-confined have shown that the prognosis may not be as dire as those with extraglandular spread (Evans 1996).
- Warthin-Like Variant
  - By light microscopy, these tumors resemble "Warthin's tumor" of the salivary gland. These tumors usually arise in a background of lymphocytic thyroiditis and show papillary architecture. The clinical course of this variant is similar to conventional papillary carcinoma (Apel et al. 1995; Baloch and LiVolsi 2000).
- Diffuse Sclerosis Variant
  - The diffuse sclerosis variant of papillary carcinoma is rare and most often affects children and young adults and may present as bilateral goiter. The tumor permeates the gland outlining the intraglandular lymphatics.
  - These lesions appear to represent 10% of the papillary carcinomas seen in children exposed to the radioactive iodine released following the Chernobyl accident.
  - These tumors often show extracapsular extension, distant and nodal metastases, and a decreased disease-free survival when compared to the usual type of papillary carcinoma; however, overall mortality is low (Chan et al. 1987; Peix et al. 1998; Santoro et al. 2000; Soares et al. 1989).
- Solid Variant of PTC
  - The solid variant of PTC is most commonly seen in children and has been reported in greater than 30% of patients with papillary carcinoma following the Chernobyl nuclear accident (Nikiforov et al. 2001; Thomas et al. 1999).
- Other Variants of PTC
  - Other rare variants of PTC which have been described include the spindle cell variant (Vergilio et al. 2002), the clear cell type (Dickersin et al. 1980), the oxyphilic (Hürthle cell) variant (Dickersin et al. 1980; Berho and Suster 1997), papillary carcinoma with lipomatous stroma (Bisi et al. 1993; Schroder and Bocker 1985), papillary carcinoma with fasciitis-like stroma (Chan et al. 1991b), and cribriform variant (Cameselle-Teijeiro and Chan 1999; Hirokawa et al. 2004). The last of these is often seen in patients with familial adenomatous polyposis although it may occur as a sporadic tumor. Recently, an aggressive form of PTC known as "hobnail" variant has been described (Lloyd et al. 2010).

Follicular Carcinoma
- Follicular carcinoma comprises about 5% of thyroid cancers; however, it is more prevalent making up 25–40% of thyroid cancers (Franssila et al. 1985; Tollefson et al. 1973) in iodide-deficient areas.
- The true incidence of follicular carcinoma is difficult to determine since the follicular variant of papillary carcinoma may still be placed into this category (LiVolsi and Asa 1994).
- Risk factors include iodine deficiency, older age, female gender, and radiation exposure (although the relationship of radiation to follicular carcinoma is far less strong than with papillary cancer) (Williams et al. 1977; Wade 1975).
- Clinically, follicular carcinoma usually presents as a solitary mass in the thyroid (Franssila et al. 1985).
- Follicular carcinoma disseminates hematogenously and metastasizes to bone, lungs, brain, and liver (Franssila et al. 1985; Jorda et al. 1993; Segal et al. 1994). Lymphatic invasion has not been reported in follicular carcinoma; however, reported cases of

follicular carcinoma with lymph node metastases most likely represent follicular variant of papillary thyroid carcinoma (LiVolsi and Asa 1994).
- Patients with widely invasive form of follicular carcinoma do poorly(Crile et al. 1985; Tollefson et al. 1973) as compared to those with encapsulated follicular tumors confined to the thyroid (prolonged survival greater than 80% at 10 years) (Schmidt and Wang 1986; Evans 1984; Thompson et al. 2001; Carcangiu 1997).
- The independent prognostic factors in follicular carcinoma include age >45, extrathyroidal extension, distant metastases, and tumor size >4 cm (Thompson et al. 2001; Jorda et al. 1993; Shaha et al. 1995).
- Anaplastic transformation has been reported in patients with follicular cancer; this may occur de novo in an untreated follicular lesion or in metastatic foci (Moore et al. 1985).
- Follicular carcinoma of the thyroid can be divided into two forms:
  – The *widely invasive follicular carcinoma* is a tumor that is clinically and surgically recognized as a cancer. Up to 80% of the patients with widely invasive cancers can develop metastases with a fatality rate of 50%.
  – The *minimally invasive follicular carcinoma* is diagnosed by examination of well-fixed histologic sections:

    It is an encapsulated tumor, which grossly resembles a follicular adenoma and only on microscopic examination shows evidence of capsular and/or vascular invasion (Fig. 5.13a, b). They can show microfollicular, trabecular, and solid growth patterns (Thompson et al. 2001; LiVolsi and Baloch 2004).

    Fine-needle aspiration cytology cannot diagnose follicular carcinoma since the diagnosis requires the demonstration of invasion at the edges of the lesion; therefore, sampling of the center, as in obtaining a cytologic sample, cannot be diagnostic (Segal et al. 1994; Franssila et al. 1985; D'Avanzo et al. 2004; Jakubiak-Wielganowicz et al. 2003; Collini et al. 2003).

    There still exists a controversy among pathologists regarding the minimum criteria for diagnosing follicular carcinoma. Is it invasion of the capsule, invasion through the capsule, and invasion into veins in or beyond the capsule? (LiVolsi and Baloch 2004; LiVolsi and Asa 1994; Thompson et al. 2001). The criterion for vascular invasion applies solely and strictly to veins in or beyond the capsule, whereas the definition of capsular invasion is controversial (LiVolsi and Baloch 2004; Williams et al. 2000). Some authors require penetration of the capsule to diagnose a follicular tumor as carcinoma, while others need tumor invasion through the capsule into the surrounding normal thyroid (Williams et al. 2000; Carcangiu 1997). Distant metastases have been reported in follicular carcinoma diagnosed only on the basis of capsular and not vascular invasion; however, in some cases, metastases were already present at initial diagnosis (Evans 1984; Kahn and Perzin 1983).

    The presence of vascular invasion is also indicative of malignancy in a follicular tumor. Invasion of vessels within or beyond the lesional capsule is necessary for a definitive diagnosis of vascular invasion (Rosai et al. 1992). We believe that the lesions with vascular invasion should be separated from the minimally invasive follicular carcinomas, which show capsular invasion only, because angioinvasive lesions have a greater probability of recurrence and metastasis (Baloch and Livolsi 2002b).

- Immunohistochemistry
  – All follicular carcinomas express thyroglobulin and show a similar cytokeratin profile to normal thyroid parenchyma. HBME1 expression can occur in 90–100% of follicular carcinomas and not adenomas; however, it is also expressed in adenomatoid nodules and follicular adenomas (Miettinen and Karkkainen 1996; van Hoeven et al. 1998; Papotti et al. 2005; Rosai 2003).
- Molecular Biology
  – A specific translocation t(2;3) leads to the expression of PAX8 peroxisome proliferator-activated receptor gamma (PPAR-gamma) chimeric protein. This has been reported in follicular carcinoma and is currently being used in a molecular assay panel for the triaging FNA specimens diagnosed as atypia/follicular lesion of undetermined significance and follicular neoplasm (Kroll et al. 2000). However, PPAR-gamma expression can occur in some cases of follicular adenoma and adenomatoid nodules (Marques et al. 2002; Gustafson et al. 2003).

5 Thyroid Pathology

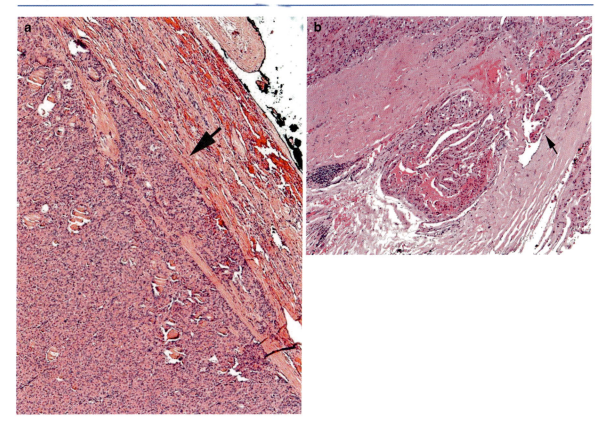

Fig. 5.13 (**a**, **b**): Follicular carcinoma. (**a**) Follicular carcinoma demonstrating invasion into tumor capsule (*arrow*). (**b**) Vascular invasion (*arrow*) by oncocytic follicular carcinoma (Hürthle cell carcinoma)

- *Ras* mutations are more frequent in follicular carcinoma as compared to follicular adenoma; some authors have found an association between *ras* mutations and clinically aggressive follicular carcinomas (Esapa et al. 1999; Basolo et al. 2000; Capella et al. 1996).
- Loss of heterozygosity on chromosome 10q and 3p can be seen in follicular carcinoma suggesting a role of tumor suppressor genes in its pathogenesis (Grebe et al. 1997; Matsuo et al. 1991).

Well-Differentiated Follicular "Tumors of Undetermined Malignant Potential"
- This designation has been proposed by some experts for follicular-patterned encapsulated tumors that have been controversial and difficult to diagnose due to questionable or minimal nuclear features of papillary thyroid carcinoma or questionable or one focus of capsular invasion that is confined to tumor capsule and does not traverse the entire thickness of capsule and lacks any nuclear features of papillary thyroid carcinoma (Williams et al. 2000).
- This terminology may be extremely helpful to pathologists in the diagnoses of certain follicular-patterned lesions; however, clinicians may find it problematic to establish treatment strategies due to lack of follow-up data (LiVolsi and Baloch 2004).

Oncocytic (Hürthle Cell) Follicular Tumors
- Oncocytic follicular (Hürthle) cells are characterized morphologically by large size, distinct cell borders, voluminous granular cytoplasm, large nucleus, and prominent nucleolus. Ultrastructural studies have shown that the cytoplasmic granularity is produced by huge mitochondria filling the cell (Nesland et al. 1985; Gonzalez-Campora et al. 1986). These can be readily found in nodular goiter, foci of nonspecific chronic thyroiditis, long-standing hyperthyroidism, and chronic lymphocytic thyroiditis (Hashimoto's disease) (Baloch and LiVolsi 1999a).
- Most Hürthle cell neoplasms of the thyroid are solitary mass lesions that show complete or partial encapsulation. They are distinguished from the

surrounding thyroid by their distinctive brown to mahogany color (LiVolsi 1990; Rosai et al. 1992; Bronner and LiVolsi 1988). Rarely, a Hürthle cell neoplasm may undergo spontaneous infarction. Extensive infarction may also be seen following fine-needle aspiration biopsy.

- To date, some clinicians and pathologists believe that oncocytic follicular tumors do not "follow the rules" for histopathologic diagnosis of malignancy. Some authors cite 80% or more of these lesions as benign, whereas others consider all such lesions malignant (Thompson et al. 1974; Gundry et al. 1983). Numerous studies throughout the world have shown that oncocytic or Hürthle cell tumors can be divided into benign and malignant categories based on pathologic criteria applied in the diagnosis of follicular carcinoma, i.e., the identification of capsular and/or vascular invasion (Carcangiu et al. 1991; Bronner and LiVolsi 1988).
- It is well known that the pathologic criterion for malignancy is more frequent in oncocytic follicular (Hürthle cell) tumors than their nononcocytic follicular (Hürthle cell) counterparts. Thus, whereas 2–3% of solitary encapsulated follicular tumors of the thyroid show invasive characteristics, 30–40% of such lesions showing Hürthle cell cytology will show such features (Bronner and LiVolsi 1988; Gonzalez-Campora et al. 1986; Chen et al. 1998).
- Approximately, 30% of oncocytic follicular (Hürthle cell) carcinomas will metastasize to the lymph nodes (Janser et al. 1989; LiVolsi 1990).
- *Immunohistochemistry.* Oncocytic follicular (Hürthle cell) lesions are positive for thyroglobulin. Carcinoembryonic antigen (CEA) expression has been described in some, but not all series. Hürthle cell lesions are positive for S100 protein (Bronner and LiVolsi 1988; Kanthan and Radhi 1998).
- *Molecular biology.* Oncocytic tumors of the thyroid are biologically different than other follicular-derived tumors. H*ras* mutations are more frequent in Hürthle cell carcinoma than follicular carcinoma (Schark et al. 1992; Bouras et al. 1998) and a high percentage of allelic alterations as compared to other follicular-derived tumors. A study by Maximo et al. showed that Hürthle cell tumors display a relatively higher percentage of common deletions of mitochondrial DNA as compared to other follicular-derived tumors. In addition, Hürthle cell tumors also showed germ line polymorphisms of ATPase 6 gene, which is required for the maintenance of mitochondrial DNA (Maximo et al. 2002).

Clear Cell Tumors

Clear cell change of the cytoplasm can occur in many follicular-derived lesions in the thyroid thyroiditis, nodules, and neoplasms (Variakojis et al. 1975; Schroder and Bocker 1985; Carcangiu et al. 1985b). Of greatest importance is the differentiation of clear cell change in follicular thyroid lesions from clear cell renal cell carcinomas metastatic to the thyroid (Lam and Lo 1998). Immunostains for thyroglobulin are usually helpful in sorting out this diagnostic problem.

Poorly Differentiated Carcinoma (Insular Carcinoma)

- This heterogeneous group of malignant thyroid tumors includes carcinomas that originate from follicular epithelium (often with evidence of coexistent papillary or follicular carcinoma). The common pathological features of poorly differentiated carcinomas are solid/trabecular/insular growth, large size, frequent extrathyroidal extension, extensive vascular invasion, presence of necrosis, and increased mitotic activity. They may be associated with well-differentiated components, of either follicular or papillary type, and less frequently with anaplastic carcinoma (Rivera et al. 2008; Volante et al. 2007). Rarely, poorly differentiated carcinoma can be seen as encapsulated tumors; in this small subset, the survival is better than expected for poorly differentiated thyroid cancer.
- Insular carcinoma is a hallmark lesion of poorly differentiated thyroid carcinoma. The term "insular" is used to describe the lesions histologic growth pattern, which is characterized by small nests of cells, which have a neuroendocrine growth pattern (carcinoid-like) (Fig. 5.14). The lesions are often large, gray-white in color, infiltrative, and show extensive necrosis, and vascular invasion is frequent. By immunohistochemistry, the tumor cells express thyroglobulin and not calcitonin. The Turin proposal suggests that the term "insular" be used to describe a pattern of growth and not a separate diagnostic term for a particular thyroid tumor; it is not uncommon to see partly "insular" growth in an otherwise solid or trabecular poorly differentiated carcinoma (Volante et al. 2007).
- A distinct molecular pathway has been reported in poorly differentiated carcinomas, which almost exclusively involves RAS gene alterations (Nikiforov et al. 2001).

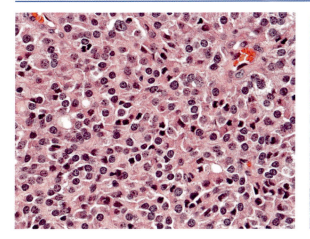

Fig. 5.14 Poorly differentiated thyroid carcinoma/insular carcinoma demonstrating tumor cell arranged in nests, i.e., neuroendocrine growth pattern

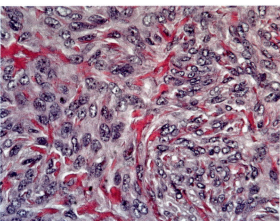

Fig. 5.15 Anaplastic carcinoma demonstrating tumor composed of pleomorphic spindle-shaped tumor cells

Anaplastic Thyroid Tumors
- Anaplastic carcinomas are a group of high-grade thyroid carcinomas, which are usually undifferentiated histologically and advertently have a lethal outcome (Carcangiu et al. 1985c; Venkatesh et al. 1990). These tumors represent approximately 10% of thyroid malignancies (Carcangiu et al. 1985c; Dumitriu et al. 1984).
- A precursor well-differentiated thyroid carcinoma (papillary, follicular, or Hürthle cell) may be observed (Chang et al. 1989).
- Grossly, the tumors are large with extensive intrathyroidal and extrathyroidal invasion.
- Histologically, a variety of patterns have been described. The tumors are usually made up of a variety of cell types. Most tumors are composed of giant cells and spindle cells (Fig. 5.15) although "squamoid" differentiation is seen in about one-third of cases (LiVolsi et al. 1987). Osteoclast-like giant cells are a common feature (Berry et al. 1990). A "paucicellular" variant of anaplastic carcinoma has been described; it is characterized by dense fibrosis, calcification, and a poor patient outcome (Wan et al. 1996). Spindle cell squamous anaplastic carcinoma may be the result of transformation of tall cell papillary carcinoma (Bronner and LiVolsi 1991; Gopal et al. 2011). Carcinosarcoma of the thyroid has been described (Giuffrida et al. 2000a; Donnell et al. 1987).
- By immunohistochemistry, anaplastic thyroid carcinomas can be positive for cytokeratin. Thyroglobulin immunostaining is often negative, and thyroid transcription factor can be rarely positive in anaplastic carcinoma (Miettinen and Franssila 2000).

Squamous Cell Carcinoma, Mucoepidermoid Carcinoma, and Intrathyroidal Thymoma-Like Neoplasms
- *Squamous cell carcinoma* in thyroid occurs usually in association with papillary or anaplastic carcinoma (Bronner and LiVolsi 1991). The primary squamous carcinoma arising de novo of the thyroid is rare and portends a poor prognosis (Sahoo et al. 2002). The major differential diagnosis is metastasis from or direct extension of squamous carcinoma originating in head and neck, lungs, or esophagus.
- *Mucoepidermoid carcinoma* is a distinctive variant of thyroid carcinoma. It is composed of solid masses of squamoid cells and mucin-producing cells, sometimes forming glands (Harach et al. 1986). All cases show thyroglobulin expression due to which some authors consider that it is a variant of papillary carcinoma (Arezzo et al. 1998; Baloch et al. 2000b). Lesions may metastasize to regional nodes and rarely distantly. Death from disease is rare (Baloch et al. 2000b).
- *Sclerosing mucoepidermoid carcinoma with eosinophilia* is usually seen in a background of lymphocytic thyroiditis and is characterized by tumor cells arranged in small sheets, anastomosing trabeculae, and narrow strands associated with dense fibrosis and numerous eosinophils. While these lesions may metastasize to lymph nodes and show extracapsular spread, vascular invasion, and perineural invasion,

death due to disease is uncommon. The tumor cells usually stain negative for thyroglobulin and calcitonin and positive for cytokeratin (Baloch et al. 2000b; Wenig et al. 1995) (Chan et al. 1991a). In lieu of their immunoprofile, it is believed that these tumors are derived from ultimobranchial body rests/solid cell nests (Baloch et al. 2000b).
- *Intrathyroidal thymoma-like neoplasms*. This group represents rare thyroid tumors which include *spindled and epithelial tumor with thymus-like differentiation* (SETTLE) *and carcinoma with thymus-like differentiation* (CASTLE). These lesions originate from branchial pouch remnants within and adjacent to the thyroid (Chan and Rosai 1991; Ahuja et al. 1998; Bayer-Garner et al. 2004; Roka et al. 2004).

Follicular-Derived Familial Tumors
- The frequency of follicular cell–derived tumors as familial events is estimated to be between 1% and 5% of all thyroid tumors (Nose 2008). This group comprises of familial nonmedullary thyroid carcinoma (FNMTC) as the predominant lesion of a familial tumor syndrome or associated with syndromes having extrathyroidal manifestations (Dotto and Nose 2008).
- PTC may occur in multiple family members. In order to be considered familial cancer, at least three first-degree relatives should be affected. The histology of these tumors is not different from nonfamilial although multifocal and bilateral lesions are found. Some series indicate that these tumors clinically behave more aggressively than sporadic tumors (Kraimps et al. 1997).Though chromosomal abnormalities have been detected in these tumors, however, specific genes need to be identified (Nose 2008).
- PTC and other follicular-derived thyroid tumors can be seen in association with PTEN hamartoma syndrome, McCune-Albright syndrome, Carney complex, Peutz-Jeghers syndrome, Werner syndrome, and MEN syndromes (Nose 2008; Dotto and Nose 2008; Fenton et al. 2001; Goto et al. 1996; Blumenthal and Dennis 2008).

Medullary Carcinoma
- Medullary thyroid carcinoma (MTC) comprises less than 10% of all thyroid malignancies (Hazard et al. 1959; Williams 1965, 1966; Block et al. 1967;Albores-Saavedra et al. 1985). This tumor is of great diagnostic importance because of its aggressiveness, its close association with multiple endocrine neoplasia syndromes (MEN IIa and IIb), and a relationship to a C-cell hyperplasia, a probable precursor lesion (Wolfe et al. 1973).
- Approximately, 10–20% of MTCs are familial (Wolfe et al. 1973). A gene associated with medullary carcinoma has been identified on chromosome 10 and involves mutations in the RET oncogene (Mulligan et al. 1993, 1994; Hofstra et al. 1994).
- It can occur at any age; however, it is more commonly reported in adults with an average age of about 50 years.
- In familial cases, children are affected; also in these instances, the age of diagnosis tends to be younger (mean age: about 20 years) (Albores-Saavedra et al. 1985; Uribe et al. 1985).
- *Clinical Presentation*
  - Most cases of MTC present as a painless but firm thyroid nodule. Lymph node metastases are seen in up to 50% of cases, whereas distant metastases such as to lung, bone, or liver may also be noted in 15–25% of cases. Some MTC can produce excess hormone other than calcitonin, the presenting symptoms may be related to that hormone hypersecretion (adrenocorticotropic hormone (ACTH), prostaglandin) (Williams et al. 1968; Kakudo et al. 1982).
  - In the familial lesions, there are associated endocrine and/or neuroendocrine lesions:
  Sipple's syndrome (multiple endocrine neoplasia (MEN) type 2 or 2A) (Sipple 1961) consists of medullary thyroid cancer and C-cell hyperplasia, adrenal pheochromocytoma and adrenal medullary hyperplasia, and parathyroid hyperplasia (Jansson et al. 1984). Studies have shown that the gene responsible for familial medullary carcinoma is RET (Eng 1996, 1999); mutations in RET (different from the RET translocation in papillary carcinoma) are found in the tumors and the germ line of patients with familial medullary carcinomas and the MEN type 2 syndromes (Eng 1996, 1999; Eng et al. 1996). Mutations in specific codons have been correlated with clinical behavior and symptomatology in some families (Eng 1999).
  MEN type 2B consists of medullary thyroid carcinoma and C-cell hyperplasia, pheochromocytoma and adrenal medullary hyperplasia, mucosal neuromas, gastrointestinal ganglioneuromas, and musculoskeletal abnormalities (Kebebew et al.

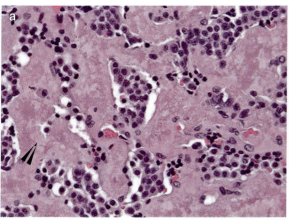 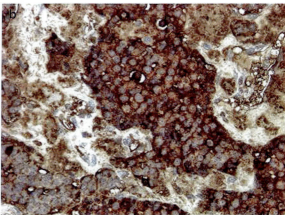

Fig. 5.16 (**a**, **b**): Medullary thyroid carcinoma. (**a**) Medullary thyroid carcinoma characterized by tumor cells arranged in nests in a background of stroma containing amyloid (*arrowhead*). (**b**) Positive calcitonin immunostaining confirming the morphologic diagnosis of medullary thyroid carcinoma

2000; Kambouris et al. 1996; Nakata et al. 2001; Nguyen et al. 2001). These patients may have familial disease (over 50% do); some cases arise apparently as spontaneous mutations. These patients have biologically aggressive medullary carcinoma and may succumb to metastases at an early age. MEN 2B shows similarity to von Recklinghausen's disease since in neurofibromatosis, similar lesions are found in the gastrointestinal tract, and pheochromocytomas are common (Nakata et al. 2001; Nguyen et al. 2001). Nerve growth factor has been identified in some medullary carcinoma of these patients; it has been postulated that this product of the tumor may be responsible for the neural lesions seen in the Men 2B patients (Marsh et al. 1997). However, the neural lesions often precede by many years the development of medullary cancer. In MEN 2B, the tumors and germ line mutations in RET are found on codon 918—an intracellular focus of the RET oncogene (Borrello et al. 1995; Eng et al. 1994).

- *Pathology*
  - MTC is usually located in the area of highest C-cell concentration, i.e., the lateral upper two-thirds of the gland.
  - In familial cases, multiple small nodules may be detected grossly, and rarely, lesions may be found in the isthmus. The tumors range in size from barely visible to several centimeters.
  - By light microscopy, MTC may be circumscribed or more likely will be infiltrating into the surrounding thyroid. The pattern of growth is of tumor cells arranged in nests separated by varying amounts of stroma. The tumor nests are composed of round, oval, or spindle-shaped cells; there often is isolated cellular pleomorphism or even multinucleated cells (Cohen et al. 2004; Asa 1997) (Fig. 5.16). The tumor stroma characteristically contains amyloid although this is not necessary for the diagnosis; about 25% of medullary carcinomas do not contain amyloid (Abrosimov 1996; Alevizaki et al. 1994; Albores-Saavedra et al. 1985). Calcifications are usually noted in the areas of amyloid deposition. The tumors commonly invade lymphatics and veins (Asa 1997).
  - Several histologic variants of medullary carcinoma on the basis of growth pattern have been described (Dominguez-Malagon et al. 1989; Harach and Williams 1983; Huss and Mendelsohn 1990; Landon and Ordonez 1985; Mendelsohn et al. 1980).
  - By immunohistochemistry, the majority of medullary carcinomas express low molecular weight cytokeratin, calcitonin, calcitonin gene-related peptide, and thyroid transcription factor (TTF1). In addition, many tumors express CEA, which may also be elevated in the serum (Kos et al. 1995; DeLilles et al. 1978; Hirsch et al. 2004). A variety of other peptides may be found in tumor cells including somatostatin, vasoactive intestinal

peptide, and synaptophysin (Matsubayashi et al. 1984; Roth et al. 1987). Some studies have also identified polysialic acid (neural cell adhesion molecule) in medullary carcinomas, but not in other thyroid tumors (Komminoth et al. 1994). Occasionally MTC (and often these are poorly differentiated/small-cell type) do not contain immunoreactive calcitonin. In order to accept a calcitonin-free MTC, it should either arise in a familial setting or occur in a thyroid with unequivocal C-cell hyperplasia (Ruppert et al. 1986).

- *Prognostic Factors*
  – From the clinical standpoint, stage is the most important variable for prognosis (Randolph and Maniar 2000; Giuffrida et al. 2000b; Gimm et al. 2001). A tumor confined to the thyroid without nodal or distant metastases is associated with prolonged survival. Several workers have found that younger patients (under age 40), especially women, fare somewhat better than the whole group of medullary cancer patients (Randolph and Maniar 2000; Gilliland et al. 1997). Patients who are discovered by screening because they are members of affected families often have very small tumors and can be cured by thyroidectomy. Patients with Sipple's syndrome tend to have less aggressive tumors than the sporadic group, whereas the patients with MEN type 2B have aggressive lesions (Randolph 1996; Brierley et al. 1996; Gimm et al. 2001). Pathologic features that have been related to prognosis include tumor pattern, amyloid content, pleomorphism, necrosis, mitotic activity, and DNA aneuploidy (Schroder et al. 1988).

Mixed Follicular and Medullary Carcinoma
- These rare and controversial tumors show thyroglobulin and calcitonin immunoreactivity and ultrastructural evidence of follicular and C-cell differentiation (Albores-Saavedra et al. 1990).

Micromedullary Carcinoma
- Micromedullary carcinoma is defined as (equivalent to micropapillary carcinoma) tumor measuring 1 cm or less and has an excellent prognosis if it is confined to the gland (Beressi et al. 1998; Guyetant et al. 1999).
- Micromedullary carcinoma can be found in glands removed prophylactically because of positive genetic testing for RET mutations (Krueger et al. 2000) or can occur as sporadic tumors. They can arise in the background of chronic thyroiditis and may be associated with C-cell hyperplasia even in the absence of familial disease (Albores-Saavedra and Krueger 2001; Kaserer et al. 2001).

Lymphoma
- Primary lymphoma of the thyroid is uncommon, but not rare. Most patients may have a history of diffuse goiter (probably the result of autoimmune thyroiditis) that has suddenly increased in size.
- Most thyroid lymphomas are diffuse type. Virtually, all examples are B-cell types; many may be extranodal lymphomas that arise in mucosa-associated lymphoid tissue (MALT) especially in GI tract
- Secondary involvement of the thyroid by lymphoma can occur in 20% of patients dying from generalized lymphoma (Kossev and Livolsi 1999; Lam et al. 1999; Yamauchi et al. 2002; Ghazanfar et al. 2002; Takano et al. 2000).

Thyroid Sarcoma
- Sarcomas of the thyroid are rare; fibrosarcomas, leiomyosarcomas, and angiosarcomas have been described (Neri et al. 1990; Tsugawa et al. 1999). Angiosarcoma of thyroid has been most commonly described from the mountainous regions of the world (Alpine regions of Europe, the Andes in South America, and the Himalayas in Asia) (Chan et al. 1986; Neri et al. 1990).

Thyroid Tumors in Unusual Locations
- *Lingual Thyroid*: Microscopic remnants of thyroid tissue have been described in 9.8% of tongues examined at autopsy. Rare cases of thyroid carcinoma arising in lingual thyroid are recorded (Diaz-Arias et al. 1992).
- *Thyroglossal Duct*
  – Most tumors arising in the remnants of thyroid tissue associated with the thyroglossal duct are papillary thyroid carcinoma (LiVolsi et al. 1974; Topf et al. 1988; Doshi et al. 2001).
  – When the diagnosis of thyroglossal cyst–associated thyroid cancer is made, the question arises: Does this tumor represent a metastasis from a primary lesion in the gland, is the primary site in the region of the gland, or is the primary site in the region of the cyst? In about 20% of cases in which the thyroid was examined pathologically were areas of papillary carcinoma found in the gland (Heshmati et al. 1997; Cignarelli et al. 2002). In those few cases where intrathyroidal tumor has been found, this was considered a

separate primary (Heshmati et al. 1997; LiVolsi et al. 1974).
- *Other Locations*: Malignant tumors arising in thyroid tissue located within the trachea or larynx are very rare but have been reported (Fih and Moore 1963). Carcinomas, usually papillary subtype, and lesions that resemble carcinoid tumors can arise in struma ovarii (Devaney et al. 1993; Kdous et al. 2003; Rosenblum et al. 1989).
- *Metastatic Neoplasms*
- Tumors metastasize to the thyroid via direct extension from tumors in adjacent structures, by retrograde lymphatic spread, or hematogenously.
- Hematogenous metastases to the thyroid vary according to tumor type (Lam and Lo 1998). Carcinomas of the kidney, lung, and colon and melanoma are most commonly found (Lam and Lo 1998). Such lesions are often solitary, circumscribed masses; they may appear quite compatible with a primary tumor (Lam and Lo 1998; Koo et al. 2004; Matias-Guiu et al. 1997; Baloch and LiVolsi 1999b).

5.4.3 Pathologic Assessment of Thyroid Specimens

In this section, the role of intraoperative assessment in surgical management of thyroid nodules, the suggested criterion for gross pathologic examination of thyroid nodule, and the essentials of the histopathologic reporting of thyroid tumors will be reviewed.

5.4.3.1 Frozen Section Diagnosis and the Thyroid

- It has been shown that though frozen section diagnosis may be specific (90–97%), it is not sensitive (60%). In addition, deferred diagnoses at frozen section do nothing to alter the operative procedure or guide the surgeon (Udelsman et al. 2001).
- In lieu of frozen sections, the initial approach to diagnose a thyroid nodule should be an aspiration biopsy (fine-needle aspiration (FNA)) (Udelsman et al. 2001; Shaha et al. 1990a, b).
For thyroid nodules that are unequivocally diagnosed as malignant, the surgeon should proceed with the appropriate surgery for that malignant diagnosis.
  - In cases where the FNA diagnosis is suspicious for malignancy and that suspected lesion is papillary carcinoma or a variant thereof, intraoperative frozen section may be useful since the diagnosis relies on the nuclear morphology and not the finding of invasion.
  - If the FNA diagnosis is "neoplasm/suspicious for neoplasm," frozen section will not provide a definitive diagnosis and therefore should not be requested (Basolo et al. 1999; Baloch and LiVolsi 2002a, b; Baloch et al. 1999b) since the limited sampling at the frozen section bench may not prove to be fruitful in finding a random microscopic focus of capsular or vascular invasion required for the diagnosis of follicular carcinoma.

5.4.3.2 Gross Examination

- As part of the macroscopic assessment of thyroid resection specimens, pertinent clinical and historical data should be provided to the pathologist. This includes:
  - Age and sex of the patient.
  - Relevant history (previous history of fine-needle aspiration biopsy and diagnosis, treatment, history of head and neck radiation, and family history of thyroid disease and identification of the procedure type (lobectomy, near total or total thyroidectomy)).
  - Radiologic, functional, and laboratory data should be included, e.g., thyroid function tests, radiologic studies (ultrasound, thyroid scan), and laboratory studies (thyroid antibodies, serum calcitonin).
- A detailed gross examination of a thyroid should be performed on the fresh specimen received, and tumor size and appearance be documented before sections are taken for frozen section or other studies.
- The specimen should be oriented spatially by the surgeon. A detailed gross examination of the specimen should include:
  - Weight and measurement (in three dimensions) of the specimen.
  - Description of the external surface and the cut surface (color, consistency).
  - Location, size, and physical characteristics (encapsulation, color, hemorrhage, FNA tracks, solid, cystic, calcified, necrosis) of the nodule (s) should be described.
  - The surgical margins should be highlighted with ink, and presence of gross extrathyroidal extension should be noted.
  - If the specimen contains regional lymph nodes, description of levels and characteristics of any

grossly involved nodes should be given. Presence of parathyroid gland(s) should be documented.
- The gross examination determines the number of sections to be taken for histopathologic evaluation.
- Diffuse lesions of the thyroid such as thyroiditis or Graves' disease without any obvious nodules, up to three sections should be submitted from each lobe and one from isthmus.
- In the case of a solitary or dominant encapsulated nodule, it is recommended that the entire circumference of the nodule be sectioned. Each section should include tumor capsule and main tumor mass with a margin of normal surrounding parenchyma if present.
- For a nonencapsulated nodule, one section per 0.5 cm should be submitted.

5.4.3.3 Histopathologic Reporting of Thyroid Tumors

- The final histopathologic report should be comprehensive and include all of the known prognostic parameters. The tumor description should include:
  - Histologic type.
  - Number/multicentricity.
  - Size, encapsulation.
  - Presence of tumor capsule and vascular invasion, perineural invasion, and extrathyroidal invasion.
  - If lymph node sampling or dissection was performed, the presence of lymph node metastases by number and size should be recorded. The identification of extranodal extension into the soft tissues should be mentioned.
  - The number of parathyroid glands removed during surgery if any should be documented and their location given if possible.
  - Additional pathologic findings in the thyroid such as nodular goiter, thyroiditis, and benign tumors should be described.
  - As additional (optional) areas to include in the report are correlation with FNA findings (especially in discrepant cases) and correlation with intraoperative diagnosis and clinical information.
  - The results of special studies (special stains (Congo-red for amyloid, elastic stain for vessels)) and immunostains (calcitonin, thyroglobulin, endothelial markers for vascular invasion), or flow cytometry, should be added as appropriate.
  - The tumor stage (Rivera et al. 2009; Lang et al. 2007).

References

Abrosimov A (1996) Histologic and immunohistochemical characterization of medullary thyroid carcinoma. Arkh Patol 58(4):43–48

Ahuja AT, Chan ES, Allen PW, Lau KY, King W, Metreweli C (1998) Carcinoma showing thymic-like differentiation (CASTLE tumor). AJNR Am J Neuroradiol 19(7):1225–1228

Akimova RN, Zotikov LA (1969) An electron microscope study of thyroid gland cells under normal conditions and during the carcinogenic process in golden hamsters. Vopr Onkol 15(11):68–75

Akslen LA, LiVolsi VA (2000a) Poorly differentiated thyroid carcinoma – it is important. Am J Surg Pathol 24(2):310–313

Akslen LA, LiVolsi VA (2000b) Prognostic significance of histologic grading compared with subclassification of papillary thyroid carcinoma [see comments]. Cancer 88(8):1902–1908

Albores-Saavedra JA, Krueger JE (2001) C-cell hyperplasia and medullary thyroid microcarcinoma. Endocr Pathol 12(4):365–377

Albores-Saavedra J, LiVolsi VA, Williams ED (1985) Medullary carcinoma. Semin Diagn Pathol 2(2):137–146

Albores-Saavedra J, Gorraez de la Mora T, de la Torre-Rendon F, Gould E (1990) Mixed medullary-papillary carcinoma of the thyroid: a previously unrecognized variant of thyroid carcinoma. Hum Pathol 21(11):1151–1155

Alevizaki M, Dai K, Grigorakis SI, Legon S, Souvatzoglou A (1994) Amylin/islet amyloid polypeptide expression in medullary carcinoma of the thyroid: correlation with the expression of the related calcitonin/CGRP genes. Clin Endocrinol (Oxf) 41(1):21–26

Alexander C, Herrara G, Jaffe K, Yu H (1985) Black thyroid. Clinical manifestations, ultrastructural findings and possible mechanisms. Hum Pathol 16:72–78

Allard R (1982) The thyroglossal cyst. Head Neck Surg 5:134–140

Amdisen A, Jensen SE, Olsen T, Schou M (1968) Development of goiter during lithium treatment. Ugeskr Laeger 130(37):1515–1518

Aozasa M, Amino N, Iwatani Y, Tamaki H, Matsuzuka F, Kuma K, Miyai K (1989) Intrathyroidal HLA-DR-positive lymphocytes in Hashimoto's disease: increases in CD8 and Leu7 cells. Clin Immunol Immunopathol 52(3):516–522

Apel RL, Asa SL, Chalvardjian A, LiVolsi VA (1994) Intrathyroidal lymphoepithelial cysts of probable branchial origin [see comments]. Hum Pathol 25(11):1238–1242

Apel RL, Asa SL, LiVolsi VA (1995) Papillary Hurthle cell carcinoma with lymphocytic stroma. "Warthin-like tumor" of the thyroid. Am J Surg Pathol 19(7):810–814

Arezzo A, Patetta R, Ceppa P, Borgonovo G, Torre G, Mattioli FP (1998) Mucoepidermoid carcinoma of the thyroid gland arising from a papillary epithelial neoplasm. Am Surg 64(4):307–311

Arnott E, Greaves D (1965) Orbital involvement in Riedel's thyroiditis. Br J Ophthalmol 491:1–5

Asa SL (1997) C-cell lesions of the thyroid. Pathol Case Rev 2:210–217

Bala TS, Janardanasarma MK, Raghunath M (1996) Dietary goitrogen-induced changes in the transport of 2-deoxy-D-glucose and amino acids across the rat blood–brain barrier. Int J Dev Neurosci 14(5):575–583

Baloch ZW, LiVolsi VA (1999a) Oncocytic lesions of the neuroendocrine system. Semin Diagn Pathol 16(2):190–199

Baloch ZW, LiVolsi VA (1999b) Tumor-to-tumor metastasis to follicular variant of papillary carcinoma of thyroid. Arch Pathol Lab Med 123(8):703–706

Baloch ZW, LiVolsi VA (2000) Warthin-like papillary carcinoma of the thyroid. Arch Pathol Lab Med 124(8):1192–1195

Baloch Z, LiVolsi VA (2002a) Pathology of the thyroid gland. Endocrine pathology. Churchill Livingstone, Philadelphia

Baloch ZW, Livolsi VA (2002b) Follicular-patterned lesions of the thyroid: the bane of the pathologist. Am J Clin Pathol 117(1):143–150

Baloch ZW, Abraham S, Roberts S, LiVolsi VA (1999a) Differential expression of cytokeratins in follicular variant of papillary carcinoma: an immunohistochemical study and its diagnostic utility. Hum Pathol 30(10):1166–1171

Baloch ZW, Gupta PK, Yu GH, Sack MJ, LiVolsi VA (1999b) Follicular variant of papillary carcinoma. Cytologic and histologic correlation. Am J Clin Pathol 111(2):216–222

Baloch ZW, Feldman MD, LiVolsi VA (2000a) Combined Riedel's disease and fibrosing Hashimoto's thyroiditis: a report of three cases with Two showing coexisting papillary carcinoma. Endocr Pathol 11(2):157–163

Baloch ZW, Solomon AC, LiVolsi VA (2000b) Primary mucoepidermoid carcinoma and sclerosing mucoepidermoid carcinoma with eosinophilia of the thyroid gland: a report of nine cases. Mod Pathol 13(7):802–807

Baloch Z, LiVolsi VA, Henricks WH, Sebak BA (2002) Encapsulated follicular variant of papillary thyroid carcinoma. Am J Clin Pathol 118(4):603–605; discussion 605–606

Baloch ZW, Barroeta JE, Walsh J, Gupta PK, Livolsi VA, Langer JE, Mandel SJ (2008) Utility of Thyroglobulin measurement in fine-needle aspiration biopsy specimens of lymph nodes in the diagnosis of recurrent thyroid carcinoma. CytoJournal 5:1

Baloch ZW, Shafique K, Flannagan M, Livolsi VA (2010) Encapsulated classic and follicular variants of papillary thyroid carcinoma: comparative clinicopathologic study. Endocr Pract 16(6):952–959. doi:7K76352100850G5K [pii] 10.4158/EP10060.OR

Bartholomew L, Cain J, Woolner L, Utz D, Ferris D (1963) Sclerosing cholangitis. Its possible association with Riedel's struma and fibrous retroperitonitis. N Engl J Med 269:8–12

Baschieri L, Castagna M, Fierabracci A, Antonelli A, Del Guerra P, Squartini F (1989) Distribution of calcitonin- and somatostatin-containing cells in thyroid lymphoma and in Hashimoto's thyroiditis. Appl Pathol 7(2):99–104

Basolo F, Baloch ZW, Baldanzi A, Miccoli P, LiVolsi VA (1999) Usefulness of Ultrafast Papanicolaou-stained scrape preparations in intraoperative management of thyroid lesions. Mod Pathol 12(6):653–657

Basolo F, Pisaturo F, Pollina LE, Fontanini G, Elisei R, Molinaro E, Iacconi P, Miccoli P, Pacini F (2000) N-ras mutation in poorly differentiated thyroid carcinomas: correlation with bone metastases and inverse correlation to thyroglobulin expression. Thyroid 10(1):19–23

Bataskis J, Nishiyama R, Schmidt R (1963) "Sproradic goiter sydrome": a clinicopathologic analysis. Am J Clin Pathol 30:241–251

Baughman R (1972) Lingual thyroid and lingual thyroglossal tract remnants. Oral Surg Oral Med Oral Pathol 34:781–798

Bayer-Garner IB, Kozovska ME, Schwartz MR, Reed JA (2004) Carcinoma with thymus-like differentiation arising in the dermis of the head and neck. J Cutan Pathol 31(9):625–629

Begum S, Rosenbaum E, Henrique R, Cohen Y, Sidransky D, Westra WH (2004) BRAF mutations in anaplastic thyroid carcinoma: implications for tumor origin, diagnosis and treatment. Mod Pathol 17(11):1359–1363

Beressi N, Campos JM, Beressi JP, Franc B, Niccoli-Sire P, Conte-Devolx B, Murat A, Caron P, Baldet L, Kraimps JL, Cohen R, Bigorgne JC, Chabre O, Lecomte P, Modigliani E (1998) Sporadic medullary microcarcinoma of the thyroid: a retrospective analysis of eighty cases. Thyroid 8(11):1039–1044

Berho M, Suster S (1997) The oncocytic variant of papillary carcinoma of the thyroid: a clinicopathologic study of 15 cases. Hum Pathol 28(1):47–53

Berry B, MacFarlane J, Chan N (1990) Osteoclastomalike anaplastic carcinoma of the thyroid. Diagnosis by fine needle aspiration cytology. Acta Cytol 34(2):248–250

Bisi H, Longatto Filho A, de Camargo RY, Fernandes VS (1993) Thyroid papillary carcinoma lipomatous type: report of two cases. Pathologica 85(1100):761–764

Block MA, Horn RC, Miller JM, Barrett JL, Brush BE (1967) Familial medullary carcinoma of the thyroid. Ann Surg 166:403–412

Blumenthal GM, Dennis PA (2008) PTEN hamartoma tumor syndromes. Eur J Hum Genet 16(11):1289–1300

Bogazzi F, Bartalena L, Gasperi M, Braverman LE, Martino E (2001) The various effects of amiodarone on thyroid function. Thyroid 11(5):511–519

Borrello MG, Smith DP, Pasini B, Bongarzone I, Greco A, Lorenzo MJ, Arighi E, Miranda C, Eng C, Alberti L et al (1995) RET activation by germline MEN2A and MEN2B mutations. Oncogene 11(11):2419–2427

Bounacer A, Wicker R, Schlumberger M, Sarasin A, Suarez HG (1997) Oncogenic rearrangements of the ret proto-oncogene in thyroid tumors induced after exposure to ionizing radiation. Biochimie 79(9–10):619–623

Bouras M, Bertholon J, Dutrieux-Berger N, Parvaz P, Paulin C, Revol A (1998) Variability of Ha-ras (codon 12) proto-oncogene mutations in diverse thyroid cancers. Eur J Endocrinol 139(2):209–216

Braga M, Graf H, Ogata A, Batista J, Hakim NC (2002) Aggressive behavior of papillary microcarcinoma in a patient with Graves' disease initially presenting as cystic neck mass. J Endocrinol Invest 25(3):250–253

Braverman LE (2001) The physiology and pathophysiology of iodine and the thyroid. Thyroid 11(5):405

Brierley J, Tsang R, Simpson WJ, Gospodarowicz M, Sutcliffe S, Panzarella T (1996) Medullary thyroid cancer: analyses of survival and prognostic factors and the role of radiation therapy in local control. Thyroid 6(4):305–310

Bronner MP, LiVolsi VA (1988) Oxyphilic (Askanazy/Hurthle cell) tumors of the thyroid: microscopic features predict biologic behavior. Surg Pathol 1:137–149

Bronner MP, LiVolsi VA (1991) Spindle cell squamous carcinoma of the thyroid: an unusual anaplastic tumor associated with tall cell papillary cancer. Mod Pathol 4(5):637–643

Cameselle-Teijeiro J, Chan JK (1999) Cribriform-morular variant of papillary carcinoma: a distinctive variant representing the sporadic counterpart of familial adenomatous polyposis-associated thyroid carcinoma? Mod Pathol 12(4):400–411

Capella G, Matias-Guiu X, Ampudia X, de Leiva A, Perucho M, Prat J (1996) Ras oncogene mutations in thyroid tumors: polymerase chain reaction-restriction-fragment-length polymorphism analysis from paraffin-embedded tissues. Diagn Mol Pathol 5(1):45–52

Carcangiu ML (1997) Minimally invasive follicular carcinoma. Endocr Path 8:231–234

Carcangiu M, Zampi G, Pupi A, Rosai J (1985a) Papillary carcinoma of the thyroid. A clinicopathologic study of 244 cases treated at the University of Florence, Italy. Cancer 55:805–828

Carcangiu ML, Sibley RK, Rosai J (1985b) Clear cell change in primary thyroid tumors. A study of 38 cases. Am J Surg Pathol 9(10):705–722

Carcangiu ML, Steeper T, Zampi G, Rosai J (1985c) Anaplastic thyroid carcinoma. A study of 70 cases. Am J Clin Pathol 83(2):135–158

Carcangiu ML, Bianchi S, Savino D, Voynick IM, Rosai J (1991) Follicular Hurthle cell tumors of the thyroid gland. Cancer 68(9):1944–1953

Carney JA, Moore SB, Northcutt RC, Woolner LB, Stillwell GK (1975) Palpation thyroiditis (multifocal granulomatour folliculitis). Am J Clin Pathol 64(5):639–647

Carney JA, Ryan J, Goellner JR (1987) Hyalinizing trabecular adenoma of the thyroid gland. Am J Surg Pathol 11(8):583–591

Carpenter GR, Emery JL (1976) Inclusions in the human thyroid. J Anat 122:77–89

Casey MB, Lohse CM, Lloyd RV (2003) Distinction between papillary thyroid hyperplasia and papillary thyroid carcinoma by immunohistochemical staining for cytokeratin 19, galectin-3, and HBME-1. Endocr Pathol 14(1):55–60

Casoli P, Tumiati B (1999) Hypoparathyroidism secondary to Riedel's thyroiditis. A case report and a review of the literature. Ann Ital Med Int 14(1):54–57

Cassano C (1971) Dyshormonogenetic goiter caused by altered synthesis of thyroglobulin. Recenti Prog Med 50(1):9–23

Cetta F, Montalto G, Petracci M, Fusco A (1997) Thyroid cancer and the Chernobyl accident. Are long-term and long distance side effects of fall-out radiation greater than estimated? J Clin Endocrinol Metab 82(6):2015–2017

Cetta F, Montalto G, Gori M, Curia MC, Cama A, Olschwang S (2000) Germline mutations of the APC gene in patients with familial adenomatous polyposis-associated thyroid carcinoma: results from a European cooperative study. J Clin Endocrinol Metab 85(1):286–292

Chan JK (1990) Papillary carcinoma of thyroid: classical and variants. Histol Histopathol 5(2):241–257

Chan JK, Rosai J (1991) Tumors of the neck showing thymic or related branchial pouch differentiation: a unifying concept. Hum Pathol 22(4):349–367

Chan YF, Ma L, Boey JH, Yeung HY (1986) Angiosarcoma of the thyroid. An immunohistochemical and ultrastructural study of a case in a Chinese patient. Cancer 57(12):2381–2388

Chan JKC, Tsui MS, Tse CH (1987) Diffuse sclerosing variant of papillary thyroid carcinoma. A histological and immunohistochemical study of three cases. Histopathology 11:191–201

Chan JK, Albores-Saavedra J, Battifora H, Carcangiu ML, Rosai J (1991a) Sclerosing mucoepidermoid thyroid carcinoma with eosinophilia. A distinctive low-grade malignancy arising from the metaplastic follicles of Hashimoto's thyroiditis. Am J Surg Pathol 15(5):438–448

Chan JK, Carcangiu ML, Rosai J (1991b) Papillary carcinoma of thyroid with exuberant nodular fasciitis-like stroma. Report of three cases. Am J Clin Pathol 95(3):309–314

Chang TC, Liaw KY, Kuo SH, Chang CC, Chen FW (1989) Anaplastic thyroid carcinoma: review of 24 cases, with emphasis on cytodiagnosis and leukocytosis. Taiwan Yi Xue Hui Za Zhi 88(6):551–556

Chen KTC, Rosai J (1977) Follicular variant of thyroid papillary carcinoma: a clinicopathologic study of six cases. Am J Surg Pathol 1:123–130

Chen H, Nicol TL, Zeiger MA, Dooley WC, Ladenson PW, Cooper DS, Ringel M, Parkerson S, Allo M, Udelsman R (1998) Hurthle cell neoplasms of the thyroid: are there factors predictive of malignancy? Ann Surg 227(4):542–546

Cheung CC, Ezzat S, Freeman JL, Rosen IB, Asa SL (2001) Immunohistochemical diagnosis of papillary thyroid carcinoma. Mod Pathol 14(4):338–342

Cignarelli M, Ambrosi A, Marino A, Lamacchia O, Cincione R, Neri V (2002) Three cases of papillary carcinoma and three of adenoma in thyroglossal duct cysts: clinical-diagnostic comparison with benign thyroglossal duct cysts. J Endocrinol Invest 25(11):947–954

Cohen Y, Xing M, Mambo E, Guo Z, Wu G, Trink B, Beller U, Westra WH, Ladenson PW, Sidransky D (2003) BRAF mutation in papillary thyroid carcinoma. J Natl Cancer Inst 95(8):625–627

Cohen EG, Shaha AR, Rinaldo A, Devaney KO, Ferlito A (2004) Medullary thyroid carcinoma. Acta Otolaryngol 124(5):544–557

Collini P, Sampietro G, Rosai J, Pilotti S (2003) Minimally invasive (encapsulated) follicular carcinoma of the thyroid gland is the low-risk counterpart of widely invasive follicular carcinoma but not of insular carcinoma. Virchows Arch 442(1):71–76

Constine L, Donaldson S, McDougall I, Cox R, Link M, Kaplan H (1984) Thyroid dysfunction after radiotherapy in children with Hodgkin's disease. Cancer 55:878–883

Crile G, Pontius K, Hawk W (1985) Factors influencing the survival of patients with follicular carcinoma of the thyroid gland. Surg Gynecol Obstet 160:409–412

D'Antonio A, Franco R, Sparano L, Terzi G, Pettinato G (2000) Amyloid goiter: the first evidence in secondary amyloidosis. Report of five cases and review of literature. Adv Clin Path 4(2):99–106

D'Avanzo A, Treseler P, Ituarte PH, Wong M, Streja L, Greenspan FS, Siperstein AE, Duh QY, Clark OH (2004) Follicular thyroid carcinoma: histology and prognosis. Cancer 100(6):1123–1129

Dahlgren M, Khosroshahi A, Nielsen GP, Deshpande V, Stone JH (2010) Riedel's thyroiditis and multifocal fibrosclerosis are part of the IgG4-related systemic disease spectrum. Arthritis Care Res (Hoboken) 62(9):1312–1318. doi:10.1002/acr.20215

Davies D, Furness P (1984) Riedel's thyroiditis with multiple organ fibrosis. Thorax 39:959–960

de los Santos ET, Keyhani-Rofagha S, Cunningham JJ, Mazzaferri EL (1990) Cystic thyroid nodules. The dilemma of malignant lesions. Arch Intern Med 150(7):1422–1427

DeLellis RA, Lloyd RD, Heitz PU, Eng C (eds) (2004) WHO: pathology and genetics. Tumours of endocrine organs. WHO classification of tumours. IARC, Lyon

DeLilles RA, Rule AH, Spiler F et al (1978) Calcitonin and carcinoembryonic antigen as tumor markers in medullary thyroid carcinoma. Am J Clin Pathol 70:587

Devaney K, Snyder R, Norris HJ, Tavassoli FA (1993) Proliferative and histologically malignant struma ovarii: a clinicopathologic study of 54 cases. Int J Gynecol Pathol 12(4):333–343

Dhillon AP, Rode J, Leathem A, Papadaki L (1982) Somatostatin: a paracrine contribution to hypothyroidism in Hashimoto's thyroiditis. J Clin Pathol 35(7):764–770

Diaz-Arias AA, Bickel JT, Loy TS, Croll GH, Puckett CL, Havey AD (1992) Follicular carcinoma with clear cell change arising in lingual thyroid. Oral Surg Oral Med Oral Pathol 74(2):206–211

Dickersin G, Vickery AL Jr, Smith S (1980) Papillary carcinoma of the thyroid, oxyphil cell type, "clear cell" variant: a light and electron microscopic study. Am J Surg Pathol 4:501–509

Dominguez-Malagon H, Delgado-Chavez R, Torres-Najera M, Gould E, Albores-Saavedra J (1989) Oxyphil and squamous variants of medullary thyroid carcinoma. Cancer 63(6):1183–1188

Donnell CA, Pollock WJ, Sybers WA (1987) Thyroid carcinosarcoma. Arch Pathol Lab Med 111(12):1169–1172

Doshi SV, Cruz RM, Hilsinger RL Jr (2001) Thyroglossal duct carcinoma: a large case series. Ann Otol Rhinol Laryngol 110(8):734–738

Dotto J, Nose V (2008) Familial thyroid carcinoma: a diagnostic algorithm. Adv Anat Pathol 15(6):332–349

Dozois RR, Beahrs OH (1977) Surgical anatomy and technique of thyroid and parathyroid surgery. Surg Clin North Am 57(4):647–661

Dralle H, Altenahr E (1979) Pituitary adenoma, primary parathyroid hyperplasia and papillary (non-medullary) thyroid carcinoma. A case of multiple endocrine neoplasia (MEN). Virchows Arch A Pathol Anat Histol 381(2):179–187

Dumitriu L, Stefaneanu L, Tasca C (1984) The anaplastic transformation of differentiated thyroid carcinoma. An ultrastructural study. Endocrinologie 22(2):91–96

Eimoto T, Naito H, Hamada S, Masuda M, Harada T, Kikuchi M (1987) Papillary carcinoma of the thyroid. A histochemical, immunohistochemical and ultrastructural study with special reference to the follicular variant. Acta Pathol Jpn 37(10): 1563–1579

Elisei R, Romei C, Vorontsova T, Cosci B, Veremeychik V, Kuchinskaya E, Basolo F, Demidchik EP, Miccoli P, Pinchera A, Pacini F (2001) RET/PTC rearrangements in thyroid nodules: studies in irradiated and not irradiated, malignant and benign thyroid lesions in children and adults. J Clin Endocrinol Metab 86(7):3211–3216

Eng C (1996) RET proto-oncogene in multiple endocrine neoplasia type 2 and Hirschsprung's disease. Semin Med (Beth Israel Hosp, Boston) 335:943–951

Eng C (1999) RET proto-oncogene in the development of human cancer. J Clin Oncol 17(1):380–393

Eng C, Smith DP, Mulligan LM, Nagai MA, Healey CS, Ponder MA, Gardner E, Scheumann GF, Jackson CE, Tunnacliffe A et al (1994) Point mutation within the tyrosine kinase domain of the RET proto-oncogene in multiple endocrine neoplasia type 2B and related sporadic tumours. Hum Mol Genet 3(2):237–241

Eng C, Clayton D, Schuffenecker I, Lenoir G, Cote G, Gagel RF, van Amstel HK, Lips CJ, Nishisho I, Takai SI, Marsh DJ, Robinson BG, Frank-Raue K, Raue F, Xue F, Noll WW, Romei C, Pacini F, Fink M, Niederle B, Zedenius J, Nordenskjold M, Komminoth P, Hendy GN, Mulligan LM et al (1996) The relationship between specific RET protooncogene mutations and disease phenotype in multiple endocrine neoplasia type 2. International RET mutation consortium analysis. JAMA 276(19):1575–1579

Esapa CT, Johnson SJ, Kendall-Taylor P, Lennard TW, Harris PE (1999) Prevalence of Ras mutations in thyroid neoplasia. Clin Endocrinol 50(4):529–535

Evans HL (1984) Follicular neoplasms of the thyroid. A study of 44 cases followed for a minimum of 10 years with emphasis on differential diagnosis. Cancer 54:535–540

Evans HL (1996) Encapsulated columnar-cell carcinoma of the thyroid. A report of four cases suggesting a favorable outcome. Am J Surg Pathol 20:1205–1211

Fatourechi V, McConahey WM, Woolner LB (1971) Hyperthyroidism associated with histologic Hashimoto's thyroiditis. Mayo Clin Proc 46(10):682–689

Fenton PA, Clarke SE, Owen W, Hibbert J, Hodgson SV (2001) Cribriform variant papillary thyroid cancer: a characteristic of familial adenomatous polyposis. Thyroid 11(2):193–197

Fenwick GR, Griffiths NM (1981) The identification of the goitrogen (−)5-vinyloxazolidine-2-thione (goitrin), as a bitter principle of cooked brussels sprouts (Brassica oleracea L. var. gemmifera). Z Lebensm Unters Forsch 172(2):90–92

Fernandez-Real JM, Ricart W (1999) Familial papillary thyroid microcarcinoma. Lancet 353(9168):1973–1974

Fialho NJ, de Oliveira CA (1971) Colloid goiter (observations on 100 operated and treated cases). Rev Bras Med 28(7):314–326

Fih J, Moore R (1963) Ectopic thyroid tissue and ectopic thyroid carcinoma. Ann Surg 157:212–222

Finkle H, Goldman F (1973) Heterotopic cartilage in the thyroid. Arch Pathol Lab Med 95:48–49

Fonseca E, Nesland J, Sobrinho-Simoes M (1997) Expression of stratified epithelial type cytokeratins in hyalinizing trabecular adenoma supports their relationship with papillary carcinoma of the thyroid. Histopathology 31:330–335

Francis IM, Das DK, Sheikh ZA, Sharma PN, Gupta SK (1995) Role of nuclear grooves in the diagnosis of papillary thyroid carcinoma. A quantitative assessment on fine needle aspiration smears. Acta Cytol 39(3):409–415

Franssila KO, Ackerman LV, Brown CL, Hedinger CE (1985) Follicular carcinoma. Semin Diagn Pathol 2(2):101–122

Fukunaga M, Shinozaki N, Endo Y, Ushigome S (1992) Atypical adenoma of the thyroid. A clinicopathologic and flow cytometric DNA study in comparison with other follicular neoplasms. Acta Pathol Jpn 42(9):632–638

Furlan JC, Bedard YC, Rosen IB (2004) Clinicopathologic significance of histologic vascular invasion in papillary and follicular thyroid carcinomas. J Am Coll Surg 198(3):341–348

Fusco A, Santoro M, Grieco M, Carlomagno F, Dathan N, Fabien N, Berlingieri MT, Li Z, De Franciscis V, Salvatore D et al (1995) RET/PTC activation in human thyroid carcinomas. J Endocrinol Invest 18(2):127–129

Fusco A, Chiappetta G, Hui P, Garcia-Rostan G, Golden L, Kinder BK, Dillon DA, Giuliano A, Cirafici AM, Santoro M, Rosai J, Tallini G (2002) Assessment of RET/PTC oncogene activation and clonality in thyroid nodules with incomplete morphological evidence of papillary carcinoma: a search for the early precursors of papillary cancer. Am J Pathol 160(6):2157–2167

Gabrilove JL, Dorrance WR, Soffer LJ (1952) Effect of corticotropin, cortisone and desoxycorticosterone on thyroid weight of the goitrogen-treated rat. Am J Physiol 169(3): 565–567

Gaitan E, Nelson NC, Poole GV (1991) Endemic goiter and endemic thyroid disorders. World J Surg 15(2):205–215

Gardner W (1956) Unusual relationships between thyroid gland and skeletal muscle in infants. Cancer 6:681–691

Gerard-Marchant R (1964) Thyroid follicle inclusions in cervical lymph nodes. Arch Pathol Lab Med 77:637–643

Ghazanfar S, Quraishy MS, Essa K, Muzaffar S, Saeed MU, Sultan T (2002) Mucosa associated lymphoid tissue lymphoma (Maltoma) in patients with cold nodule thyroid. J Pak Med Assoc 52(3):131–133

Ghossein RA, Rosai J, Heffess C (1997) Dyshormonogenetic goiter: a clinicopathologic study of 56 cases. Endocr Pathol 8(4):283–292

Gibson W, Peng T, Croker B (1980) C-cell nodules in adult human thyroid: a common autopsy finding. Am J Clin Pathol 73:347–351

Gilliland FD, Hunt WC, Morris DM, Key CR (1997) Prognostic factors for thyroid carcinoma. A population-based study of 15,698 cases from the Surveillance, Epidemiology and End Results (SEER) program 1973–1991. Cancer 79(3):564–573

Gimm O, Sutter T, Dralle H (2001) Diagnosis and therapy of sporadic and familial medullary thyroid carcinoma. J Cancer Res Clin Oncol 127(3):156–165

Giordano TJ, Kuick R, Thomas DG, Misek DE, Vinco M, Sanders D, Zhu Z, Ciampi R, Roh M, Shedden K, Gauger P, Doherty G, Thompson NW, Hanash S, Koenig RJ, Nikiforov YE (2005) Molecular classification of papillary thyroid carcinoma: distinct BRAF, RAS, and RET/PTC mutation-specific gene expression profiles discovered by DNA microarray analysis. Oncogene 24(44):6646–6656

Giuffrida D, Attard M, Marasa L, Ferrau F, Marletta F, Restuccia N, Gambino L, Janni F, Failla G (2000a) Thyroid carcinosarcoma, a rare and aggressive histotype: a case report. Ann Oncol 11(11):1497–1499

Giuffrida D, Ferrau F, Bordonaro R, Mattina M, Priolo D, Aiello RA, Cordio S, Motta S, Failla G (2000b) Medullary carcinoma of the thyroid: diagnosis and therapy. Clin Ter 151(1): 29–35

Goldsmith JD, Lai ML, Daniele GM, Tomaszewski JE, LiVolsi VA (2000) Amyloid goiter: report of two cases and review of the literature. Endocr Pract 6(4):318–323

Golshan MM, McHenry CR, de Vente J, Kalajyian RC, Hsu RM, Tomashefski JF (1997) Acute suppurative thyroiditis and necrosis of the thyroid gland: a rare endocrine manifestation of acquired immunodeficiency syndrome. Surgery 121(5):593–596

Gonzalez-Campora R, Herrero-Zapatero A, Lerma E, Sanchez F, Galera H (1986) Hurthle cell and mitochondrion-rich cell tumors. A clinicopathologic study. Cancer 57(6):1154–1163

Gopal PP, Montone KT, Baloch Z, Tuluc M, Livolsi V (2011) The variable presentations of anaplastic spindle cell squamous carcinoma associated with tall cell variant of papillary thyroid carcinoma. Thyroid 21(5):493–499. doi:10.1089/thy.2010.0338

Gordon G, Sparano B, Kramer A, Kelly R, Latropoulos M (1984) Thyroid gland pigmentation and minocycline therapy. Am J Pathol 117:98–109

Goto M, Miller RW, Ishikawa Y, Sugano H (1996) Excess of rare cancers in Werner syndrome (adult progeria). Cancer Epidemiol Biomarkers Prev 5(4):239–246

Grebe SK, McIver B, Hay ID, Wu PS, Maciel LM, Drabkin HA, Goellner JR, Grant CS, Jenkins RB, Eberhardt NL (1997) Frequent loss of heterozygosity on chromosomes 3p and 17p without VHL or p53 mutations suggests involvement of unidentified tumor suppressor genes in follicular thyroid carcinoma. J Clin Endocrinol Metab 82(11):3684–3691

Greer MA, Studer H, Kendall JW (1967) Studies on the pathogenesis of colloid goiter. Endocrinology 81(3):623–632

Grieco M, Santoro M, Berlingieri MT, Melillo RM, Donghi R, Bongarzone I, Pierotti MA, Della Porta G, Fusco A, Vecchio G (1990) PTC is a novel rearranged form of the ret proto-oncogene and is frequently detected in vivo in human thyroid papillary carcinomas. Cell 60(4):557–563

Gundry S, Burney R, Thompson N, Lloyd R (1983) Total thyroidectomy for Hürthle cell neoplasm of the thyroid gland. Arch Surg 118:529–553

Gustafson KS, LiVolsi VA, Furth EE, Pasha TL, Putt ME, Baloch ZW (2003) Peroxisome proliferator-activated receptor gamma expression in follicular-patterned thyroid lesions. Caveats for the use of immunohistochemical studies. Am J Clin Pathol 120(2):175–181

Guyetant S, Rousselet MC, Durigon M, Chappard D, Franc B, Guerin O, Saint-Andre JP (1997) Sex-related C cell hyperplasia in the normal human thyroid: a quantitative autopsy study. J Clin Endocrinol Metab 82(1):42–47

Guyetant S, Dupre F, Bigorgne JC, Franc B, Dutrieux-Berger N, Lecomte-Houcke M, Patey M, Caillou B, Viennet G, Guerin O, Saint-Andre JP (1999) Medullary thyroid microcarcinoma: a clinicopathologic retrospective study of 38 patients with no prior familial disease. Hum Pathol 30(8):957–963

Haggitt RC, Reid BJ (1986) Hereditary gastrointestinal polyposis syndromes. Am J Surg Pathol 10(12):871–887

Harach H (1986) Solid cell nests of the human thyroid in early stages of postnatal life. Acta Anat (Basel) 127(2):62–264

Harach HR (1987) Mixed follicles of the human thyroid gland. Acta Anat (Basel) 129(1):27–30

Harach H (1988) Solid cell nests of the thyroid. J Pathol 155:191–200

Harach HR (1993) Palpation thyroiditis resembling C cell hyperplasia. Usefulness of immunohistochemistry in their differential diagnosis. Pathol Res Pract 189(4):488–490

Harach HR, Williams ED (1983) Glandular (tubular and follicular) variants of medullary carcinoma of the thyroid. Histopathology 7(1):83–97

Harach HR, Williams ED (1990) The pathology of granulomatous diseases of the thyroid gland. Sarcoidosis 7(1):19–27

Harach HR, Day ES, de Strizic NA (1986) Mucoepidermoid carcinoma of the thyroid. Report of a case with immunohistochemical studies. Medicina 46(2):213–216

Harach HR, Vujanic GM, Jasani B (1993) Ultimobranchial body nests in human fetal thyroid: an autopsy, histological, and immunohistochemical study in relation to solid cell nests and mucoepidermoid carcinoma of the thyroid. J Pathol 169(4):465–469

Harach HR, Soubeyran I, Brown A, Bonneau D, Longy M (1999) Thyroid pathologic findings in patients with Cowden disease. Ann Diagn Pathol 3(6):331–340

Harach HR, Escalante DA, Day ES (2002) Thyroid cancer and thyroiditis in Salta, Argentina: a 40-yr study in relation to iodine prophylaxis. Endocr Pathol 13(3):175–181

Hay ID, Grant CS, van Heerden JA, Goellner JR, Ebersold JR, Bergstralh EJ (1992) Papillary thyroid microcarcinoma: a study of 535 cases observed in a 50-year period. Surgery 112(6):1139–1146; discussion 1146–1137

Hayashi Y, Tamai H, Fukata S, Hirota Y, Katayama S, Kuma K, Kumagai LF, Nagataki S (1985) A long term clinical, immunological, and histological follow-up study of patients with goitrous chronic lymphocytic thyroiditis. J Clin Endocrinol Metab 61(6):1172–1178

Hazard JB, Kenyon R (1954) Atypical adenoma of the thyroid. Arch Pathol 58:554–563

Hazard JB, Hawk WA, Crile G (1959) Medullary (solid) carcinoma of the thyroid. A clinicopathologic entity. J Clin Endocrinol Metab 19:152–161

Heshmati HM, Fatourechi V, van Heerden JA, Hay ID, Goellner JR (1997) Thyroglossal duct carcinoma: report of 12 cases. Mayo Clin Proc 72(4):315–319

Hirokawa M, Kuma S, Miyauchi A, Qian ZR, Nakasono M, Sano T, Kakudo K (2004) Morules in cribriform-morular variant of papillary thyroid carcinoma: immunohistochemical characteristics and distinction from squamous metaplasia. APMIS 112(4–5):275–282

Hirosawa H, Noguchi M, Sakata N, Tanaka S, Miyazaki I (1983) Adenoma or adenomatous goiter with the clinical symptoms of hyperthyroidism. Horumon To Rinsho 31(Suppl):95–98

Hirota Y, Tamai H, Hayashi Y, Matsubayashi S, Matsuzuka F, Kuma K, Kumagai LF, Nagataki S (1986) Thyroid function and histology in forty-five patients with hyperthyroid Graves' disease in clinical remission more than ten years after thionamide drug treatment. J Clin Endocrinol Metab 62(1):165–169

Hirsch MS, Faquin WC, Krane JF (2004) Thyroid transcription factor-1, but not p53, is helpful in distinguishing moderately differentiated neuroendocrine carcinoma of the larynx from medullary carcinoma of the thyroid. Mod Pathol 17(6):631–636

Hnilica P, Nyulassy S (1985) Plasma cells in aspirates of goitre and overt permanent hypothyroidism following subacute thyroiditis. Preliminary report. Endocrinol Exp 19(4):221–226

Hofstra RM, Landsvater RM, Ceccherini I, Stulp RP, Stelwagen T, Luo Y, Pasini B, Hoppener JW, van Amstel HK, Romeo G et al (1994) A mutation in the RET proto-oncogene associated with multiple endocrine neoplasia type 2B and sporadic medullary thyroid carcinoma [see comments]. Nature 367(6461):375–376

Hosoya T, Sakamoto A, Kasai N, Sakurai K (1983) Nodal psammoma body in thyroid cancer as an indicator of cancer metastasis to the lymph node. Gan No Rinsho 29(11):1336–1339

Hunt JL, Barnes EL (2003) Non-tumor-associated psammoma bodies in the thyroid. Am J Clin Pathol 119(1):90–94

Hunt JL, Baloch Z, Barnes EL, Swalsky PA, Trusky CL, Sasatomi E, Finkelstein S, LiVolsi VA (2003a) Loss of heterozygosity of tumor suppressor genes in cytologically atypical areas in Hashimoto's thyroiditis. Am J Surg Pathol 27:159–166

Hunt JL, LiVolsi VA, Baloch ZW, Barnes EL, Swalsky PA, Niehouse L, Finkelstein SD (2003b) Microscopic papillary thyroid carcinoma compared with clinical carcinomas by loss of heterozygosity mutational profile. Am J Surg Pathol 27(2):159–166

Huss LJ, Mendelsohn G (1990) Medullary carcinoma of the thyroid gland: an encapsulated variant resembling the hyalinizing trabecular (paraganglioma-like) adenoma of thyroid. Mod Pathol 3(5):581–585

Imai C, Kakihara T, Watanabe A, Ikarashi Y, Hotta H, Tanaka A, Uchiyama M (2002) Acute suppurative thyroiditis as a rare complication of aggressive chemotherapy in children with acute myelogenous leukemia. Pediatr Hematol Oncol 19(4):247–253

Ivanova R, Soares P, Castro P, Sobrinho-Simoes M (2002) Diffuse (or multinodular) follicular variant of papillary thyroid carcinoma: a clinicopathologic and immunohistochemical analysis of ten cases of an aggressive form of differentiated thyroid carcinoma. Virchows Arch 440(4):418–424

Iwatani Y, Amino N, Mori H, Asari S, Izumiguchi Y, Kumahara Y, Miyai K (1983) T lymphocyte subsets in autoimmune thyroid diseases and subacute thyroiditis detected with monoclonal antibodies. J Clin Endocrinol Metab 56(2):251–254

Iwatani Y, Hidaka Y, Matsuzuka F, Kuma K, Amino N (1993) Intrathyroidal lymphocyte subsets, including unusual CD4+ CD8+ cells and CD3loTCR alpha beta lo/-CD4-CD8- cells, in autoimmune thyroid disease. Clin Exp Immunol 93(3):430–436

Jakubiak-Wielganowicz M, Kubiak R, Sygut J, Pomorski L, Kordek R (2003) Usefulness of galectin-3 immunohistochemistry in differential diagnosis between thyroid follicular carcinoma and follicular adenoma. Pol J Pathol 54(2):111–115

Janser JC, Pusel J, Rodier JF, Navarrete E, Rodier D (1989) Hurthle cell tumor of the thyroid gland. Analysis of a series of 33 cases. J Chir (Paris) 126(11):619–624

Jansson S, Hansson G, Salander H, Stenstrom G, Tisell L (1984) Prevalence of C-cell hyperplasia and medullary thyroid carcinoma in a consecutive series of pheochromocytoma patients. World J Surg 8:493–500

Johnson THLR, Thompson NW, Beierwalters WH, Sisson JC (1988) prognostic implications of the tall cell variant of papillary carcinoma. Am J Surg Pathol 12:22–27

Jorda M, Gonzalez-Campora R, Mora J, Herrero-Zapatero A, Otal C, Galera H (1993) Prognostic factors in follicular carcinoma of the thyroid. Arch Pathol Lab Med 117(6):631–635

Kahn NF, Perzin KH (1983) Follicular carcinoma of the thyroid: an evaluation of the histologic criteria used for diagnosis. Pathol Annu 18(Pt 1):221–253

Kakudo K, Miyauchi A, Ogihara T et al (1982) Medullary carcinoma of the thyroid with ectopic ACTH syndrome. Acta Pathol Jpn 32:793–800

Kambouris M, Jackson CE, Feldman GL (1996) Diagnosis of multiple endocrine neoplasia [MEN] 2A, 2B and familial medullary thyroid cancer [FMTC] by multiplex PCR and heteroduplex analyses of RET proto-oncogene mutations. Hum Mutat 8(1):64–70

Kantelip B, Lusson JR, deRiberolles C, Lamaison D, Bailly P (1986) Intracardiac ectopic thyroid. Hum Pathol 17:1293–1296

Kanthan R, Radhi JM (1998) Immunohistochemical analysis of thyroid adenomas with Hurthle cells. Pathology 30(1):4–6

Kaplan M, Kauli R, Lubin E et al (1978) Ectopic thyroid gland. J Pediatr 92:205

Kaserer K, Scheuba C, Neuhold N, Weinhausel A, Haas OA, Vierhapper H, Niederle B (2001) Sporadic versus familial medullary thyroid microcarcinoma: a histopathologic study of 50 consecutive patients. Am J Surg Pathol 25(10):1245–1251

Katsikas D, Shorthouse A, Taylor S (1976) Riedel's thyroiditis. Br J Surg 63:929–931

Katz AD, Hachigian M (1988) Thyroglossal duct cysts. A thirty year experience with emphasis on occurrence in older patients. Am J Surg 155(6):741–744

Katz SM, Vickery AL Jr (1974) The fibrous variant of Hashimoto's thyroiditis. Hum Pathol 5(2):161–170

Kawai K, Tamai H, Mori T, Morita T, Matsubayashi S, Katayama S, Kuma K, Kumagai LF (1993) Thyroid histology of hyperthyroid Graves' disease with undetectable thyrotropin receptor antibodies. J Clin Endocrinol Metab 77(3):716–719

Kdous M, Hachicha R, Gamoudi A, Boussen H, Benna F, Hechiche M, Attia I, Rahal K (2003) Struma ovarii. Analysis of a series of 7 cases and review of the literature. Tunis Med 81(8):571–576

Kebebew E, Ituarte PH, Siperstein AE, Duh QY, Clark OH (2000) Medullary thyroid carcinoma: clinical characteristics, treatment, prognostic factors, and a comparison of staging systems. Cancer 88(5):1139–1148

Kennedy J, Thomson J, Buchannan W (1972) Amyloid in the thyroid. QJ Med 43:127–143

Komminoth P, Roth J, Saremasiani P et al (1994) Polysialic acid of the neural cell adhesion molecule in the human thyroid: a marker for medullary carcinoma and primary C-cell hyperplasia. An immunohistochemical study on 79 thyroid lesions. Am J Surg Pathol 18:399

Komorowski R, Hanson G (1977) Morphologic changes in the thyroid following low-dose childhood radiation. Arch Pathol Lab Med 101:36–39

Kondalenko VF, Kalinin AP, Odinokova VA (1970) Ultrastructure of the normal and pathologic human thyroid gland. Arkh Patol 32(4):25–34

Koo HL, Jang J, Hong SJ, Shong Y, Gong G (2004) Renal cell carcinoma metastatic to follicular adenoma of the thyroid gland. A case report. Acta Cytol 48(1):64–68

Kos M, Separovic V, Sarcevic B (1995) Medullary carcinoma of the thyroid: histomorphological, histochemical and immunohistochemical analysis of twenty cases. Acta Med Croatica 49(4–5):195–199

Kossev P, Livolsi V (1999) Lymphoid lesions of the thyroid: review in light of the revised European-American lymphoma classification and upcoming World Health Organization classification. Thyroid 9(12):1273–1280

Kovalenko AE (1999) Contemporary concepts of embryology and surgical anatomy of the thyroid gland. Klin Khir 8:38–42

Kraimps JL, Bouin-Pineau MH, Amati P, Mothes D, Bonneau D, Marechaud R, Barbier J (1997) Familial papillary carcinoma of the thyroid. Surgery 121(6):715–718

Kroll TG, Sarraf P, Pecciarini L, Chen CJ, Mueller E, Spiegelman BM, Fletcher JA (2000) PAX8-PPAR[gamma] 1 fusion in oncogene human thyroid carcinoma. Science 289:1357–1360

Krueger JE, Maitra A, Albores-Saavedra J (2000) Inherited medullary microcarcinoma of the thyroid: a study of 11 cases. Am J Surg Pathol 24(6):853–858

La Vecchia C, Ron E, Franceschi S, Dal Maso L, Mark SD, Chatenoud L, Braga C, Preston-Martin S, McTiernan A, Kolonel L, Mabuchi K, Jin F, Wingren G, Galanti MR, Hallquist A, Lund E, Levi F, Linos D, Negri E (1999) A pooled analysis of case–control studies of thyroid cancer. III. Oral contraceptives, menopausal replacement therapy and other female hormones. Cancer Causes Control 10(2):157–166

Lam KY, Lo CY (1998) Metastatic tumors of the thyroid gland: a study of 79 cases in Chinese patients. Arch Pathol Lab Med 122(1):37–41

Lam KY, Lo CY, Kwong DL, Lee J, Srivastava G (1999) Malignant lymphoma of the thyroid. A 30-year clinicopathologic experience and an evaluation of the presence of Epstein-Barr virus. Am J Clin Pathol 112(2):263–270

Lambert MJ 3rd, Johns ME, Mentzer R (1980) Acute suppurative thyroiditis. Am Surg 46(8):461–463

Landon G, Ordonez NG (1985) Clear cell variant of medullary carcinoma of the thyroid. Hum Pathol 16:844

Lang W, Georgii A, Atay Z (1977) Differential diagnosis between atypical adenoma and follicular carcinoma of the thyroid gland (author's transl). Verh Dtsch Ges Pathol 61:275–279

Lang B, Lo CY, Chan WF, Lam KY, Wan KY (2007) Restaging of differentiated thyroid carcinoma by the sixth edition AJCC/UICC TNM staging system: stage migration and predictability. Ann Surg Oncol 14(5):1551–1559. doi:10.1245/s10434-006-9242-2

Leesen E, Janssen L, Smet M, Breysem L (2001) Acute suppurative thyroiditis. JBR-BTR 84(2):68

Lindsay S (1960) Carcinoma of the thyroid gland: a clinical and pathologic study of 239 patients at the University of California Hospital. Charles C. Thomas, Sprigfield

Liu J, Singh B, Tallini G, Carlson DL, Katabi N, Shaha A, Tuttle RM, Ghossein RA (2006) Follicular variant of papillary thyroid carcinoma: a clinicopathologic study of a problematic entity. Cancer 107(6):1255–1264. doi:10.1002/cncr.22138

LiVolsi VA (1990) Surgical pathology of the thyroid. Saunders, Philadelphia

LiVolsi VA (1992) Papillary neoplasms of the thyroid. Pathologic and prognostic features. Am J Clin Pathol 97(3):426–434

LiVolsi VA (1993) Postpartum thyroiditis. The pathology slowly unravels. Am J Clin Pathol 100(3):193–195

LiVolsi VA (1994) The pathology of autoimmune thyroid disease: a review. Thyroid 4(3):333–339

LiVolsi VA (1996) Well differentiated thyroid carcinoma. Clin Oncol (R Coll Radiol) 8(5):281–288

LiVolsi VA (2000) Hyalinizing trabecular tumor of the thyroid: adenoma, carcinoma, or neoplasm of uncertain malignant potential? Am J Surg Pathol 24(12):1683–1684

LiVolsi VA, Asa SL (1994) The demise of follicular carcinoma of the thyroid gland. Thyroid 4(2):233–236

LiVolsi VA, Baloch ZW (2004) Follicular neoplasms of the thyroid: view, biases, and experiences. Adv Anat Pathol 11(6):279–287

LiVolsi VA, Feind CR (1976) Parathyroid adenoma and non-medullary thyroid carcinoma. Cancer 38(3):1391–1393

LiVolsi VA, Merino MJ (1994) Worrisome histologic alterations following fine-needle aspiration of the thyroid (WHAFFT). Pathol Annu 29(Pt 2):99–120

LiVolsi VA, Perzin KH, Savetsky L (1974) Carcinoma arising in median ectopic thyroid (including thyroglossal duct tissue). Cancer 34(4):1303–1315

LiVolsi VA, Brooks JJ, Arendash-Durand B (1987) Anaplastic thyroid tumors. Immunohistology. Am J Clin Pathol 87(4):434–442

Lloyd RV, Erickson LA, Asioli S (2010) Papillary thyroid carcinoma with prominent hobnail features: a New aggressive variant of moderately differentiated papillary carcinoma. A clinicopathologic, immunohistochemical, and molecular study of 8 cases. Am J Surg Pathol. doi:10.1097/PAS.0b013e3181d85d94

Lupoli G, Vitale G, Caraglia M, Fittipaldi MR, Abbruzzese A, Tagliaferri P, Bianco AR (1999) Familial papillary thyroid microcarcinoma: a new clinical entity. Lancet 353(9153):637–639

Mai KT, Landry DC, Thomas J, Burns BF, Commons AS, Yazdi HM, Odell PF (2001) Follicular adenoma with papillary architecture: a lesion mimicking papillary thyroid carcinoma. Histopathology 39(1):25–32

Maloof F, Wang CA, Vickery AL Jr (1975) Nontoxic goiter-diffuse or nodular. Med Clin North Am 59(5):1221–1232

Mansberger AR Jr, Wei JP (1993) Surgical embryology and anatomy of the thyroid and parathyroid glands. Surg Clin North Am 73(4):727–746

Marasini B, Massarotti M, Cossutta R (2005) Thyroid function, pulmonary arterial hypertension and scleroderma. Am J Med 118(3):322–323. doi:S0002-9343(04),00750-8 [pii] 10.1016/j.amjmed.2004.09.020

Marques AR, Espadinha C, Catarino AL, Moniz S, Pereira T, Sobrinho LG, Leite V (2002) Expression of PAX8-PPAR gamma 1 rearrangements in both follicular thyroid carcinomas and adenomas. J Clin Endocrinol Metab 87(8):3947–3952

Marsh DJ, Zheng Z, Arnold A, Andrew SD, Learoyd D, Frilling A, Komminoth P, Neumann HP, Ponder BA, Rollins BJ, Shapiro GI, Robinson BG, Mulligan LM, Eng C (1997) Mutation analysis of glial cell line-derived neurotrophic factor, a ligand for an RET/coreceptor complex, in multiple endocrine neoplasia type 2 and sporadic neuroendocrine tumors. J Clin Endocrinol Metab 82(9):3025–3028

Matias-Guiu X, LaGuette J, Puras-Gil AM, Rosai J (1997) Metastatic neuroendocrine tumors to the thyroid gland mimicking medullary carcinoma: a pathologic and immunohistochemical study of six cases. Am J Surg Pathol 21(7):754–762

Matsubayashi S, Yanaihara C, Ohkubo M et al (1984) Gastrin-releasing peptide immunoreactivity in medullary thyroid carcinoma. Cancer 53:2472

Matsuo K, Tang SH, Fagin JA (1991) Allelotype of human thyroid tumors: loss of chromosome 11q13 sequences in follicular neoplasms. Mol Endocrinol 5(12):1873–1879

Maximo V, Soares P, Lima J, Cameselle-Teijeiro J, Sobrinho-Simoes M (2002) Mitochondrial DNA somatic mutations (point mutations and large deletions) and mitochondrial DNA variants in human thyroid pathology: a study with emphasis on Hurthle cell tumors. Am J Pathol 160(5):1857–1865

Mazzaferri EL (1987) Papillary thyroid carcinoma: factors influencing prognosis and current therapy. Semin Oncol 14(3):315–332

Mazzaferri EL (1999) An overview of the management of papillary and follicular thyroid carcinoma. Thyroid 9(5):421–427

Mazzaferri E, Young RL (1981) Papillary thyroid carcinoma: a 10-year follow-up report of the impact of therapy in 576 patients. Am J Med 70:511–518

Meachim G, Young M (1963) De Quervain's subacute granulomatous thyroiditis: histological identification and incidence. J Clin Pathol 16:189–199

Meij S, Hausman R (1978) Occlusive phlebitis, a diagnostic feature in Riedel's thyroiditis. Virchows Arch [A] 377:339–349

Mendelsohn G, Baylin SB, Bigner SH, Wells SA Jr, Eggleston JC (1980) Anaplastic variants of medullary thyroid carcinoma: a light-microscopic and immunohistochemical study. Am J Surg Pathol 4(4):333–341

Meshikhes AW, Butt MS, Al-Saihati BA (2004) Combined parathyroid adenoma and an occult papillary carcinoma. Saudi Med J 25(11):1707–1710

Meyer J, Steinberg L (1969) Microscpically benign thyroid follicles in cervical lymph nodes. Cancer 24:301–311

Miettinen M, Franssila KO (2000) Variable expression of keratins and nearly uniform lack of thyroid transcription factor 1 in thyroid anaplastic carcinoma. Hum Pathol 31(9):1139–1145

Miettinen M, Karkkainen P (1996) Differential reactivity of HBME-1 and CD15 antibodies in benign and malignant thyroid tumours. Preferential reactivity with malignant tumours. Virchows Arch 429(4–5):213–219

Mikhailov IG, Vasil'ev NB, Smirnova EA (1980) Comparative quantitative electron-microscopic study of the nucleoli of human thyroid oncocytes and follicular cells. Arkh Patol 42(4):32–36

Miller FR (2003) Surgical anatomy of the thyroid and parathyroid glands. Otolaryngol Clin North Am 36(1):1–7, vii

Mills SE, Allen MS Jr (1986) Congenital occult papillary carcinoma of the thyroid gland. Hum Pathol 17(11):1179–1181

Mitchell JD, Kirkham N, Machin D (1984) Focal lymphocytic thyroiditis in Southampton. J Pathol 144(4):269–273

Mizukami Y, Michigishi T, Kawato M et al (1982) Chronic thyroiditis: thyroid function and histologic correlations in 601 cases. Hum Pathol 23:980

Mizukami Y, Funaki N, Hashimoto T, Kawato M, Michigishi T, Matsubara F (1988a) Histologic features of thyroid gland in a patient with bromide-induced hypothyroidism. Am J Clin Pathol 89(6):802–805

Mizukami Y, Michigishi T, Hashimoto T et al (1988b) Silent thyroiditis: a histologic and immunohistochemical study. Hum Pathol 19:423–431

Mizukami Y, Nonomura A, Michigishi T, Ohmura K, Noguchi M, Ishizaki T (1995) Diffuse follicular variant of papillary carcinoma of the thyroid. Histopathology 27(6):575–577

Moore JH Jr, Bacharach B, Choi HY (1985) Anaplastic transformation of metastatic follicular carcinoma of the thyroid. J Surg Oncol 29(4):216–221

Mulligan LM, Kwok JB, Healey CS, Elsdon MJ, Eng C, Gardner E, Love DR, Mole SE, Moore JK, Papi L et al (1993) Germ-line mutations of the RET proto-oncogene in multiple endocrine neoplasia type 2A. Nature 363(6428):458–460

Mulligan LM, Eng C, Healey CS, Clayton D, Kwok JB, Gardner E, Ponder MA, Frilling A, Jackson CE, Lehnert H et al (1994) Specific mutations of the RET proto-oncogene are related to disease phenotype in MEN 2A and FMTC. Nat Genet 6(1):70–74

Murray D (1998) The thyroid gland. Functional endocrine pathology. Blackwell Science, Malden

Nair K (1951) Adenoma of thyroid; simple adenomatous goiter. Antiseptic 48(9):716–724

Nakamura N, Carney JA, Jin L, Kajita S, Pallares J, Zhang H, Qian X, Sebo TJ, Erickson LA, Lloyd RV (2005) RASSF1A and NORE1A methylation and BRAFV600E mutations in thyroid tumors. Lab Invest 85(9):1065–1075

Nakata S, Okugi H, Saitoh Y, Takahashi H, Shimizu K (2001) Multiple endocrine neoplasia type 2B. Int J Urol 8(7):398–400

Namba H, Nakashima M, Hayashi T, Hayashida N, Maeda S, Rogounovitch TI, Ohtsuru A, Saenko VA, Kanematsu T, Yamashita S (2003) Clinical implication of hot spot BRAF mutation, V599E, in papillary thyroid cancers. J Clin Endocrinol Metab 88(9):4393–4397

Neri A, Aldovini D, Leonardi E, Giampiccolo M, Pedrolli C (1990) Primary angiosarcoma of the thyroid gland.

Presentation of a clinical case. Recenti Prog Med 81(5): 318–321
Nesland JM, Sobrinho-Simoes MA, Holm R, Sambade MC, Johannessen JV (1985) Hurthle-cell lesions of the thyroid: a combined study using transmission electron microscopy, scanning electron microscopy, and immunocytochemistry. Ultrastruct Pathol 8(4):269–290
Nguyen L, Niccoli-Sire P, Caron P, Bastie D, Maes B, Chabrier G, Chabre O, Rohmer V, Lecomte P, Henry JF, Conte-Devolx B (2001) Pheochromocytoma in multiple endocrine neoplasia type 2: a prospective study. Eur J Endocrinol 144(1): 37–44
Nikiforov YE (2002) RET/PTC rearrangement in thyroid tumors. Endocr Pathol 13(1):3–16
Nikiforov YE, Rowland JM, Bove KE, Monforte-Munoz H, Fagin JA (1997) Distinct pattern of ret oncogene rearrangements in morphological variants of radiation-induced and sporadic thyroid papillary carcinomas in children. Cancer Res 57(9):1690–1694
Nikiforov YE, Erickson LA, Nikiforova MN, Caudill CM, Lloyd RV (2001) Solid variant of papillary thyroid carcinoma: incidence, clinical-pathologic characteristics, molecular analysis, and biologic behavior. Am J Surg Pathol 25(12): 1478–1484
Nikiforov YE, Steward DL, Robinson-Smith TM, Haugen BR, Klopper JP, Zhu Z, Fagin JA, Falciglia M, Weber K, Nikiforova MN (2009) Molecular testing for mutations in improving the fine needle aspiration diagnosis of thyroid nodules. J Clin Endocrinol Metab 94(6):2092–2098, Epub 2009 Mar 24
Nikiforova MN, Caudill CM, Biddinger P, Nikiforov YE (2002) Prevalence of RET/PTC rearrangements in Hashimoto's thyroiditis and papillary thyroid carcinomas. Int J Surg Pathol 10(1):15–22
Nikiforova MN, Kimura ET, Gandhi M, Biddinger PW, Knauf JA, Basolo F, Zhu Z, Giannini R, Salvatore G, Fusco A, Santoro M, Fagin JA, Nikiforov YE (2003) BRAF mutations in thyroid tumors are restricted to papillary carcinomas and anaplastic or poorly differentiated carcinomas arising from papillary carcinomas. J Clin Endocrinol Metab 88(11):5399–5404
Nose V (2008) Familial Non-medullary thyroid carcinoma: an update. Endocr Pathol 19(4):226–240
O'Toole K, Fenoglio-Preiser C, Pushparaj N (1985) Endocrine changes associated with the human aging process. III. Effect of age on the number of calcitonin immunoreactive cells in the thyroid gland. Hum Pathol 16:991–1000
Pacini F, Vorontsova T, Molinaro E, Shavrova E, Agate L, Kuchinskaya E, Elisei R, Demidchik EP, Pinchera A (1999) Thyroid consequences of the Chernobyl nuclear accident. Acta Paediatr Suppl 88(433):23–27
Papi G, Corrado S, Cesinaro AM, Novelli L, Smerieri A, Carapezzi C (2002) Riedel's thyroiditis: clinical, pathological and imaging features. Int J Clin Pract 56(1): 65–67
Papi G, Corrado S, Carapezzi C, Corsello SM (2003a) Postpartum thyroiditis presenting as a cold nodule and evolving to Graves' disease. Int J Clin Pract 57(6):556–558
Papi G, Corrado S, Carapezzi C, De Gaetani C, Carani C (2003b) Riedel's thyroiditis and fibrous variant of Hashimoto's thyroiditis: a clinicopathological and immunohistochemical study. J Endocrinol Invest 26(5):444–449

Papotti M, Volante M, Giuliano A et al (2000) RET/PTC activation in hyalinizing trabecular tumors of the thyroid. Am J Surg Pathol 24:1615–1621
Papotti M, Rodriguez J, Pompa RD, Bartolazzi A, Rosai J (2005) Galectin-3 and HBME-1 expression in well-differentiated thyroid tumors with follicular architecture of uncertain malignant potential. Mod Pathol 18(4):541–546
Peix JL, Mabrut JY, Van Box SP, Berger N (1998) Thyroid cancer in children and adolescents. Clinical aspects, diagnostic problems and special therapeutics. Ann Endocrinol (Paris) 59(2):113–120
Petkov R, Gavrailov M, Mikhailov I, Todorov G, Kutev N (1995) Differentiated thyroid cancer – a study of the pathomorphological variants in 216 patients. Khirurgiia 48(2):11–12
Petrova GV, Tereshchenko VP, Avetis'ian IL (1996) The dynamics of thyroid diseases in the inhabitants of Kiev and Kiev Province after the accident at the Chernobyl Atomic Electric Power Station. Lik Sprava 5–6:67–70
Prasad ML, Pellegata NS, Huang Y, Nagaraja HN, Chapelle Ade L, Kloos RT (2005) Galectin-3, fibronectin-1, CITED-1, HBME1 and cytokeratin-19 immunohistochemistry is useful for the differential diagnosis of thyroid tumors. Mod Pathol 18(1):48–57
Puxeddu E, Moretti S, Elisei R, Romei C, Pascucci R, Martinelli M, Marino C, Avenia N, Rossi ED, Fadda G, Cavaliere A, Ribacchi R, Falorni A, Pontecorvi A, Pacini F, Pinchera A, Santeusanio F (2004) BRAF(V599E) mutation is the leading genetic event in adult sporadic papillary thyroid carcinomas. J Clin Endocrinol Metab 89(5):2414–2420
Ramelli F, Studer H, Bruggisser D (1982) Pathogenesis of thyroid nodules in multinodular goiter. Am J Pathol 109:215–223
Randolph GW (1996) Medullary carcinoma of the thyroid: subtypes and current management. Compr Ther 22(4):203–210
Randolph GW, Maniar D (2000) Medullary carcinoma of the thyroid. Cancer Control 7(3):253–261
Rao C, Ferguson G, Kyle V (1973) Retroperitoneal fibrosis associated with Riedel's struma. Can Med Assoc J 108:1019–1021
Riazmontazer N, Bedayat G (1991) Psammoma bodies in fine needle aspirates from thyroids containing nontoxic hyperplastic nodular goiters. Acta Cytol 35(5):563–566
Rivera M, Ghossein RA, Schoder H, Gomez D, Larson SM, Tuttle RM (2008) Histopathologic characterization of radioactive iodine-refractory fluorodeoxyglucose-positron emission tomography-positive thyroid carcinoma. Cancer 113(1):48–56
Rivera M, Tuttle RM, Patel S, Shaha A, Shah JP, Ghossein RA (2009) Encapsulated papillary thyroid carcinoma: a clinicopathologic study of 106 cases with emphasis on its morphologic subtypes (histologic growth pattern). Thyroid 19(2):119–127
Rodriguez JM, Moreno A, Parrilla P, Sola J, Soria T, Tebar FJ, Aranda F (1997) Papillary thyroid microcarcinoma: clinical study and prognosis. Eur J Surg 163(4):255–259
Roka S, Kornek G, Schuller J, Ortmann E, Feichtinger J, Armbruster C (2004) Carcinoma showing thymic-like elements – a rare malignancy of the thyroid gland. Br J Surg 91(2):142–145
Ron E, Kleinerman RA, Boice JD, LiVolsi VA, Flannery JT, Fraumeni JF (1987) A population-based case–control study of thyroid cancer. J Natl Cancer Inst 79(1):1–12
Rosai J (2003) Immunohistochemical markers of thyroid tumors: significance and diagnostic applications. Tumori 89(5): 517–519

Rosai J, Carcangui ML, DeLellis RA (1992) Tumors of the thyroid gland, vol 3rd Series, Fascicle 5. Atlas of tumor pathology. Armed Forces Institute of Pathology, Washington, DC

Rosenblum NG, LiVolsi VA, Edmonds PR, Mikuta JJ (1989) Malignant struma ovarii. Gynecol Oncol 32(2):224–227

Rosenthal D, Carvalho-Guimaraes DP, Knobel M, Medeiros-Neto GA (1990) Dyshormonogenetic goiter: presence of an inhibitor of normal human thyroid peroxidase. J Endocrinol Invest 13(11):901–904

Roth L (1965) Inclusions of nonneoplastic thyroid tissue within cervical lymph nodes. Cancer 18:105–111

Roth KA, Bensch KG, Hoffman AR (1987) Characterization of opioid peptides in human thyroid medullary carcinoma. Cancer 59:1594

Roti E, Uberti ED (2001) Iodine excess and hyperthyroidism. Thyroid 11(5):493–500

Ruiz-Velasco R, Waisman J, Van Herle AJ (1978) Cystic papillary carcinoma of the thyroid gland. Diagnosis by needle aspiration with transmission electron microscopy. Acta Cytol 22(1):38–42

Ruppert JM, Eggleston JC, de Bustros A, Baylen SB (1986) Disseminated calcitonin-poor medullary thyroid carcinoma in a patient with calcitonin-rich primary tumor. Am J Surg Pathol 10:513–518

Sahoo M, Bal CS, Bhatnagar D (2002) Primary squamous-cell carcinoma of the thyroid gland: new evidence in support of follicular epithelial cell origin. Diagn Cytopathol 27(4):227–231

Santoro M, Rosati R, Grieco M, Berlingieri MT, D'Amato GL, de Franciscis V, Fusco A (1990) The ret proto-oncogene is consistently expressed in human pheochromocytomas and thyroid medullary carcinomas. Oncogene 5(10):1595–1598

Santoro M, Dathan NA, Berlingieri MT, Bongarzone I, Paulin C, Grieco M, Pierotti MA, Vecchio G, Fusco A (1994) Molecular characterization of RET/PTC3; a novel rearranged version of the RETproto-oncogene in a human thyroid papillary carcinoma. Oncogene 9(2):509–516

Santoro M, Thomas GA, Vecchio G, Williams GH, Fusco A, Chiappetta G, Pozcharskaya V, Bogdanova TI, Demidchik EP, Cherstvoy ED, Voscoboinik L, Tronko ND, Carss A, Bunnell H, Tonnachera M, Parma J, Dumont JE, Keller G, Hofler H, Williams ED (2000) Gene rearrangement and Chernobyl related thyroid cancers. Br J Cancer 82(2):315–322

Schark C, Fulton N, Yashiro T, Stanislav G, Jacoby R, Straus FH 2nd, Dytch H, Bibbo M, Kaplan EL (1992) The value of measurement of ras oncogenes and nuclear DNA analysis in the diagnosis of Hurthle cell tumors of the thyroid. World J Surg 16(4):745–751; discussion 752

Schmidt RJ, Wang CA (1986) Encapsulated follicular carcinoma of the thyroid: diagnosis, treatment, and results. Surgery 100(6):1068–1077

Schottenfeld D, Gershman ST (1977) Epidemiology of thyroid cancer – Part II. Clin Bull 7(3):98–104

Schroder S, Bocker W (1985) Lipomatous lesions of the thyroid gland: a review. Appl Pathol 3(3):140–149

Schroder S, Bocker W, Baisch H, Burk CG, Arps H, Meiners I, Kastendieck H, Heitz PU, Kloppel G (1988) Prognostic factors in medullary thyroid carcinomas. Survival in relation to age, sex, stage, histology, immunocytochemistry, and DNA content. Cancer 61(4):806–816

Schwaegerle S, Bauer T, Esselstyn C (1988) Riedel's thyroiditis. Am J Clin Pathol 90:715–722

Segal K, Arad A, Lubin E, Shpitzer T, Hadar T, Feinmesser R (1994) Follicular carcinoma of the thyroid. Head Neck 16(6):533–538

Shaha A, Gleich L, Di Maio T, Jaffe BM (1990a) Accuracy and pitfalls of frozen section during thyroid surgery. J Surg Oncol 44(2):84–92

Shaha AR, DiMaio T, Webber C, Jaffe BM (1990b) Intraoperative decision making during thyroid surgery based on the results of preoperative needle biopsy and frozen section. Surgery 108(6):964–967; discussion 970–961

Shaha AR, Loree TR, Shah JP (1995) Prognostic factors and risk group analysis in follicular carcinoma of the thyroid. Surgery 118(6):1131–1136; discussion 1136–1138

Sheils O, Smyth P, Finn S, Sweeney EC, O'Leary JJ (2002) RET/PTC rearrangements in Hashimoto's thyroiditis. Int J Surg Pathol 10(2):167–168; discussion 168–169

Sipple JH (1961) The association of pheochromocytoma with carcinoma of the thyroid gland. Am J Med 31:163–166

Soares J, Limbert E, Sobrinho-Simoes M (1989) Diffuse sclerosing variant of papillary thyroid carcinoma. A clinicopathologic study of 10 cases. Pathol Res Pract 185(2):200–206

Soares P, Trovisco V, Rocha AS, Feijao T, Rebocho AP, Fonseca E, Vieira de Castro I, Cameselle-Teijeiro J, Cardoso-Oliveira M, Sobrinho-Simoes M (2004) BRAF mutations typical of papillary thyroid carcinoma are more frequently detected in undifferentiated than in insular and insular-like poorly differentiated carcinomas. Virchows Arch 444(6):572–576

Sobrinho-Simoes M, Nesland JM, Johannessen JV (1988) Columnar-cell carcinoma. Another variant of poorly differentiated carcinoma of the thyroid. Am J Clin Pathol 89(2):264–267

Sobrinho-Simoes M, Sambade C, Nesland JM, Johannessen JV (1989) Tall cell papillary carcinoma. Am J Surg Pathol 13(1):79–80

Strauss A, Trujillo M (1986) Lithium-induced goiter and voice changes. J Clin Psychopharmacol 6(2):120–121

Struder H, Peter H, Gerber H (1987) Morphologic and functional changes in developing goiters. In: Hall R, Kobberling J (eds) Thyroid disorders associated with iodine deficiency and excess. Raven, New York

Sugiyama S (1971) The embryology of the human thyroid gland including ultimobranchial body and others related. Ergeb Anat Entwicklungsgesch 44(2):3–111

Tachikawa T, Kumazawa H, Kyomoto R, Yukawa H, Yamashita T, Nishikawa M (2001) Clinical study on prognostic factors in thyroid carcinoma. Nippon Jibiinkoka Gakkai Kaiho [J Otorhinolaryngol Soc Jpn] 104(2):157–164

Takano T, Miyauchi A, Matsuzuka F, Yoshida H, Kuma K, Amino N (2000) Diagnosis of thyroid malignant lymphoma by reverse transcription-polymerase chain reaction detecting the monoclonality of immunoglobulin heavy chain messenger ribonucleic acid. J Clin Endocrinol Metab 85(2):671–675

Tallini G (2011) Poorly differentiated thyroid carcinoma. Are we these yet. Endocr Pathol 22(4):190–194

Tamimi DM (2002) The association between chronic lymphocytic thyroiditis and thyroid tumors. Int J Surg Pathol 10(2):141–146

Thomas GA, Bunnell H, Cook HA, Williams ED, Nerovnya A, Cherstvoy ED, Tronko ND, Bogdanova TI, Chiappetta G, Viglietto G, Pentimalli F, Salvatore G, Fusco A, Santoro M,

Vecchio G (1999) High prevalence of RET/PTC rearrangements in Ukrainian and Belarussian post-Chernobyl thyroid papillary carcinomas: a strong correlation between RET/PTC3 and the solid-follicular variant. J Clin Endocrinol Metab 84(11):4232–4238

Thompson N, Dun E, Batsakis J, Nishiyama R (1974) Hürthle cell lesions of the thyroid gland. Surg Gynecol Obstet 139:555–560

Thompson LD, Wieneke JA, Paal E, Frommelt RA, Adair CF, Heffess CS (2001) A clinicopathologic study of minimally invasive follicular carcinoma of the thyroid gland with a review of the English literature. Cancer 91(3):505–524

Tielens ET, Sherman SI, Hruban RH, Ladenson PW (1994) Follicular variant of papillary thyroid carcinoma. A clinicopathologic study. Cancer 73(2):424–431

Tollefson HR, Shah JP, Huvos AG (1973) Follicular carcinoma of the thyroid. Am J Surg 126:523–528

Tomer Y, Ban Y, Concepcion E, Barbesino G, Villanueva R, Greenberg DA, Davies TF (2003) Common and unique susceptibility loci in Graves and Hashimoto diseases: results of whole-genome screening in a data set of 102 multiplex families. Am J Hum Genet 73(4):736–747

Topf P, Fried MP, Strome M (1988) Vagaries of thyroglossal duct cysts. Laryngoscope 98(7):740–742

Tsugawa K, Koyanagi N, Nakanishi K, Wada H, Tanoue K, Hashizume M, Sugimachi K (1999) Leiomyosarcoma of the thyroid gland with rapid growth and tracheal obstruction: a partial thyroidectomy and tracheostomy using an ultrasonically activated scalpel can be safely performed with less bleeding. Eur J Med Res 4(11):483–487

Udelsman R, Westra WH, Donovan PI, Sohn TA, Cameron JL (2001) Randomized prospective evaluation of frozen-section analysis for follicular neoplasms of the thyroid. Ann Surg 233(5):716–722

Uribe M, Fenoglio-Preiser CM, Grimes M, Feind C (1985) Medullary carcinoma of the thyroid gland. Clinical, pathological and immunohistochemical features with review of the literature. Am J Surg Pathol 9:577–594

van Hoeven KH, Kovatich AJ, Miettinen M (1998) Immunocytochemical evaluation of HBME-1, CA 19–9, and CD-15 (Leu-M1) in fine-needle aspirates of thyroid nodules. Diagn Cytopathol 18(2):93–97

Variakojis D, Getz ML, Paloyan E, Straus FH (1975) Papillary clear cell carcinoma of the thyroid gland. Hum Pathol 6(3):384–390

Venkatesh YS, Ordonez NG, Schultz PN, Hickey RC, Goepfert H, Samaan NA (1990) Anaplastic carcinoma of the thyroid. A clinicopathologic study of 121 cases. Cancer 66(2):321–330

Vergilio J, Baloch ZW, LiVolsi VA (2002) Spindle cell metaplasia of the thyroid arising in association with papillary carcinoma and follicular adenoma. Am J Clin Pathol 117(2):199–204

Vickery AL Jr (1981) The diagnosis of malignancy in dyshormonogenetic goitre. Clin Endocrinol Metab 10(2):317–335

Volante M, Collini P, Nikiforov YE, Sakamoto A, Kakudo K, Katoh R, Lloyd RV, LiVolsi VA, Papotti M, Sobrinho-Simoes M, Bussolati G, Rosai J (2007) Poorly differentiated thyroid carcinoma: the Turin proposal for the use of uniform diagnostic criteria and an algorithmic diagnostic approach. Am J Surg Pathol 31(8):1256–1264

Vollenweider R, Stolkin I, Hedinger C (1982) Focal lymphocytic thyroiditis and iodized salt prophylaxis. Comparative studies on goiter specimens at the Institute of Pathology of Zurich University. Schweiz Med Wochenschr 112(14):482–488

Wade JS (1975) The aetiology and diagnosis of malignant tumours of the thyroid gland. Br J Surg 62(10):760–764

Wan SK, Chan JK, Tang SK (1996) Paucicellular variant of anaplastic thyroid carcinoma. A mimic of Riedel's thyroiditis. Am J Clin Pathol 105(4):388–393

Weetman AP, Fung HY, Richards CJ, McGregor AM (1990) IgG subclass distribution and relative functional affinity of thyroid microsomal antibodies in postpartum thyroiditis. Eur J Clin Invest 20(2):133–136

Weiss ML, Deckart H, Pilz R, Deckart E, Kleinau E (1984) Oncocytes in thyroid gland aspirates – differential diagnostic problem: tumor/thyroiditis. Radiobiol Radiother (Berl) 25(5):765–768

Wenig BM, Adair CF, Heffess CS (1995) Primary mucoepidermoid carcinoma of the thyroid gland: a report of six cases and a review of the literature of a follicular epithelial-derived tumor. Hum Pathol 26(10):1099–1108

Wenig BM, Thompson LDR, Adair CF, Shmookler B, Heffess CF (1998) Thyroid papillary carcinoma of columnar cell type. A clinicopathologic study of 16 cases. Cancer 82:740–753

Williams ED (1965) A review of 17 cases of carcinoma of the thyroid and pheochromocytoma. J Clin Pathol 18:288–292

Williams ED (1966) Histogenesis of medullary carcinoma of the thyroid. J Clin Pathol 19:114–118

Williams E, Karim S, Sandler M (1968) Prostaglandin secretion by medullary carcinoma of the thyroid: a possible cause of the associated diarrhea. Lancet 1:22–23

Williams ED, Doniach I, Bjarnason O, Michie W (1977) Thyroid cancer in an iodide rich area: a histopathological study. Cancer 39(1):215–222

Williams ED, Abrosimov A, Bogdanova TI, Roasi J, Sidorov Y, Thomas GA (2000) Two proposals regarding the terminology of thyroid tumors. Guest Editorial. Int J Surg Pathol 8(3):181–183

Wirtschafter A, Schmidt R, Rosen D, Kundu N, Santoro M, Fusco A, Multhaupt H, Atkins JP, Rosen MR, Keane WM, Rothstein JL (1997) Expression of the RET/PTC fusion gene as a marker for papillary carcinoma in Hashimoto's thyroiditis [see comments]. Laryngoscope 107(1):95–100

Wolfe HJ, Melvin KE, Cervi-Skinner SJ, Saadi AA, Juliar JF, Jackson CE, Tashjian AH Jr (1973) C-cell hyperplasia preceding medullary thyroid carcinoma. N Engl J Med 289(9):437–441

Wolfe H, DeLellis R, Voelkel E, Tashjian A (1975) Distribution of calcitonin containing cells in the normal neonatal human thyroid gland: a correlation of morphology with peptide content. J Clin Endocrinol Metab 41:1076–1081

Wreesmann VB, Ghossein RA, Hezel M, Banerjee D, Shaha AR, Tuttle RM, Shah JP, Rao PH, Singh B (2004) Follicular variant of papillary thyroid carcinoma: genome-wide appraisal of a controversial entity. Genes Chromosomes Cancer 40(4):355–364

Xing M (2005) BRAF mutation in thyroid cancer. Endocr Relat Cancer 12(2):245–262

Xing M, Tufano RP, Tufaro AP, Basaria S, Ewertz M, Rosenbaum E, Byrne PJ, Wang J, Sidransky D, Ladenson PW (2004) Detection of BRAF mutation on fine needle aspiration biopsy specimens: a new diagnostic tool for papillary thyroid cancer. J Clin Endocrinol Metab 89(6):2867–2872

Yamauchi A, Tomita Y, Takakuwa T, Hoshida Y, Nakatsuka S, Sakamoto H, Aozasa K (2002) Polymerase chain reaction-based clonality analysis in thyroid lymphoma. Int J Mol Med 10(1):113–117

Zampi G, Bianchi S, Amorosi A, Vezzosi V (1994) Thyroid cancer: anatomy and pathologic histology. Chir Ital 46(4):4–7

Zhu Z, Gandhi M, Nikiforova MN, Fischer AH, Nikiforov YE (2003) Molecular profile and clinical-pathologic features of the follicular variant of papillary thyroid carcinoma. An unusually high prevalence of ras mutations. Am J Clin Pathol 120(1):71–77

Energy Devices in Minimally Invasive Thyroidectomy

6

Pier Francesco Alesina and Martin K. Walz

6.1 Introduction

An accurate haemostasis is essential during any surgical procedure. This problem is well known for thyroid surgery since over one century when Billroth, considered one of the best surgeons in Europe, reported a mortality of 40% on a series of 20 patients in 1869. Few decades later, in the hands of Theodor Kocher, thyroidectomy developed into a safe operation with a mortality rate of 0.5% by 1898 (Richard 1990). The key for these extraordinary results was the technique he introduced which first ligated the major arteries and veins followed by identifying and isolating the recurrent laryngeal nerve (Kocher 1883). Since that time, suture ligation has continued to be the gold standard of obtaining haemostasis. The introduction of the minimally invasive thyroid surgery poses the problem to break this 100-year-old rule. The impossibility to ligate is obvious for the purely endoscopic operations such as the endoscopic neck, thoracic and axillary approach (Henry and Segab 2006; Strik et al. 2007; Kang et al. 2009), but also the video-assisted operation due to the limited working space permits conventional ligatures only after the extraction of the thyroid lobe through the skin incision (Miccoli et al. 2006). Many instruments are now available for this use and have been demonstrated to be at least as safe as the knot-and-tie technique.

6.2 Energy Devices

6.2.1 Ultrasound Dissection

The first description of the use of an energy device for thyroidectomy was published in 1999 (Takami et al. 1999). The authors used the ultrasonically activated shears (Ultracision, Ethicon Endo-Surgery, Cincinnati, Ohio) that allows simultaneous cutting and coagulation of blood vessels by using mechanical vibration at a frequency of 55.5 kHz. This causes the rupture of hydrogen bonds of the proteins, and thus proteins are denatured to form a coagulum, which seals the vessels and assures hemostasis at temperatures between 50°C and 100°C (Bandi et al. 2008). Speed of cutting and effectivity of coagulation can be adjusted by the power setting of the generator and the pressure applied on the shears. The transmitted energy is related to the pressure on the tissue and the vibrating blade and to the heat between the two blades which may achieve more than 200°C (Emam and Cuschieri 2003). In their observational study, Takami and coauthors compared the safety and effectiveness of the Ultracision device with conventional ligatures. In a group of 28 patients affected by Graves' disease, half of the subtotal thyroidectomies were performed by the new device causing a significant reduction of the operating time and loss of blood. In 2000, these results were confirmed in a well-designed prospective randomized study showing that the use of ultrasonic dissection reduces significantly the operating time without increasing the complications rate (Voutilainen and Haglund 2000). Afterward, many studies on the use of harmonic scalpel in conventional and minimally invasive thyroid surgery have been published and are summarized in Table 6.1.

P.F. Alesina, M.D. (✉) • M.K. Walz, M.D.
Clinic for Surgery and Centre of Minimal Invasive Surgery, Kliniken Essen-Mitte, Academic Hospital of the University of Duisburg-Essen, Henricistrasse 92, D-45136 Essen, Germany
e-mail: pieroalesina@yahoo.it; mkwalz@kliniken-essen-mitte.de

Table 6.1 Ultracision vs. conventional vessel ligature

Author	Study	Patients	Type of surgery	Operative time	Bleeding	Significant differences	Complication	Cost
Takami (1999)	Observational	14 vs. 14	Subtotal thyroidectomy	76 vs. 98	No	Shorter operative time, less intra- and postoperative blood loss	No difference	Not analyzed
Voutilainen (2000)	Prospective randomized	19 vs. 17	Total thyroidectomy Lobectomy	99.1 vs. 134.9	0 vs. 1	Shorter operative time	No difference	Slightly higher ($10) for ligature
Meurisse (2000)	Prospective randomized	17 vs. 17	Total thyroidectomy	70.7 vs. 96.5	–	Significant reduction in operating time, blood loss, postoperative analgesic consumption	Lower incidence of transient hypoparathyroidism	Same costs
Miccoli (2002)	Retrospective case–control	26 vs. 26	Total thyroidectomy Lobectomy (MIVAT)	53.9 vs. 90.6 37.3 vs. 49.4	No	Shorter operative time	No difference	Not analyzed
Siperstein (2002)	Retrospective case–control	47 vs. 36 38 vs. 49	Total thyroidectomy Lobectomy	132 vs. 161 89 vs. 115	No	Shorter operative time for uni- and bilateral surgery	No difference	Not analyzed
Defechereux (2003)	Prospective randomized	17 vs. 17	Total thyroidectomy	70.7 vs. 96.5	No	Significant reduction in operating time, blood loss, and maybe in transitory hypoparathyroidism	No difference	Same costs
Mantke (2003)	Prospective non-randomized	11 vs. 13 5 vs. 3	Bilateral resection Unilateral resection	64.6 vs. 143.1 (for both procedures)	No	Shorter operative time	No difference	Not analyzed
Marchesi (2003)	Prospective randomized	72 vs. 70	Total thyroidectomy	–	–	Shorter operative time, less blood loss	Higher incidence of nerve palsy	Not analyzed
Ortega (2004)	Prospective randomized	100 vs. 100	Total thyroidectomy (57 vs. 57) Lobectomy (43 vs. 43)	86 vs. 101 61 vs. 78	0 vs. 2	Shorter operative time	No difference	More cost for ligature
Cordon (2005)	Prospective randomized	7 vs. 12 23 vs. 18	Total thyroidectomy Partial thyroidectomy	104 vs. 136 93 vs. 112	No	Operative time not different if adjusted for the type of procedure	No difference	Not analyzed
Karvounaris (2006)	Prospective	150 vs. 150	Total thyroidectomy Lobectomy	50 vs. 83 36 vs. 52	No	Shorter operative time	No difference	Not analyzed
Miccoli (2006)	Prospective randomized	50 vs. 50	Total thyroidectomy	40.0 vs. 46.7	No	Shorter operative time, less pain, less drainage volume	Lower incidence of transient hypoparathyroidism	Not analyzed
Koutsoumanis (2007)	Prospective	71 vs. 81 vs. 98 6 vs. 7 vs. 9	Total thyroidectomy Partial thyroidectomy	65 vs. 70.5 vs. 124	0 vs. 0 vs. 2	Shorter operative time	No difference	Ultracision more expensive

Kilic (2007)	Prospective randomized	40 vs. 40	Total thyroidectomy	–	Significant differences in terms of operative time, number of ligatures, amount of bleeding, average length of incision, total amount of drainage fluid, and cosmetic satisfaction	–	–
Leonard (2008)	Prospective	21 vs. 31	Lobectomy	63 vs. 59	No difference	No difference	Not analyzed
Lombardi (2008)	Prospective randomized	100 vs. 100	Total thyroidectomy	53.1 vs. 75.8	Shorter operative time	No difference, No difference also for the incision length	No differences concerning the charges of the hospitalization
Hallgrimsson (2008)	Prospective randomized	27 vs. 24	Total thyroidectomy	121 vs. 172	Shorter operative time, less ligatures	No difference	No difference
Barczyński (2008)	Prospective randomized	38 vs. 38	Lobectomy (MIVAT)	31.4 vs. 47.5	Shorter operative time, less intraoperative blood loss, shorter scar, and higher cosmetic satisfaction in the short follow-up		Slightly higher ($30)
Yildirim (2008)	Prospective randomized	50 vs. 54	Total thyroidectomy	77.9 vs. 105	Shorter operative time, less ligatures and blood loss, less drains	No difference	Not analyzed
Koh (2008)	Prospective randomized	31 vs. 34	Total thyroidectomy with central neck dissection	98 vs. 141	Shorter operative time	No difference	Not analyzed
Foreman (2009)	Retrospective	106 vs. 77	Total thyroidectomy Lobectomy	82.8 vs. 94.0 61.7 vs. 66.7	Shorter operative time for total thyroidectomy, reduced hypocalcaemia	No difference	Not analyzed
Sebag (2009)	Prospective randomized	50 vs. 50	Total thyroidectomy	84 vs. 104	Shorter operative time	No difference	Slightly higher
Papavramidis (2010)	Prospective randomized	45 vs. 45	Total thyroidectomy	76.67 vs. 101.74	Duration of surgery, operative difficulty, postoperative pain	No difference	Not analyzed
Miccoli (2010)	Prospective randomized	31 vs. 31	Total thyroidectomy	33.4 vs. 47.2	Shorter operative time, less ligatures and clips, less pain and less suction volume	No difference	Not analyzed

Group I comprised the conventional knot-and-tie technique, group II comprised the ligation of all but the superior thyroid vessels with a scalpel, and group III comprised patients in whom the device was used exclusively

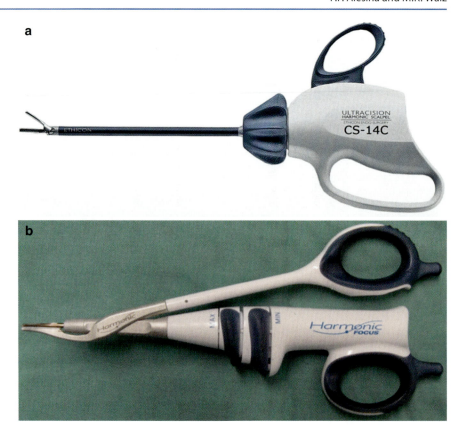

Fig. 6.1 (a) Harmonic® (CS14C) shear and (b) Harmonic FOCUS® shear (Ethicon Endo-Surgery, Cincinnati, Ohio)

Among the 13 prospective randomized studies, all except one confirm a shorter-operative-time ultrasonic dissection compared with conventional ligatures. Other advocated advantages are less blood loss, less postoperative analgesic consumption, decreased incidence of transient hypoparathyroidism, lower total amount of drainage fluid, and improved cosmetic satisfaction. A cost analysis was performed in eight studies. Despite the costs of the disposable instrument, overall costs of the operation seem to be at least not higher due to the shortened operative time. Two studies concentrated their attention on the use of ultrasonic shear during minimally invasive video-assisted thyroidectomy (MIVAT) (Miccoli et al. 2002; Barczyński et al. 2008). Both studies demonstrate a shorter operative time compared to conventional dissection with clip application. Beside that, use of harmonic scalpel is associated with a shortened scar and therefore higher cosmetic satisfaction (Barczyński et al. 2008). Actually, two different ultrasonic devices are available for thyroid surgery (Fig. 6.1): the Harmonic® (CS14C) Shear and the Harmonic FOCUS® Shear (Ethicon Endo-Surgery, Cincinnati, Ohio). As recently demonstrated in a prospective randomized study (Miccoli et al. 2010), the Harmonic FOCUS® Shear seems to have the same advantage as the previous model in term of time saving and efficacy. Due to its configuration, the Harmonic CS14C is the preferred instrument for MIVAT. Obviously, the ultrasonic technology is essential for the purely endoscopic operations with infraclavicular approach where conventional ligature is impossible at all and clip application is extremely time consuming.

6.2.2 Bipolar Vessel Sealer

More recently, a bipolar vessel sealer (LigaSure®; Covidien, Boulder, Colorado) has also been demonstrated to be equally safe and effective in thyroid surgery as conventional vessel division (Kiriakopoulos et al. 2004). This instrument permits vessels sealing with bipolar electrocautery and pressure (Fig. 6.2). It denatures collagen and elastin fibers and creates a seal of tissue and vessels reaching a temperature of 70–90°C between the blades. (Heniford et al. 2001; Kim et al. 2008). A feedback-controlled response automatically discontinues energy delivery when the seal cycle is complete. Thereby, only a minimal lateral thermic

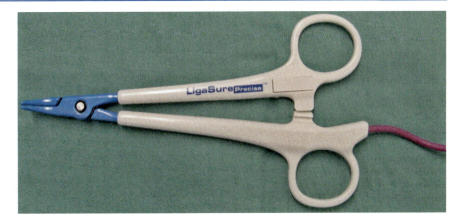

Fig. 6.2 LigaSure® (Covidien, Boulder, Colorado)

spread is provided. Coagulated tissue has to be divided by scissor. The studies focusing on the use of LigaSure in conventional thyroid surgery are summarized in Table 6.2. All except one could demonstrate a shorter operative time for LigaSure®, associated in two studies also to a shorter hospital stay. The cost analysis, performed in three series, showed increased costs due to the use of a disposable device. Unfortunately, studies on the use of LigaSure® during minimally invasive thyroid surgery are missing. The integration of a cutting device has been recently introduced, and this will represent the key to allow for even more time saving and could improve its use during minimally invasive surgery.

Recently, a new reusable device based on bipolar thermofusion coagulation (BiClamp®, ERBE, Tuebingen, Germany) has become available (Fig. 6.3). Comparable to LigaSure®, the output of power is measured and calculated during the activation of the device. After reaching a high resistance between the blades, power is terminated. The attraction of that device is its serviceability for at least 30 procedures. Thereby, costs can be minimized (Alesina et al. 2010). Initially, the efficacy of this system was demonstrated on a porcine model (Richter et al. 2006). In a prospective study, the BiClamp was supposed to reduce the operative time and the severity of postoperative hypocalcemia compared to LigaSure (Oussoultzoglou et al. 2008). We reported our experience with BiClamp® in a recent prospective non-randomized study on 186 patients showing that the mean operative time for total thyroidectomy was significantly shorter in the energy device group (73 min) than in the conventional ligatures group (81 min). Shortening the operative time of about 10 min was traduced in a costs saving of 10% in our setting.

6.2.3 Ultrasound Dissection Versus Bipolar Vessel Sealer

In the comparisons between Ultracision® and LigaSure®, the harmonic device seems to show the shortest operative time (Table 6.3). Both Ultracision® and LigaSure® are disposable instruments and therefore usually increase the costs of the operation. Despite the well-documented safety of all energy-based devices, they have the potential for invisible and undesirable heat-related collateral/proximity iatrogenic injury to adjacent structures. The unquestioned advantage in terms of operative time should be balanced with the possible increased complication rate, especially when total thyroidectomy is requested. To date, improved postoperative complication rates have rarely been cited as a major advantage of use of the ultrasonic dissector. In 2000 and 2003, Meurisse et al. reported a non-significant decrease in the incidence of transient hypoparathyroidism among patients treated using Ultracision® (Meurisse et al. 2000; Defechereux et al. 2003). These results have been not confirmed by Sartori et al. who showed that the use of LigaSure® or Ultracision® is associated with a significantly higher hypocalcaemia rate (Sartori et al. 2008). Basically, the most critical aspect of using the new energy devices in thyroid surgery is the damage of the RLN by lateral thermic spread. To avoid RLN palsy by heat application, two surgical options are possible: first, the use of clips and conventional sutures near to the nerve, or second, a dissection through the thyroid tissue near Barry's ligament leaving a small thyroid remnant.

Table 6.2 LigaSure vs. conventional vessel ligature

Author	Study	Patients	Type of surgery	Operative time	Bleeding	Significant differences	Complications	Cost
Kiriakopoulos (2004)	Case–control	40 vs. 40	Total thyroidectomy	84 vs. 89	No	None	No difference	Increased costs
Petrakis (2004)	Retrospective	270 vs. 247	Total thyroidectomy	71 vs. 86	1 vs. 8	Shorter operative time and postoperative drain volume	Less laryngeal nerve palsy, hematoma, and hypocalcemia, shorter hospital stay	Not analyzed
Lachanas (2005)	Case–control	72 vs. 72	–	–	–	Shorter operative time	No difference	Not analyzed
Kirdak (2005)	Retrospective non-randomized	30 vs. 28	Total thyroidectomy (8 vs. 9) Subtotal thyroidectomy (14 vs. 9) Lobectomy (8 vs. 10)	102.5 vs. 128.8 103.3 vs. 119.3 77.3 vs. 99.8	No	Shorter operative time for total thyroidectomy and lobectomy	No difference	Not analyzed
Parmeggiani (2005)	Retrospective	70 vs. 120	Total thyroidectomy	72.2 vs. 91.3	1 vs. 2	Shorter operative time (about 20 min)	Lesser transient hypoparathyroidism	Increased costs
Fujita (2006)	Retrospective	22 vs. 30	All kind of procedures	135.3 vs. 100.6	No	Shorter hospital stay	No difference	Not analyzed
Barbaros (2006)	Case–control	50 vs. 50	Thyroidectomy	58 vs. 75	No	Shorter operative time, shorter hospital stay	No difference	Not analyzed
Lepner (2007)	Retrospective non-randomized	204 vs. 199	Total thyroidectomy (143 vs. 121) Subtotal thyroidectomy (11 vs. 26) Lobectomy (50 vs. 52)	78.3 vs. 104.8 64 vs. 106 54 vs. 75.3	3 vs. 7	Shorter operative time for all types of procedure	Lesser hypoparathyroidism, no differences for RLN palsy and bleeding	Not analyzed
Saint Marc (2007)	Prospective randomized	100 vs. 100	Total thyroidectomy	41.5 vs. 48.8	1 vs. 2	Shorter operative time	No difference	Additional costs for LigaSure
Marrazzo (2007)	Prospective randomized	25 vs. 25	Thyroidectomy	60 vs. 92.4	1 vs. 0	Shorter operative time, shorter hospital stay	No difference	Not analyzed
Musunuru (2008)	Retrospective non-randomized	51 vs. 99	Lobectomy	52 vs. 92	No	Shorter operative time	No difference	Not analyzed

Fig. 6.3 BiClamp® (ERBE, Tuebingen, Germany)

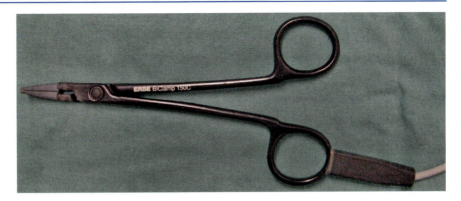

Table 6.3 Ultracision vs. LigaSure vs. conventional ligature

Author	Study	Patients	Type of surgery	Operative time	Bleeding	Significant differences	Complications	Cost
Sartori (2008)	Prospective randomized	50 vs. 50 vs. 50	Total thyroidectomy	94 vs. 129 vs. 118	1 vs. 0 vs. 0	Shorter operative time for Ultracision	Higher morbidity for both	Not analyzed
Manouras (2008)	Retrospective	144 vs. 148 vs. 90	Total thyroidectomy	73.8 vs. 74.3 vs. 93.3	1 vs. 1 vs. 0	Shorter operative time for both	No difference	Not analyzed
Pons (2009)	Prospective randomized	20 vs. 20 vs. 20	Total thyroidectomy	114 vs. 122 vs. 151	No	Shorter operative time for Ultracision, less pain for both	No difference	Higher for both
Di Rienzo (2010)	Prospective randomized	31 vs. 31 vs. 31	Total thyroidectomy	62.7 vs. 68.9 vs. 72.7	No	Shorter operative time for Ultracision	No difference	Not analyzed
Rahbari (2010)	Prospective randomized	45 vs. 45	Total thyroidectomy	184.2 vs. 187.6	?	No difference	No difference	No difference
Zarebczan (2010)	Retrospective		Total thyroidectomy Lobectomy			Shorter operative time for Ultracision	No difference	

6.3 Conclusion

In minimally invasive thyroid surgery, the new energy devices have demonstrated safety and efficiency. They may increase costs but shorten operating times.

References

Alesina PF, Rolfs T, Walz MK (2010) Bipolar thermofusion vessel sealing system (TVS) versus conventional vessel ligation (CVL) in thyroid surgery – results of a prospective study. Langenbecks Arch Surg 395:115–119

Bandi G, Wen CC, Wilkinson EA et al (2008) Comparison of blade temperature dynamics after activation of Harmonic Ace scalpel and the Ultracision Harmonic Scalpel LCS-K5. J Endourol 22:333–336

Barbaros U, Erbil Y, Bozbora A et al (2006) The use of LigaSure in patients with hyperthyroidism. Langenbecks Arch Surg 391:575–579

Barczyński M, Konturek A, Cichoń S (2008) Minimally invasive video-assisted thyroidectomy (MIVAT) with and without use of harmonic scalpel – a randomized study. Langenbecks Arch Surg 393:647–654

Cordón C, Fajardo R, Ramírez J et al (2005) A randomized, prospective, parallel group study comparing the Harmonic Scalpel to electrocautery in thyroidectomy. Surgery 137:337–341

Defechereux T, Rinken F, Maweja S et al (2003) Evaluation of the ultrasonic dissector in thyroid surgery. A prospective randomised study. Acta Chir Belg 103:274–277

Di Rienzo RM, Bove A, Bongarzoni G et al (2010) Comparison of conventional technique, Ligasure Precise and Harmonic Focus in total thyroidectomy. G Chir 31:296–298

Emam TA, Cuschieri A (2003) How safe is high-power ultrasonic dissection? Ann Surg 237:186–191

Foreman E, Aspinall S, Bliss RD et al (2009) The use of the harmonic scalpel in thyroidectomy: 'beyond the learning curve'. Ann R Coll Surg Engl 91:214–216

Fujita T, Doihara H, Ogasawara Y et al (2006) Utility of vessel-sealing systems in thyroid surgery. Acta Med Okayama 60:93–98

Hallgrimsson P, Lovén L, Westerdahl J et al (2008) Use of the harmonic scalpel versus conventional haemostatic techniques in patients with Grave disease undergoing total thyroidectomy: a prospective randomised controlled trial. Langenbecks Arch Surg 393:675–680

Heniford BT, Matthews BD, Sing RF et al (2001) Initial results with an electrothermal bipolar vessel sealer. Surg Endosc 15:799–801

Henry JF, Segab F (2006) Lateral endoscopic approach for thyroid and parathyroid surgery. Ann Chir 131:51–56

Kang SW, Lee SC, Lee SH et al (2009) Robotic thyroid surgery using a gasless, transaxillary approach and the da Vinci S system: the operative outcomes of 338 consecutive patients. Surgery 146:1048–1055

Karvounaris DC, Antonopoulos V, Psarras K et al (2006) Efficacy and safety of ultrasonically activated shears in thyroid surgery. Head Neck 28:1028–1031

Kilic M, Keskek M, Ertan T et al (2007) A prospective randomized trial comparing the harmonic scalpel with conventional knot tying in thyroidectomy. Adv Ther 24:632–638

Kim FJ, Chammas MF Jr, Gewehr E et al (2008) Temperature safety profile in laparoscopic devices: Harmonic Ace (ACE), Ligasure V (LV) and plasma trisector (PT). Surg Endosc 22:1464–1469

Kirdak T, Korun N, Ozguc H (2005) Use of ligasure in thyroidectomy procedures: results of a prospective comparative study. World J Surg 29:771–774

Kiriakopoulos A, Dimitrios T, Dimitrios L et al (2004) Use of a diathermy system in thyroid surgery. Arch Surg 139:997–1000

Kocher T (1883) Ueber Kropfextirpation und ihre Folgen. Arch Klin Chir 29:254–335

Koh YW, Park JH, Lee SW et al (2008) The harmonic scalpel technique without supplementary ligation in total thyroidectomy with central neck dissection: a prospective randomized study. Ann Surg 247:945–949

Koutsoumanis K, Koutras AS, Drimousis PG et al (2007) The use of a harmonic scalpel in thyroid surgery: report of a 3-year experience. Am J Surg 193:693–696

Lachanas VA, Prokopakis EP, Mpenakis AA et al (2005) The use of Ligasure Vessel Sealing System in thyroid surgery. Otolaryngol Head Neck Surg 132:487–489

Leonard DS, Timon C (2008) Prospective trial of the ultrasonic dissector in thyroid surgery. Head Neck 30:904–908

Lepner U, Vaasna T (2007) Ligasure vessel sealing system versus conventional vessel ligation in thyroidectomy. Scand J Surg 96:31–34

Lombardi CP, Raffaelli M, Cicchetti A et al (2008) The use of "harmonic scalpel" versus "knot tying" for conventional "open" thyroidectomy: results of a prospective randomized study. Langenbecks Arch Surg 393:627–631

Manouras A, Markogiannakis H, Koutras AS et al (2008) Thyroid surgery: comparison between the electrothermal bipolar vessel sealing system, harmonic scalpel, and classic suture ligation. Am J Surg 195:48–52

Mantke R, Pross M, Klose S et al (2003) The harmonic scalpel in conventional thyroid surgery. Possibilities and advantages. Chirurg 74:739–742

Marchesi M, Biffoni M, Cresti R et al (2003) Ultrasonic scalpel in thyroid surgery. Chir Ital 55:299–308

Marrazzo A, Casà L, David M et al (2007) Thyroidectomy with LigaSure versus traditional thyroidectomy: our experience. Chir Ital 59:361–365

Meurisse M, Defechereux T, Maweja S et al (2000) Evaluation of the ultracision ultrasonic dissector in thyroid surgery. Prospective randomized study. Ann Chir 125:468–472

Miccoli P, Berti P, Raffaelli M et al (2002) Impact of harmonic scalpel on operative time during video-assisted thyroidectomy. Surg Endosc 16:663–666

Miccoli P, Berti P, Frustaci GL et al (2006) Video-assisted thyroidectomy: indications and results. Langenbecks Arch Surg 391:68–71

Miccoli P, Materazzi G, Miccoli M et al (2010) Evaluation of a new ultrasonic device in thyroid surgery: comparative randomized study. Am J Surg 199:736–740

Musunuru S, Schaefer S, Chen H (2008) The use of the Ligasure for hemostasis during thyroid lobectomy. Am J Surg 195: 382–384; discussion 384–385

Ortega J, Sala C, Flor B et al (2004) Efficacy and cost-effectiveness of the UltraCision harmonic scalpel in thyroid surgery: an analysis of 200 cases in a randomized trial. J Laparoendosc Adv Surg Tech A 14:9–12

Oussoultzoglou E, Panaro F, Rosso E et al (2008) Use of BiClamp decreased the severity of hypocalcemia after total thyroidectomy compared with LigaSure: a prospective study. World J Surg 32:1968–1973

Papavramidis TS, Sapalidis K, Michalopoulos N et al (2010) UltraCision harmonic scalpel versus clamp-and-tie total thyroidectomy: a clinical trial. Head Neck 32:723–727

Parmeggiani U, Avenia N, De Falco M et al (2005) Major complications in thyroid surgery: utility of bipolar vessel sealing (Ligasure Precise). G Chir 26:387–394

Petrakis IE, Kogerakis NE, Lasithiotakis KG et al (2004) LigaSure versus clamp-and-tie thyroidectomy for benign nodular disease. Head Neck 26:903–909

Pons Y, Gauthier J, Ukkola-Pons E et al (2009) Comparison of LigaSure vessel sealing system, harmonic scalpel, and conventional hemostasis in total thyroidectomy. Otolaryngol Head Neck Surg 141:496–501

Rahbari R, Mathur A, Kitano M et al (2010) Prospective randomized trial of ligasure versus harmonic hemostasis technique in thyroidectomy. Ann Surg Oncol. doi:10.1245/s10434-010-1251-5

Richard B (1990) Welbourn: the history of endocrine surgery. Praegel, New York

Richter S, Kollmar O, Neunhoeffer E et al (2006) Differential response of arteries and veins to bipolar vessel sealing: evaluation of a novel reusable device. J Laparoendosc Adv Surg Tech A 16:149–155

Saint Marc O, Cogliandolo A, Piquard A et al (2007) LigaSure vs clamp-and-tie technique to achieve hemostasis in total thyroidectomy for benign multinodular goiter: a prospective randomized study. Arch Surg 142:150–156; discussion 157

Sartori PV, De Fina S, Colombo G et al (2008) Ligasure versus ultracision in thyroid surgery: a prospective randomized study. Langenbecks Arch Surg 393:655–658

Sebag F, Fortanier C, Ippolito G et al (2009) Harmonic scalpel in multinodular goiter surgery: impact on surgery and cost analysis. J Laparoendosc Adv Surg Tech A 19:171–174

Siperstein AE, Berber E, Morkoyun E (2002) The use of the harmonic scalpel vs conventional knot tying for vessel ligation in thyroid surgery. Arch Surg 137:137–142

Strik MW, Anders S, Barth M et al (2007) Total videoendoscopic thyroid resection by the axillobilateral breast approach. Operative method and first results. Chirurg 78: 1139–1144

Takami H, Ikeda Y, Niimi M (1999) Ultrasonically activated scalpel for subtotal thyroidectomy in Graves' disease. Am J Surg 178:433–434

Voutilainen PE, Haglund CH (2000) Ultrasonically activated shears in thyroidectomies: a randomized trial. Ann Surg 231:322–328

Yildirim O, Umit T, Ebru M et al (2008) Ultrasonic harmonic scalpel in total thyroidectomies. Adv Ther 25: 260–265

Zarebczan B, Mohanty D, Chen H (2010) A comparison of the LigaSure and harmonic scalpel in thyroid surgery: a single institution review. Ann Surg Oncol. doi:10.1245/s10434-010-1334-1343

Local Anesthesia in MIT

Leon Kushnir and William B. Inabnet

7.1 History of Using Local Anesthesia in Thyroid Surgery

Thyroid and parathyroid surgery was historically performed under local anesthesia. Due to the significant morbidity and mortality of general anesthesia and the absence of adequate medications for hyperthyroid conditions, local anesthesia was widely used to safely manage elderly and medically compromised patients and those with complicated thyrotoxicosis and large goiters. Sir Thomas Peel (TP) Dunhill, in 1912, is generally credited with being the first surgeon to use local anesthesia for thyroid surgery. As anesthesiologist experience grew and safe general anesthesia techniques were developed and refined, the practice of local anesthesia for thyroid surgery receded. During this time, local anesthesia in thyroid surgery was primarily being used in centers outside of the United States as a necessity rather than choice (i.e., lack of adequate resources or trained personnel, inability to provide postoperative care for critically ill patients).

Almost a century later, the development of minimally invasive surgical techniques, the introduction of effective medical management of hyperthyroidism, and a preference for outpatient surgery prompted renewed interest in the techniques of local anesthesia for thyroid surgery. Several well-designed studies published early in 2000s demonstrated safety and feasibility of this approach, and today an increasing number of thyroid and parathyroid surgery are being performed using local anesthesia in an outpatient setting.

7.2 Anatomy and Definition

Thyroid surgery using regional/local anesthesia involves the use of intravenous sedation combined with a locally injected anesthetic solution to achieve cervical plexus blockade. This approach depends upon accurate localization of the nerves that supply the intended surgical field.

Motor and sensory innervation to the neck and the posterior scalp is supplied by the nerve roots of the second, third, and fourth cervical vertebrae. The fibers emerge between the anterior and the middle scalene muscles and divide into *superficial* (sensory) and *deep* (motor and sensory) plexus.

The *superficial cervical plexus* fibers extend laterally until they emerge at the midway point between the mastoid process and C6 transverse process along the posterior border of the sternocleidomastoid (SCM) muscle. These fibers then divide into four distinct nerves to provide sensory innervation to the anterior and posterior skin of the neck.

The *deep cervical plexus* fibers extend medially and have a more complex architecture which bears some importance to the thyroid surgeon. The deep plexus braches contain both motor and sensory fibers, supplying the deep structures of the neck such as the trapezius and the anterior neck muscles, and contributing motor fibers to the phrenic nerve to innervate the ipsilateral diaphragm. In addition, the third and fourth cervical

---

L. Kushnir, M.D. (✉) • W.B. Inabnet, M.D.
Division of Metabolic, Endocrine and Minimally Invasive Surgery, Mount Sinai Medical Center,
5 East 98th Street 15th floor, Box 1259,
New York, NY 10029, USA
e-mail: leonkushnir@yahoo.com; william.inabnet@mountsinai.org

nerves typically send a branch to the spinal accessory nerve, while the fourth and fifth nerves may contribute fibers to the brachial plexus. Due to this proximity, motor fibers can inadvertently become anesthetized during deep cervical block, producing temporary brachial plexus or ipsilateral diaphragm paresis.

7.3 Medications

The efficacy of a regional block is directly dependent on the proximity of the local anesthetic agent to the target nerve; therefore, a thorough knowledge of cervical plexus anatomy is vital to administering an effective block. The *duration* of the block is mainly affected by the drug clearance rate from the local environment and the total dose, rather than volume or concentration, of the anesthetic. All local anesthetics will demonstrate shorter duration of action compared to other peripheral sites due to the high vascularity of the neck.

The choice of anesthetic agent is dictated by individual preference and the anticipated procedure duration. Intermediate- (i.e., lidocaine, mepivacaine) and long-acting (i.e., bupivacaine, ropivacaine, etidocaine, tetracaine,) hydrophobic anesthetic agents are commonly used for regional anesthesia. Lidocaine is widely available and commonly used. Plain lidocaine produces approximately 1–3 h of sensory blockade, while addition of epinephrine slightly prolongs its duration. Mepivacaine causes a mild vasoconstriction and hence has a 25% longer duration of action compared to lidocaine. Bupivacaine, a long-acting anesthetic agent, provides a sensory block of 6–12 h when injected peripherally for regional anesthesia.

Several adjuncts are sometimes added to local anesthetic agents to enhance or alter their activity. Addition of epinephrine, usually at a concentration of 5 mcg/mg, reliably produces vasoconstriction which slows drug clearance and prolongs block duration. Moreover, peak plasma concentration is lowered, thus decreasing the risk of systemic toxicity and allowing the use of a higher anesthetic dose. It is important to note that addition of epinephrine will not provide protection from toxic side-effects of an accidental intravascular injection. Sodium bicarbonate is sometimes added to increase the speed of onset of local anesthetic agents. Several studies have failed to conclusively prove this effect. In fact, overalkalinizing the solution by adding too much bicarbonate may precipitate the anesthetic thus inactivating it.

7.4 Technique

7.4.1 Overview

It is the Mount Sinai Hospital standard practice for the surgeon to perform the cervical block in the operating room prior to prepping the skin and draping the patient. Alternatively, a dedicated anesthesiologist with specialty training in regional anesthesia can be used.

Intravenous sedation administered by a trained anesthesiologist is very helpful to ensure patient cooperation and decrease patient discomfort and anxiety. The specific technique of monitored anesthesia care (MAC) is beyond the scope of this chapter, but a combination of a sedative, such as a benzodiazepine or propofol, combined with a fast-acting narcotic, such as remifentanil, is often used. The patient is positioned supine with a shoulder roll to extend the neck, and both arms tucked and secured to the patient's side. The head is turned to expose the injection site and held in place by the assistant to prevent inadvertent movement during block administration.

Superficial and deep cervical block is performed on the side of the proposed operation (i.e., hemithyroidectomy, localized parathyroidectomy). In addition, a unilateral superficial block on the contralateral side is then performed. If bilateral neck surgery is anticipated, such as a total thyroidectomy, bilateral deep and superficial cervical block is performed. The skin of the proposed incision site is also injected subcutaneously in all cases.

A word of caution is warranted at this point. Since fibers from C3 to C5 nerve roots combine to form the phrenic nerve, temporary bilateral diaphragmatic paralysis from bilateral deep cervical block is theoretically possible. In fact, patients with known neurological disorders and especially those with unilateral diaphragmatic paralysis should be approached with caution and offered only general anesthesia. The true incidence, however, of respiratory arrest due to bilateral phrenic nerve paralysis from bilateral deep cervical block is extremely rare. Vast majority of phrenic nerve blocks are asymptomatic since many patients have adequate tidal volumes from their intercostal muscles. The senior author has not seen this complication during more than 10 years of practice.

Our anesthetic agents of choice are 30 mL of 0.5% lidocaine and 30 mL of 0.25% bupivacaine drawn into a 60 mL syringe, producing a 50:50 solution. A small gauge (i.e., 22G) needle is used to inject approximately 8–10 mL of the local anesthetic at each injection site. Any remaining solution is passed to the sterile field for possible intraoperative use to augment the block.

7.4.2 Superficial Block

The purpose of the superficial cervical block is to anesthetize the superficial cervical plexus nerves as they emerge deep to the sternocleidomastoid muscle (SCM).

A midway point between the mastoid process and the clavicular head along the anterior border of the SCM is identified. This area is then cleaned with an antiseptic solution. The local anesthetic is then injected in a subplatysmal plane along the anterior border of the SCM, 3–4 cm above and below the needle insertion site. Prior to injection, aspiration is performed to prevent intravascular injection. This technique will adequately anesthetize ipsilateral platysma and strap muscles.

It is also our standard practice to augment the superficial cervical plexus block by a subcutaneous injection of 5–10 mL of the local anesthetic at the proposed incision site. This adjunct blocks the complex sensory innervation of the anterior neck which is supplied by nerves originating from both sides of the neck.

7.4.3 Deep Block

The purpose of the deep cervical blockade is to anesthetize the deep cervical plexus fibers as they emerge near the transverse process of the C2–C4 cervical vertebrae.

The mastoid process is palpated and a point 2 cm (approximately two finger breadths) caudal along the cervical spine selected. This area corresponds to the C2 cervical vertebrae, while C3 and C4 are located approximately 4 and 6 cm, respectively, caudally along the bony cervical spine. The needle is carefully inserted perpendicular to the skin, aiming at the transverse process until bone contact is felt. This occurs in most patients at a depth of 1–2 cm. If the needle is advanced past 2 cm without bone contact, it should be withdrawn, insertion site identified again, and the needle reinserted under a slightly different angle. After bone contact is made, the needle is withdrawn 1–2 mm and aspirated to rule out intravascular injection. Next, 8–10 mL of the solution is slowly injected and the needle withdrawn. This process is then repeated approximately 2 cm caudal along the bony cervical spine, at the level of C3 transverse process. This technique provides excellent deep cervical blockade and minimized the potential for brachial plexus injury that can occur during lower (5–7 cm caudal to mastoid process) injection.

7.5 Surgical Technique Adjuncts

Standard surgical technique should not be altered regardless of which type of anesthesia is used. Certain consideration pertaining to thyroid surgery under local anesthesia, however, must be kept in mind during these procedures. Because the patient is not under general anesthesia, he or she may move suddenly. This will cause a shift in the surgical field which may have significant consequences if it occurs during a critical junction of the dissection (i.e., RLN or EBSLN dissection, carotid artery or jugular vein mobilization, etc.). The surgeon must be aware of this possibility and be extra vigilant during these crucial portions of the procedure.

In addition, mobilization of the upper pole of the thyroid gland under local anesthesia is sometimes challenging. This area has innervation from the cranial nerves and is not adequately blocked by the deep cervical block. A previously comfortable, cooperative patient may suddenly move due to significant ear and jaw pain during this dissection. He or she may require additional intravenous sedation or an injection of the local anesthetic directly into the upper pole and/or the surrounding strap muscles. Our usual practice is to warn the anesthesia team of a possible need for increased sedation prior to upper pole mobilization. In addition, we routinely place the incision slightly higher to facilitate upper pole mobilization and decrease patient discomfort.

An anesthesiologist must be continually present during the case since patients' response to sedative medication varies substantially. The respiratory drive may be suppressed even after a small dose and protective airway reflexes may be significantly diminished. Frequently, maneuvers such as head tilt/chin lift and jaw thrust are required during surgery even with minimally sedated patients or those with sleep apnea or obesity. An ether screen is essential in these situations since it allows the anesthesiologist easy, quick, and safe access to the airway. In addition, the surgical drapes are kept off the patients' face during the surgery, decreasing the sense of claustrophobia and discomfort for the semi-awake patient. This arrangement also decreases oxygen trapping under the surgical drapes, thus minimizing the fire hazard.

The level of sedation must be carefully monitored and titrated by an experienced anesthesiologist. Oversedation will lead to hypoventilation, airway obstruction, and a disinhibited, noncooperative patient. This will make the operation unsafe and may require conversion to a general anesthesia with endotracheal intubation.

Nerve monitoring of the external branch of the superior laryngeal nerve is another possible and rather simple adjunct that can be used during regional blockade. As described by Lifante and colleagues, this technique involves percutaneous placement of electrodes into right and left cricothyroid muscle and using nerve monitoring probe to stimulate the nerve or the cricothyroid muscle. The authors showed improvement in nerve visualization and subjective voice-quality outcomes with this technique.

7.6 Patient Selection

To ensure safe surgery, satisfied patient, and good outcomes, careful patient selection is crucial. Absolute contraindications for thyroid surgery under cervical plexus blockade include patient refusal to regional anesthesia, true allergy to local anesthetic, and communication barriers such as mental retardation, dementia, or language barrier. Extensive or complicated surgery (i.e., cervical lymphadenectomy, preoperative surgical field, potential for sternotomy, large goiters) and presence of locally invasive cancer should also preclude the use of regional anesthesia. Local anesthetic agents such as lidocaine and bupivacaine lower the seizure threshold and increase the chance of a perioperative seizure. Therefore, patients with a history of a seizure disorder must be advised to undergo surgery under general anesthesia rather than regional blockade.

Certain patient-specific factors must be kept in mind when selecting the appropriate anesthetic option. Obesity, while not prohibitive, does increase the complexity of regional blockade anesthesia. Surface landmarks are often obscured, and studies have shown that patients with a body mass index (BMI) greater than or equal to 30 kg/m^2 are 1.62 times more likely to have a failed block. In addition, obesity is associated with sleep apnea, more rapid oxygen desaturation due to reduced functional residual capacity, difficult intubations, and airway obstruction. Despite these challenges, an experienced anesthesiologist/surgeon team can safely administer regional anesthesia, and the obese population should not be excluded from this anesthetic option.

The elderly patient also presents certain unique physiological challenges. Age-related changes in systemic absorption, distribution, and clearance of a local anesthetic cause an increased sensitivity, decreased dose requirements, and a change in onset and duration of action. Due to these physiologic changes, the senior author found elderly patients to be most amenable to this approach, with decreased drug requirements, increased tolerance, and easier regional block administration.

Systemic anticoagulation must be reversed prior to administration of cervical regional blockade. Oral anticoagulants such as aspirin, warfarin, clopidogrel, and others must be discontinued prior to surgery.

7.7 Complications

True rate of complications during regional anesthesia is very difficult to assess. The low incidence of complications makes almost any study underpowered and the data difficult to extrapolate and apply to clinical practice. In addition, most of the large studies are retrospective reviews or voluntary reports, which are inherently wrought with flaws. Despite these facts, regional anesthesia is considered safe, with a very low incidence of significant injuries. A large French study

Table 7.1 Regional block complications

Complication		Solution
Local	Bleeding	• Use small needle (22G)
		• Do not advance needle past 2 cm during deep block
		• Compress all vascular punctures for >20 s
		• Assure normal coagulation preoperatively
	Infection	• Use aseptic technique
	Nerve injury/neurotrauma	• Know your anatomy and surface landmarks
		• Monitor for paresthesia
Systemic	Allergy	• Switch to different anesthetic class
	Drug toxicity	• Avoid intravascular injection
		– Aspirate plunger prior to every injection
		– Slow injection
		• Respiratory and cardiovascular support
		• Benzodiazepines and/or muscle relaxants for tonic-clonic muscle activity
		• Intravenous fat emulsion (Intralipid®) for refractory cases
		– 1 mL/kg bolus of 20% solution followed by 0.25 m/kg infusion with a repeat bolus if necessary (maximum total dose = 8 mL/kg)

of almost 160,000 regional blocks demonstrated a major complication rate of 3.5/10,000 procedures and a four deaths.

Regional block complications can be broadly separated into two categories: local and systemic (Table 7.1). Local complications during cervical regional block include bleeding, infection, nerve injury, and neurotrauma. The risk of bleeding is very low in cervical regional anesthesia. This risk can be minimized further by using a small gauge needle, not advancing the needle past 2 cm deep during deep cervical blockade, compressing any vascular punctures, and assuring normal coagulation profile prior to surgery. The risk of infection during a "single-shot" peripheral block using aseptic technique is extremely rare.

All local anesthetic agents are inherently neurotoxic, and permanent nerve damage is possible if the dose/concentration is high enough. The risk however is low, and permanent or temporary injury caused by the local anesthetic is very uncommon. Neurotrauma due to needle injury or intraneural injection is another potential cause of nerve injury during regional blockade. While recent studies have shown that intraneural injection or nerve impalement can occur without producing significant neural injury, this practice should obviously be avoided. Iatrogenic injury is possible as well. Thyroid gland injection producing local hematoma formation, vagus nerve involvement leading to temporary recurrent laryngeal nerve paralysis, or intravascular injection into the thyroid or jugular vein or the carotid artery causing systemic effects has been reported. Careful attention to detail, knowledge of surface landmarks and cervical anatomy, and good technique will minimize most of the above risks.

Systemic complications include (a) allergic reaction to the local anesthetic and (b) drug toxicity. True allergic reaction to local anesthetic agents is extremely low and is usually a normal side effect from intravascular injection, epinephrine-associated tachyarrhythmias, vasovagal reactions, etc. A switch between anesthetic classes (amide to ester, or vice versa) is usually sufficient to eliminate this problem.

Drug toxicity usually manifests as central nervous system (CNS) and cardiovascular (CV) toxicity (Table 7.2). These are the two most common and most serious systemic complications and are almost always due to an inadvertent intravascular injection. CNS and CV toxicity is dependent on the local agent plasma concentration, which varies linearly with the dose: doubling of the dose leads to a doubling of the peak plasma concentration. When the plasma levels rise slowly, CNS toxicity usually progresses through a well-described sequence of symptoms. Tinnitus, tongue numbness, muscular twitching, and lightheadedness are followed by seizures, coma, respiratory arrest, and eventually cardiovascular collapse. These stages may be "skipped," however, during a rapid rise in plasma levels (i.e., intravascular injection), and

Table 7.2 Central nervous system and cardiovascular drug toxicity following cervical regional anesthesia

Central nervous system (CNS) toxicity	Early signs
	• Metallic taste
	• Tongue numbness
	• Dizziness
	CNS excitability
	• Restlessness
	• Agitation
	CNS depression
	• Slurred speech
	• Drowsiness
	Respiratory arrest
	Coma
	Seizure
Cardiovascular (CV) toxicity	Sympathetic discharge
	• Hypertension
	• Tachycardia
	Moderate myocardial depression
	• Decreased cardiac output
	• Moderate hypertension
	Severe myocardial depression
	• Profound hypotension
	• Myocardial conduction abnormalities
	• Dysrhythmias (ventricular fibrillation and/or pulseless electrical activity)

Note: Symptoms of local anesthetic systemic toxicity often do not progress in the order described above. Patient may manifest any combination of symptoms in almost any order. Sound clinical judgment, high index of suspicion, and prompt intervention are essential

seizures may be the first manifestation of CNS toxicity. All local anesthetic agents have the same propensity for causing seizures.

Cardiovascular toxicity can usually be achieved only during an intravascular injection. The plasma levels needed to produce cardiac symptoms are approximately three times higher than the minimal level necessary to achieve CNS toxicity. Cardiac toxicity manifests initially as sympathetic discharge (i.e., hypertension with tachycardia), followed by myocardial depression with a decreased cardiac output and moderate hypertension, and eventually progresses to profound hypotension, myocardial conduction abnormalities, and dysrhythmias such as ventricular fibrillation and/or pulseless electrical activity (PEA).

Prevention is the best treatment for systemic local anesthetic toxicity. Because most events are due to accidental intravascular injection, every effort must be made to avoid this event by aspiration prior to local injection. Using small doses of the local anesthetic and injecting slowly are also good ways to minimize systemic toxicity from accidental intravascular injection. Treatment of CNS toxicity centers on supportive measures of airway managements and cardiovascular support until plasma levels fall below toxic levels. As with most seizures, tonic-clonic muscle activity can be controlled with sedatives, such as benzodiazepines, or muscle relaxants, such as succinylcholine. Cardiovascular depression must be treated promptly and ACLS protocol initiated as necessary. Intralipid®, a fat emulsion used in total parenteral nutrition (TPN), has been described as an effective treatment of local anesthetic-induced cardiovascular depression refractory to other treatments. Recommended dose is 1 mL/kg bolus of 20% intralipid solution followed by 0.25 mL/kg infusion with a repeat bolus if necessary, and a maximum total dose of 8 mL/kg.

7.8 Summary

Regional cervical blockade is a safe and effective anesthetic choice for thyroid surgery. Careful patient selection, a thorough knowledge of cervical anatomy, ability to troubleshoot possible complications, and good surgical technique will produce excellent surgical results and high level of patient satisfaction.

Bibliography

Arora N, Dhar P et al (2006) Seminars: local and regional anesthesia for thyroid surgery. J Surg Oncol 94(8):708–713

Auroy Y, Benhamou D et al (2002) Major complications of regional anesthesia in France: the SOS Regional Anesthesia Hotline Service. Anesthesiology 97(5):1274–1280

Bigeleisen PE (2006) Nerve puncture and apparent intraneural injection during ultrasound-guided axillary block does not invariably result in neurologic injury. Anesthesiology 105(4): 779–783

Chassard D, Berrada K et al (1996) Alkalinization of local anesthetics: theoretically justified but clinically useless. Can J Anaesth 43(4):384–393

Dunhill TP (1912) A discussion on partial thyroidectomy under local anaesthesia, with special reference to exophthalmic goitre: an address introductory to a discussion on the subject. Proc R Soc Med 5(Surg Sect):61–69

Finucane BT, SpringerLink (Online service) (2007) Complications of regional anesthesia. Springer Science+Business Media, LLC, New York

Hadzic A, New York School of Regional Anesthesia (2007) Textbook of regional anesthesia and acute pain management. McGraw-Hill, Medical Pub. Division, New York

Hisham AN, Aina EN (2002) A reappraisal of thyroid surgery under local anaesthesia: back to the future? ANZ J Surg 72(4):287–289

Inabnet WB, Shifrin A et al (2008) Safety of same day discharge in patients undergoing sutureless thyroidectomy: a comparison of local and general anesthesia. Thyroid 18(1):57–61

Lifante JC, McGill J et al (2009) A prospective, randomized trial of nerve monitoring of the external branch of the superior laryngeal nerve during thyroidectomy under local/regional anesthesia and IV sedation. Surgery 146(6):1167–1173

Litz RJ, Popp M et al (2006) Successful resuscitation of a patient with ropivacaine-induced asystole after axillary plexus block using lipid infusion. Anaesthesia 61(8):800–801

Mulroy MF (2009) A practical approach to regional anesthesia. Wolters Kluwer/Lippincott Williams & Wilkins, Philadelphia

Nielsen KC, Guller U et al (2005) Influence of obesity on surgical regional anesthesia in the ambulatory setting: an analysis of 9,038 blocks. Anesthesiology 102(1):181–187

Rosenblatt MA, Abel M et al (2006) Successful use of a 20% lipid emulsion to resuscitate a patient after a presumed bupivacaine-related cardiac arrest. Anesthesiology 105(1):217–218

Snyder SK, Roberson CR et al (2006) Local anesthesia with monitored anesthesia care vs general anesthesia in thyroidectomy: a randomized study. Arch Surg 141(2):167–173

Spanknebel K, Chabot JA et al (2005) Thyroidectomy using local anesthesia: a report of 1,025 cases over 16 years. J Am Coll Surg 201(3):375–385

Stevens RA, Chester WL et al (1989) The effect of pH adjustment of 0.5% bupivacaine on the latency of epidural anesthesia. Reg Anesth 14(5):236–239

Weinberg G (2006) Lipid infusion resuscitation for local anesthetic toxicity: proof of clinical efficacy. Anesthesiology 105(1):7–8

Weinberg G, Ripper R et al (2003) Lipid emulsion infusion rescues dogs from bupivacaine-induced cardiac toxicity. Reg Anesth Pain Med 28(3):198–202

Endoscopic Thyroidectomy in the Neck

Konstantinos P. Economopoulos and Dimitrios Linos

8.1 Introduction

The first endoscopic operation in the neck was described for the surgery of the parathyroids by Gagner (1996), 15 years after the other surgical specialties discovered the advantages of endoscopic techniques in natural cavities. The first complete endoscopic thyroidectomy was performed 1 year later by Huscher and coworkers in Italy (Huscher et al. 1997). The relative delay in the inception of endoscopic procedures on the neck could be explained by the narrow operative field and numerous vital structures of this anatomical region, as well as the fact that there were no easily accepted benefits compared to the traditional approach except the potential better esthetics from the small incisions.

Henry et al. defined endoscopic thyroidectomy as "a surgical technique in which dissection of the thyroid gland is entirely performed with the help of an endoscope, in a closed area maintained by insufflation or mechanical retraction" (Slotema et al. 2008; Henry and Sebag 2006). Therefore, endoscopic thyroidectomy techniques do not include semi-open procedures or partially endoscopic procedures like the well-known video-assisted thyroidectomy developed by Miccoli (Miccoli et al. 1999) and Bellantone (Bellantone et al. 1999). In addition, endoscopic thyroidectomy techniques can be subdivided into cervical and extracervical approaches. The aim of this chapter is to present the existing cervical endoscopic techniques and discuss the advantages and disadvantages of their implementation.

8.2 Anterior Cervical Approach

Three nonrandomized studies have been published describing anterior cervical approach of endoscopic thyroidectomy (Table 8.1). Gagner et al. (2003) compared the results of 18 cases with solitary nodules treated by the anterior cervical approach with 18 consecutive conventional thyroidectomies. Feasibility and safety were confirmed, cosmetic results were superior for endoscopic thyroidectomy, and convalescence was reduced compared with conventional approach. In Gagner's technique, the main incision is in the midline just above the sternal notch through which the 5-mm trocar for the endoscope is placed. An additional 5-mm trocar is inserted at the superior medial border of the sternocleidomastoid muscle and two 2-mm trocars are also used as shown in the Fig. 8.1. The final specimen is extracted in a plastic bag from the 5-mm incision at superior medial border of the sternocleidomastoid muscle. Identification and dissection of all vital structures is done by the use of the Ultracision (Ethicon Endosurgery Cincinnati, OH, USA).

K.P. Economopoulos, M.D., Ph.D. (✉)
Department of Surgery, Massachusetts General Hospital, Harvard Medical School, 2 Hawthorne Place, Unit 6G, Boston, MA 02114, USA
e-mail: economopoulos@gmail.com

D. Linos, M.D., Ph.D.
Professor of Surgery, St. George's University of London Medical School at the University of Nicosia, Nicosia, Cyprus

Department of Surgery, Hygeia Hospital,
7 Fragoklisias St., Marousi, Athens 15125, Greece
e-mail: dlinos@hms.harvard.edu

Table 8.1 Patient characteristics and operative details of published studies

First author (reference)	Country	Surgical approach	Number of patients (male/female)	Mean age (range) (years)	Mean nodule diameter (range) (mm)	Mean operating time (range) (min)	Conversion rate (%)	Complications
Gagner (Gagner et al. 2003)	USA	Anterior cervical	18 (2/16)	43 (17–66)	27 (6–70)	220 (120–330)	2/18 (11.1)	3 hypercarbia, 1 parathyroidectomy
Cougard (Cougard et al. 2005)	France	Anterior cervical	40 (4/36)	46	24	89	8/24 (33.3), 0/16 (0)[a]	0
Yeung (Yeung and Wong 2003)	Hong Kong	Anterior cervical	18	42 (28–72)	25 (12–38)	185 (105–330)	4/18 (22.2)	0
Henry and Palazzo and Sebag (Henry and Sebag 2006; Palazzo et al. 2006; Sebag et al. 2006)	France	Lateral cervical	38 (5/33)	45 (20–69)	22 (7–47)	99 (64–150)	2/38 (5.2)	0
Inabnet (Inabnet et al. 2003)	USA	Lateral cervical	38	–	25 (6–70)	190 (105–330)	3/38 (7.9)	1 permanent laryngeal nerve palsy
Slotema (Slotema et al. 2008)	France	Lateral cervical	112	–	–	98 (46–190)	10/112 (8.9)	1 permanent laryngeal nerve palsy, 1 hematoma

[a]Without and with the use of ultracision

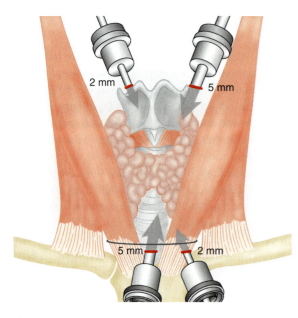

Fig. 8.1 The Gagner anterior endoscopic approach

A slightly different approach was proposed by (Cougard et al. 2005) in 40 patients using a 15-mm middle incision above the suprasternal notch, one 3-mm trocar on the side of the lesion, and one 5-mm trocar at the opposite side (Fig. 8.2). A Veress needle is added in the upper midline whenever it was necessary to improve the working space. The final specimen was extracted through the median incision. Feasibility and safety of this approach were confirmed, and conversion rate was reduced with the use of ultrasonic shears (Cougard et al. 2005).

Finally, Yeung et al. (Yeung 1998; Yeung and Wong 2003) presented the results from 18 patients who underwent endoscopic thyroidectomy by the anterior cervical approach using the same anatomical landmarks with Cougard's technique. However, the conversion rate to classical cervicotomy was the highest reported in the literature for the anterior cervical approach.

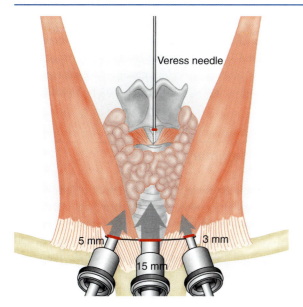

Fig. 8.2 The Cougard anterior endoscopic approach

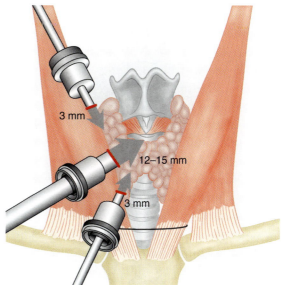

Fig. 8.3 The Henry lateral endoscopic approach

8.3 Lateral Cervical Approach

Five nonrandomized studies have been published describing lateral cervical approach of endoscopic thyroidectomy (Table 8.1); four of them are from the same institution (Henry and Sebag 2006; Palazzo et al. 2006; Sebag et al. 2006). Henry and colleagues developed an endoscopic thyroidectomy based on the same approach and principles of the successful endoscopic parathyroidectomy performed in their institution (Henry and Sebag 2006). This "back door" approach to the thyroid lobe places three trocars on the anterior border of the sternocleidomastoid muscle on the side of the lesion. A 12- to 15-mm skin crease incision at the level of the isthmus is used for the insertion of the endoscope, and two 3-mm trocars are then placed 4 cm below and 6 cm above the main optic trocar incision (Fig. 8.3). The indications of this lateral endoscopic technique are: (1) a solitary thyroid nodule smaller than 3 cm in diameter, (2) small toxic nodules, and (3) small follicular lesions of undetermined cytology. Main contraindications are previous neck surgery and neck irradiation. Conversion rate to open thyroidectomy and mean operating time were better to those reported after anterior endoscopic thyroidectomy procedures (Table 8.1). They have reported 38 initial endoscopic thyroidectomies with no recurrent laryngeal nerve injury and two conversions to open thyroidectomy (Palazzo et al. 2006) and an additional 112 cases with one recurrent laryngeal nerve palsy. Their mean operative time was 98 min (Slotema et al. 2008).

Inabnet and colleagues (Inabnet et al. 2003) have applied a slightly different lateral endoscopic approach in 38 patients. Early in their experience, a totally endoscopic approach was performed. After the initial 10- to 15-mm superolateral incision, a working space was created by CO_2 insufflation. Later, this technique was modified to allow identification and ligation of the superior thyroid vessels directly through their initial incision. Three additional trocars (two 3 mm and one 5 mm) were used (Fig. 8.4). Of the 38 cases, 35 were completed endoscopically. They report one permanent recurrent laryngeal nerve palsy most likely due to collateral energy from the ultrasonic scalpel (Inabnet et al. 2003).

8.4 Commentary

It appears that endoscopic thyroidectomy in the neck has been substituted by semi-open, partially endoscopic or extracervical surgical techniques since there is no

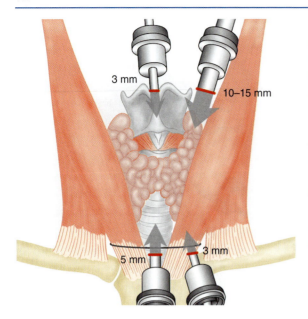

Fig. 8.4 The Inabnet lateral endoscopic approach

report published after 2008. These "historical" techniques maintained the surgical working space by using gas inflation techniques. However, the insufflation of CO_2 in the neck was related with several complications to the initial patients including massive subcutaneous emphysema (Gottlieb et al. 1997), arterial and venous injuries, pneumomediastinum, and gas embolism (Muenscher et al. 2011). In addition, special training and special equipment were needed both for anterior and lateral endoscopic approaches in the neck (Muenscher et al. 2011).

The main indications for endoscopic thyroidectomy using a cervical access were restricted to solitary nodules smaller than 3 cm in diameter and to thyroid lobes up to 20 mL in volume (Cougard et al. 2005; Gagner et al. 2003; Henry and Sebag 2006; Inabnet et al. 2003; Palazzo et al. 2006; Sebag et al. 2006; Slotema et al. 2008; Yeung and Wong 2003). Contraindications include the large goiters, previous neck surgery, neck irradiation, and invasive malignant tumors (Slotema et al. 2008). Given that benign nodules, which are less than 3 cm, do not necessarily require surgical excision, only small toxic adenomas and follicular nodules were eligible for endoscopic cervical thyroidectomy (Slotema et al. 2008).

The operative time ranged from 64 to 330 min, and the conversion rate ranged from 5.2 % to 33.3 %. Higher conversion rates were noticed with the anterior cervical endoscopic approaches, while complications were limited after both anterior and lateral endoscopic procedures (Table 8.1). Reasons of conversion to classical thyroidectomy were histological diagnosis of malignancy, hemorrhage, large lesions, concurrent thyroiditis, injuries of adjacent anatomical structures, and difficulty in dissection (Slotema et al. 2008).

8.5 Summary

Endoscopic thyroidectomy in the neck is feasible and safe for solitary nodules smaller than 3 cm in diameter and thyroid lobes up to 20 mL in volume. It is characterized by higher cost, longer operative time, and severe limitations in the extent of thyroidectomy and surgical indications.

Although minimally invasive thyroidectomy started as a "closed" purely endoscopic thyroidectomy with incisions in the neck, today, these techniques are not widely practiced. They are mentioned though for their historical interest and potential lessons for other similar future endoscopic attempts.

References

Bellantone R, Lombardi CP, Raffaelli M et al (1999) Minimally invasive, totally gasless video-assisted thyroid lobectomy. Am J Surg 177(4):342–343

Cougard P, Osmak L, Esquis P et al (2005) Endoscopic thyroidectomy. A preliminary report including 40 patients. Ann Chir 130(2):81–85

Gagner M (1996) Endoscopic subtotal parathyroidectomy in patients with primary hyperparathyroidism. Br J Surg 83(6):875

Gagner M, Inabnet BW 3rd, Biertho L (2003) Endoscopic thyroidectomy for solitary nodules. Ann Chir 128(10):696–701

Gottlieb A, Sprung J, Zheng XM et al (1997) Massive subcutaneous emphysema and severe hypercarbia in a patient during endoscopic transcervical parathyroidectomy using carbon dioxide insufflation. Anesth Analg 84(5):1154–1156

Henry JF, Sebag F (2006) Lateral endoscopic approach for thyroid and parathyroid surgery. Ann Chir 131(1):51–56

Huscher CS, Chiodini S, Napolitano C et al (1997) Endoscopic right thyroid lobectomy. Surg Endosc 11(8):877

Inabnet WB 3rd, Jacob BP, Gagner M (2003) Minimally invasive endoscopic thyroidectomy by a cervical approach. Surg Endosc 17(11):1808–1811

Miccoli P, Berti P, Conte M et al (1999) Minimally invasive surgery for thyroid small nodules: preliminary report. J Endocrinol Invest 22(11):849–851

Muenscher A, Dalchow C, Kutta H et al (2011) The endoscopic approach to the neck: a review of the literature, and overview of the various techniques. Surg Endosc 25(5):1358–1363

Palazzo FF, Sebag F, Henry JF (2006) Endocrine surgical technique: endoscopic thyroidectomy via the lateral approach. Surg Endosc 20(2):339–342

Sebag F, Palazzo FF, Harding J et al (2006) Endoscopic lateral approach thyroid lobectomy: safe evolution from endoscopic parathyroidectomy. World J Surg 30(5):802–805

Slotema ET, Sebag F, Henry JF (2008) What is the evidence for endoscopic thyroidectomy in the management of benign thyroid disease? World J Surg 32(7):1325–1332

Yeung GH (1998) Endoscopic surgery of the neck: a new frontier. Surg Laparosc Endosc 8(3):227–232

Yeung GH, Wong HW (2003) Videoscopic thyroidectomy: the uncertain path to practicality. Asian J Surg 26(3):133–138

Minimally Invasive Video-Assisted Thyroidectomy

9

Paolo Miccoli and Gabriele Materazzi

9.1 Introduction

The first endoscopic procedures proposed to reduce the invasiveness of surgery in the neck were the endoscopic and video-assisted parathyroidectomies because it was quite evident that parathyroid adenomas were ideal candidates for a minimal access surgery, being these tumors mostly benign and characterized by their limited size. Later on, the same accesses proved to be suitable also for removing small thyroid nodules, and new approaches were soon proposed, in some cases, also modifying the old ones. At present, some controversies still exist about what should be considered a real minimally invasive operation for thyroid. Although the concern raised by some about the possible adverse effect of CO_2 insufflation in the neck was probably over evaluated, the procedure we set up in 1998, minimally invasive video-assisted thyroidectomy (MIVAT), was characterized by the use of an external retraction avoiding any gas inflation which is not necessary to create an adequate operative space in the neck. This approach to the thyroid has been used in our Department of Surgery for the last 8 years on more than 2,500 patients with results that can successfully rival those of standard open surgery also in terms of operative time. Of course, this is not an operation which might be proposed for any patient: its main limit is represented by the necessity of a severe selection of the patients undergoing surgery. Only 10–30% of the cases, according to different authors, fulfill the inclusion criteria for a MIVAT.

9.2 Preoperative Evaluation and Anesthesia

The most relevant limit is represented by the size of both the nodule and the gland as measured by means of an accurate ultrasonographic study to be performed preoperatively. In endemic goiter countries, indeed, the gland volume can be relevant independently from the nodule volume, and this aspect might be responsible for the necessity of converting the procedure. Ultrasonography can also be useful to exclude the presence of a thyroiditis, which might make the dissection troublesome. In case ultrasonography only gives the suspicion of thyroiditis, of course, autoantibodies should be measured in the serum. In any case when a correct diagnosis is performed preoperatively, thyroiditis must be considered a contraindication.

One of the most controversial aspects in terms of indications is the opportunity of treating malignancies. No doubt "low risk" papillary carcinomas constitute an ideal indication for MIVAT, but a good selection has to take into account the exact profile of possible lymph node involvement in the neck. In fact, although the completeness of a total thyroidectomy achievable with video-assisted procedures is beyond debate, the greatest caution should be taken when approaching a disease involving either metastatic lymph nodes or an extracapsular invasion of the gland. In these cases, an

P. Miccoli, M.D., Ph.D., FACS (✉)
Dipartimento di Chirurgia,
Ed 30E, Via Paradisa 2, Pisa 56100, Italia
e-mail: p.miccoli@med.unipi.it

G. Materazzi, M.D.
Department of Surgery, University of Pisa,
Ed 30E 2nd floor, Via Paradisa 2, Pisa 5600, Italy
e-mail: gmaterazzi@yahoo.com

endoscopic approach might be inadequate to obtain a full clearance of the nodes or the complete removal of the neoplastic tissue (infiltration of the trachea or the esophagus). Again, an accurate echographic study is of paramount importance in order to select the right cases undergoing video-assisted surgery.

The operation is generally performed with patient under general anesthesia, but also local anesthesia (deep bilateral cervical block) can be used.

All patients should be rendered euthyroid before surgery. Preoperative preparation of patients with thyrotoxicosis is particularly critical to avoid operative or postoperative thyroid storm. The planned procedure should be discussed with the patient and informed consent must be obtained, particularly focusing on the convenience of converting to open, traditional cervicotomy, in case of locally advanced cancer, difficult endoscopic dissection due to thyroiditis, and intraoperative bleeding.

Routine preoperative laryngoscopy is strongly recommended in all patients undergoing thyroid surgery in order to identify preoperatively asymptomatic vocal cord hypomotility or palsy.

9.3 Surgical Technique

9.3.1 Operating Room Setup

9.3.1.1 Patient
- Supine position without neck hyperextension
- Conventional neck preparation and draping
- A sterile drape covering the skin

9.3.1.2 Team (Fig. 9.1)
- The surgeon is on the right side of the table.
- The first assistant is on the left side of the table (opposite the surgeon).
- The second assistant is at the head of the table.
- The third assistant is on the left side of the table.
- The scrub nurse is behind the surgeon on the right side of the table.

9.3.1.3 Instrumentation (Fig. 9.2)
9.3.1.4 MIVAT Kit
1. Forward-oblique telescope: 30°, diameter 5 mm, length 30 cm
2. Suction dissector: with cutoff hole, with stylet, blunt, length 21 cm
3. Ear forceps: very thin, serrated, working length 12.5 cm
4. Conventional tissue retractor: army/navy type
5. Small tissue retractor: double-ended, length 12 cm
6. Clip applier for vascular clips
7. Straight scissors: length 12.5 cm
   - Ultrasound generator
   - Single screen (double screen can be useful but is not mandatory)
   - Electrocautery (monopolar)

9.3.2 Operative Technique

9.3.2.1 Preparation of the Operative Space
The patient is positioned in supine position with his neck not extended. Hyperextension must be avoided because it would reduce the operative space (Fig. 9.3). The skin is protected by means of a sterile film (Tegaderm®). A 1.5-cm horizontal skin incision is performed 2 cm above the sternal notch in the central cervical area. Subcutaneous fat and platysma are carefully dissected so as to avoid any minimum bleeding. During this step, the surgeon should use the electrocautery with its blade protected with a thin film of sterile drape, leaving just the tip able to coagulate in order to avoid damage to the skin or the superficial planes. Two small retractors are used to expose the midline which has to be incised for 2–3 cm on an absolutely bloodless plane (Figs. 9.4 and 9.5).

The blunt dissection of the thyroid lobe from the strap muscles is completely carried out through the skin incision by gentle retraction and using tiny spatulas. When the thyroid lobe is almost completely dissected from the strap muscles, larger and deeper retractors (army/navy type) can be inserted, and they will maintain the operative space during all the endoscopic part of the procedure (Figs. 9.6 and 9.7). Then, a 30° 5- or 7-mm endoscope is introduced through the skin incision: from this moment on, the procedure is entirely endoscopic until the extraction of the lobe of the gland. Preparation of the thyrotracheal groove is completed under endoscopic vision by using small (2 mm in diameter) instruments like spatulas, forceps, spatula sucker, or scissors.

9.3.2.2 Ligature of the Main Thyroid Vessels
Avoiding the electrocautery (neither bipolar nor monopolar) is particularly important at this point in

9 Minimally Invasive Video-Assisted Thyroidectomy

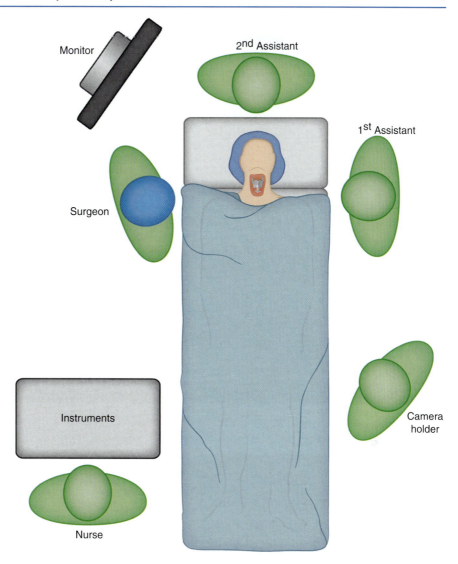

Fig. 9.1 Operating room setup, team

time when both laryngeal nerves are not yet exposed. Harmonic® device is utilized for almost all the vascular structures, but if the vessel to be coagulated is running particularly close to the inferior laryngeal nerve, then hemostasis is achieved by means of small vascular clips applied by a disposable or reusable clip applier.

The first vessel to be ligated is the middle vein, when present, or the small veins between jugular vein and thyroid capsule. This step allows a better preparation of the thyrotracheal groove where the recurrent nerve will be later searched.

During this step, the endoscope has to be held inside the camera with the 30° tip looking downward and in an orthogonal axis with the thyroid lobe and trachea.

A further step is represented by the exposure of the upper pedicle, which must be carefully prepared, until an optimal visualization of the different branches is achieved. During this step, the endoscope should be rotated of 180° with the 30° tip looking upward and held in a parallel direction with the thyroid lobe and trachea, in order to better visualize the upper portion of the operative camera where the superior thyroid vein and artery are running.

The upper pedicle is then prepared by retracting downward and medially the thyroid lobe by means of the retractor and the assistant spatula. The correct position of the retractors (both the first one on the strap muscles and the second one on the upper part of the thyroid lobe) is very important during this step in

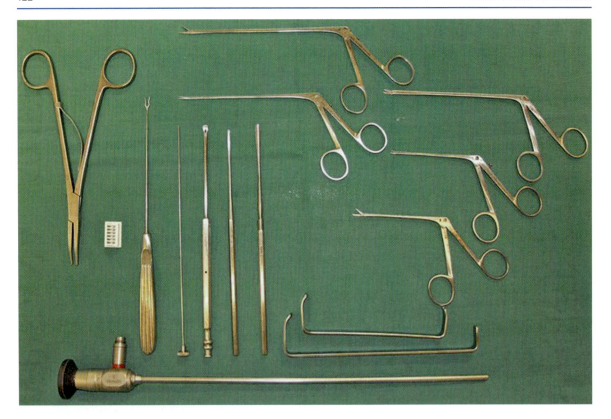

Fig. 9.2 Instrumentation for MIVAT

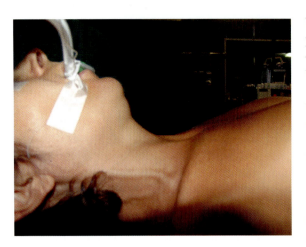

Fig. 9.3 MIVAT position of the patient on the operating table. The neck is not extended

order to obtain the best visualization of the vessels. A further spatula can be used to pull the vessels laterally. This will allow the external branch of the superior laryngeal nerve to be easily identified during most procedures (Fig. 9.8). Its injury can be avoided by keeping the inactive blade of Harmonic® in the posterior position so as to not transmit the heat to this delicate structure. At this point in time, section of the upper pedicle can be obtained by harmonic scalpel "en bloc" or selectively, depending on the diameter of the single vessels and/or the anatomical situation (Figs. 9.9 and 9.10).

9.3.2.3 Inferior Laryngeal Nerve and Parathyroid Glands Identification and Dissection

After retracting medially and lifting up the thyroid lobe, the fascia can be opened by a gentle spatula retraction. During this step, the endoscope should be repositioned in an orthogonal axis with the thyroid lobe and trachea, looking downward with its 30° angle. The recurrent laryngeal nerve appears generally at this point in time, lying in the thyrotracheal groove, posterior to the Zuckerkandl tuberculum (posterior lobe) which constitutes an important landmark in this phase. This way, the recurrent nerve and the parathyroid glands are dissected and freed from the thyroid (Fig. 9.11).

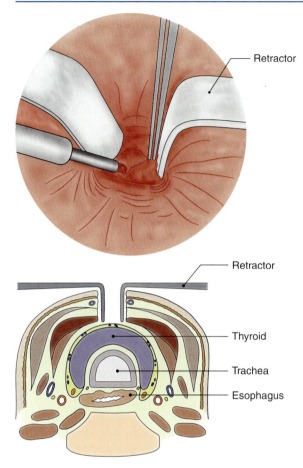

Fig. 9.4 Access to the operative space during MIVAT: after having incised the skin (1.5-cm transversal incision two fingers above the sternal notch), two small retractors open the space. The midline is localized and opened by means of cautery (see also anatomical section schema showing how to put retractors)

Dissection of the entire nerve from the mediastinum to its entrance into the larynx is not mandatory and might result in a time waste during the endoscopic phase. It is correct and very safe to identify the laryngeal nerve, to free it from the thyroid capsule as much as possible, but it is important to stress that the complete dissection of the nerve can be more easily obtained, during the further step, under direct vision, when the thyroid lobe has already been extracted. Also, both parathyroid glands are generally easily visualized during the endoscopic step, thanks to the camera magnification. Their vascular supply is preserved by selective section of the branches of the inferior thyroid artery. During dissection, when dealing with large vessels or small vessels close to the nerve, hemostasis can be achieved by 3-mm titanium vascular clips.

9.3.2.4 Extraction of the Lobe and Resection

At this point in time, the lobe is completely freed. The endoscope and the retractors can be removed, and the upper portion of the gland rotated and pulled out using conventional forceps. A gentle traction over the lobe allows the complete exteriorization of the gland. The operation is now conducted as in open surgery under direct vision. The lobe is freed from the trachea by ligating the small vessels and dissecting the Berry ligament. It is very important to check once again the laryngeal nerve at this point in time, so to avoid its injury before the final step. The isthmus is then dissected from the trachea and divided. After completely exposing the trachea, the lobe is finally removed.

Drainage is not necessary. The midline is then approached by a single stitch; platysma is closed by a subcuticular suture, and a cyanoacrylate sealant is used for the skin.

If total thyroidectomy is the planned operation, the same procedure is to be performed on the opposite side after the first lobe has been removed.

9.4 Postoperative Treatment

After surgery, patients undergoing MIVAT require strict observation during the first 5–10 h on the ward. Dysphonia, airway obstruction, and neck swelling must be carefully checked. No drain is left, so careful surveillance for postoperative hematomas is required during the immediate postoperative period. Postoperative bleeding risk is very low and dramatically decreases after 5 h.

In case of postoperative hematoma, if compressive symptoms and airway obstruction are present, reintervention and immediate hematoma evacuation are strongly required.

Patients can start oral intake since the evening on the operative day and will be discharged the day after. On the first and second postoperative day, serum calcium must be checked in order to control hypoparathyroidism by substitutive therapy, as described in Table 9.1.

Wound care is not really necessary after MIVAT, because of the glue covering the skin and postoperative pain will be controlled by means of both IV or oral analgesics.

Voice impairments and subjective or objective dysphonia require immediate postoperative vocal cord check by and ENT doctor. In case of normal postoperative course, vocal cord check can be delayed after 3 months.

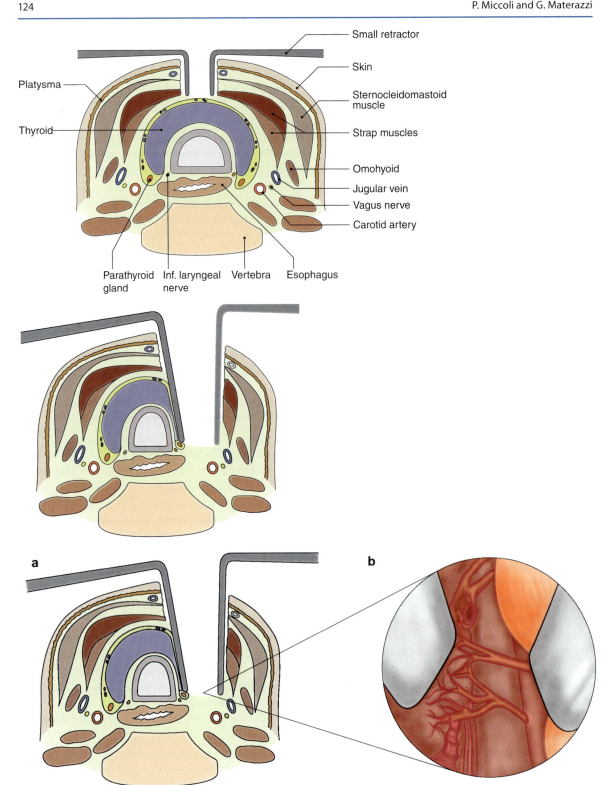

Figs. 9.5, 9.6, and 9.7 Access to the operative space during MIVAT: when the thyroid lobe is almost completely dissected from the strap muscles, larger and deeper retractors (**a**, **b**) (army/navy type) can be inserted, and they will maintain the operative space during all the endoscopic part of the procedure

9 Minimally Invasive Video-Assisted Thyroidectomy

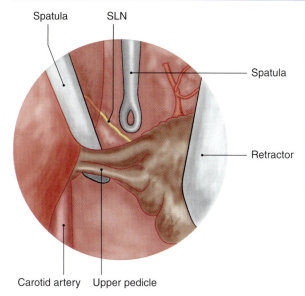

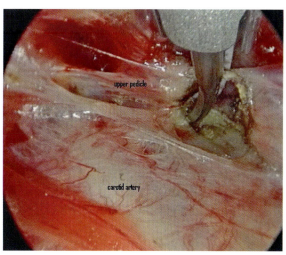

Fig. 9.10 Endoscopic vision: section of the upper pedicle by Harmonic. Carotid artery is well visible and under control

Fig. 9.8 Endoscopic vision. Dissection of the upper pedicle (*right side*) during MIVAT: the upper pedicle is prepared by retracting downward and medially the thyroid lobe by means of the retractor and the assistant spatula. The correct position of the retractors (both the first one on the strap muscles and the second one on the upper part of the thyroid lobe) is very important during this step in order to obtain the best visualization of the vessels. A further spatula can be used to pull the vessels laterally. This will allow the external branch of the superior laryngeal nerve (*SLN*) to be easily identified

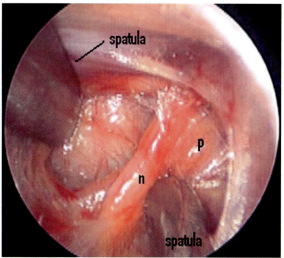

Fig. 9.11 MIVAT endoscopic vision. Dissection of the inferior laryngeal nerve. The recurrent laryngeal nerve (*n*) appears lying in the thyrotracheal groove. Parathyroid gland is also well visible (*p*)

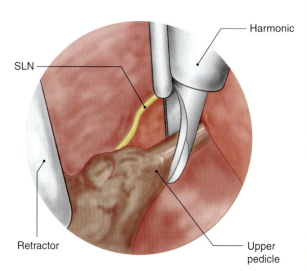

Table 9.1 Management of postoperative hypocalcemia

Management of hypocalcemia following thyroidectomy on the first postoperative day	
Acute symptomatic	Calcium gluconate IV
Asymptomatic calcium ≤7.5[a] mg/dL	Calcium (3 g) + vitamin D (0.5 µg) per os daily
Asymptomatic calcium 7.5–7.9 mg/dL	Calcium (1.5 g) per os daily

[a]Normal range: 8–10 mg/dL

Fig. 9.9 MIVAT endoscopic vision. Section of the upper pedicle (*left side*) during MIVAT: section of the upper pedicle can be obtained by harmonic scalpel "en bloc" or selectively, depending on the diameter of the single vessels and/or the anatomical situation. External branch of the superior laryngeal nerve (*SLN*) injury can be avoided by keeping the inactive blade of Harmonic® in the posterior position so as to not transmit the heat to this delicate structure

Additional Readings

Barczyński M, Konturek A, Cichoń S (2008) Minimally invasive video-assisted thyroidectomy (MIVAT) with and without use of harmonic scalpel – a randomized study. Langenbecks Arch Surg 393(5):647–654

Del Rio P, Berti M, Sommaruga L, Arcuri MF, Cataldo S, Sianesi M (2008) Pain after minimally invasive videoassisted and after minimally invasive open thyroidectomy – results of a prospective outcome study. Langenbecks Arch Surg 393(3): 271–273, Epub 2007 Oct 2

Gourakis G, Sotiropoulos GC, Neuhäuser M, Musholt TJ, Karaliotas C, Lang H (2008) Comparison between minimally invasive video-assisted thyroidectomy and conventional thyroidectomy: is there any evidence-based information? Thyroid 18(7):721–727

Lombardi CP, Raffaelli M, D'alatri L, De Crea C, Marchese MR, Maccora D, Paludetti G, Bellantone R (2008) Video-assisted thyroidectomy significantly reduces the risk of early postthyroidectomy voice and swallowing symptoms. World J Surg 32(5):693–700

Miccoli P, Materazzi G (2004) Minimally invasive video assisted thyroidectomy (MIVAT). Surg Clin North Am 84:735–741

Miccoli P, Elisei R, Materazzi G, Capezzone M, Galleri D, Pacini F, Berti P, Pinchera A (2002) Minimally invasive video assisted thyroidectomy for papillary carcinoma: a prospective study about its completeness. Surgery 132: 1070–1074

Miccoli P, Berti P, Ambrosini CE (2008a) Perspectives and lessons learned after a decade of minimally invasive video-assisted thyroidectomy. ORL J Otorhinolaryngol Relat Spec 70(5):282–286

Miccoli P, Minuto MN, Ugolini C, Pisano R, Fosso A, Berti P (2008b) Minimally invasive video-assisted thyroidectomy for benign thyroid disease: an evidence-based review. World J Surg 32(7):1333–1340, Review

Miccoli P, Pinchera A, Materazzi G, Biagini A, Berti P, Faviana P, Molinaro E, Viola D, Elisei R (2009) Surgical treatment of low- and intermediate-risk papillary thyroid cancer with minimally invasive video-assisted thyroidectomy. J Clin Endocrinol Metab 94(5):1618–1622

Terris DJ, Angelos P, Steward DL, Simental AA (2008) Minimally invasive video-assisted thyroidectomy: a multi-institutional North American experience. Arch Otolaryngol Head Neck Surg 134(1):81–84

Minimally Invasive Video-Assisted Thyroidectomy

10

Pier Francesco Alesina and Martin K. Walz

10.1 Introduction

The minimally invasive video-assisted approach was first described in 1996 for parathyroid (Miccoli et al. 1997) and few years later for thyroid surgery (Bellantone et al. 1999; Miccoli et al. 1999). In the same period following the enthusiastic results of laparoscopic abdominal surgery, a purely endoscopic parathyroidectomy and thyroidectomy with multiple trocars placement and CO_2 insufflation were also performed (Gagner 1996; Huscher et al. 1997). The innovation of the video-assisted technique consisted of a gasless procedure performed through a single 1.5–2 cm central access and use of an endoscope for magnification. Because of its similarity to conventional surgery, this method gained quickly a quite large acceptance (Miccoli et al. 2002). Moreover, the attraction of the mini-incision has been supposed in earlier studies to be coupled with an advantage in terms of postoperative pain and cosmetic result in favour of MIVAT when compared to conventional thyroidectomy (Miccoli et al. 2001; Bellantone et al. 2002). Our experience with MIVAT is based on more than 1,500 procedures performed over more than 10 years experience in a tertiary referral centre for endocrine surgery.

P.F. Alesina, M.D. (✉) • M.K. Walz, M.D.
Clinic for Surgery and Centre of Minimal Invasive Surgery,
Kliniken Essen-Mitte, Academic Hospital
of the University of Duisburg-Essen,
Essen, Germany
e-mail: pieroalesina@yahoo.it; mkwalz@kliniken-essen-mitte.de

10.2 Patients' Selection: Indications for Surgery

The indications for minimally invasive thyroid surgery are summarized in Table 10.1. A careful preoperative evaluation is essential for adequate patients' selection. After clinical examination and thyroid function tests, neck ultrasonography is crucial as the diameter of the main thyroid nodule and the overall thyroid volume are the most relevant selections criteria for MIVAT. Beside a solitary thyroid nodule with uncertain cytology and multinodular goitre, also low-risk papillary thyroid carcinomas without evidence of local invasion and lymph nodes metastases are ideal indications for this procedure as the thyroid volume is normal and therefore suitable for mini-incision and precise endoscopic dissection (Miccoli et al. 2009). Patients with thyroiditis or Graves' disease represent a challenge for the endocrine surgeon because of the difficult dissection and risk of bleeding and therefore should be not considered suitable for MIVAT during the learning period. In experienced hands, the video-assisted approach has been demonstrated to be feasible and safe even in cases of Graves' disease (Alesina et al. 2011). During the last years, we extended the indication for video-assisted thyroidectomy also on thyroid glands of 35–100 ml. Contraindications of MIVAT are listed in Table 10.2. Apart from redo-surgery and large multinodular goitres, medullary and high-risk differentiated thyroid cancers remain a contraindication to MIVAT because of the need for extensive lymph node dissection.

Table 10.1 MIVAT: indications

Thyroid nodule <35 mm
Multinodular goitre with thyroid volume <100 mL
Follicular or indeterminate lesions
Low-risk differentiated thyroid carcinoma
RET-oncogene mutation (prophylactic surgery)
Graves' disease (after learning phase)
Thyroiditis (after learning phase)
Previous neck irradiation (after learning phase)

Table 10.2 MIVAT: contraindications

Previous neck surgery
Large multinodular goitre
Differentiated carcinoma >2 cm
Local advanced cancer (lymph node metastases or local infiltration)

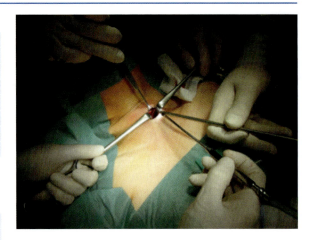

Fig. 10.1 A 5-mm 30° endoscope and a spatula are inserted through the minicervicotomy

10.3 Operative Technique

Thyroid surgery is always performed under general anaesthesia. The neck is not hyperextended. MIVAT is performed through a 1.5- to 3-cm skin incision according to the volume of the thyroid gland. For thyroid volume >50 ml, generally 3.5–4 cm is necessary. In our experience, there is no standard for positioning the incision, and generally, the presence of a skin crease indicates the most suitable cosmetic incision. Subcutaneous fatty tissue and platysma are divided, and the strap muscles are separated in the midline (3–4 cm longitudinally). The strap muscles are then retracted laterally with conventional retractors (Langenbeck retractors), and the thyroid is gently retracted medially to create the working space. A 5-mm 30° endoscope (Karl Storz Endoskope®, Tuttlingen) is inserted, and the thyroid mobilization is completed laterally (Fig. 10.1). Micro-dissecting instruments (spatulas and spatula-aspirator, as well as small forceps and scissors) are used for the endoscopic part of the procedure (Fig. 10.2). Generally, this step of the procedure can be performed with a blunt dissection, as the only important vessel to be divided at this step is the middle thyroid vein. Then, the thyroid lobe is retracted downward with the retractor, and the upper thyroid vessels (superior artery and vein) are isolated (Fig. 10.3) and coagulated using haemostatic device or clips. Alternatively, especially when the skin incision is very low in the neck, it is possible to grasp the lobe and gently retract it caudally and laterally with a forceps and use the two retractors respectively laterally and cranially on the strap muscles (Fig. 10.4). According to the position of the skin incision could be also necessary at this step to rotate the angle of the 30° endoscope and looking from above. Rotation of the angle of view will also allow for the identification of the superior laryngeal nerve. Afterwards, the thyroid lobe is retracted again medially and pulled up with the tip of the retractor to expose the thyrotracheal grove for the visualization of the inferior laryngeal nerve (Figs. 10.5 and 10.6). The endoscopic identification of the inferior laryngeal nerve is useful to completely mobilize the thyroid lobe dorsally, but a failed endoscopic visualization of the nerve should not be considered a reason for conversion, as it is possible to identify the nerve during the "open" part of the procedure. The thyroid lobe is then pulled through the skin incision in cephalad direction applying traction to the upper portion of the gland; division of the thyroid isthmus may facilitate extraction of larger thyroid lobes. The dissection of the nerve is then continued under direct vision, and finally, the lobe is separated from the trachea. Conventional ligations of small vessels running around Berry's ligament are a typical step of our operation. For total thyroidectomy, the procedure is conducted on the same way on the opposite side. Drainage is generally not indicated. We do not use to suture the strap muscles on the midline. The procedure is completed by horizontal stitches of the platysma with absorbable suture and intradermic skin closure.

Fig. 10.2 Surgical instrumentarium

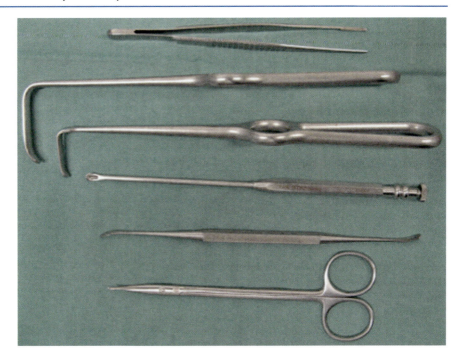

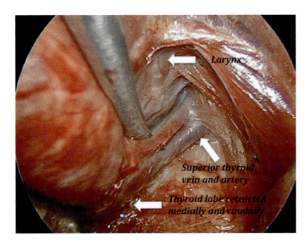

Fig. 10.3 Dissection of the upper pole

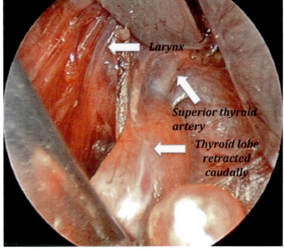

Fig. 10.4 Thyroid lobe retracted caudally with a grasp

10.4 Personal Experience

Our experience with the video-assisted thyroid surgery started in 1999. The early results on 18 patients that underwent hemithyroidectomy between November 1999 and November 2000 confirmed safety and feasibility of the technique (Walz et al. 2001). Since then, MIVAT has become a routine operation and has been performed in 1,637 patients (1,302 women, 335 men; mean age, 46.7 ± 13.5 years). Indications for surgery and surgical procedures are summarized in Tables 10.3 and 10.4, respectively. The mean operative time ranged from 55 min for lobectomy to 78 min for a total thyroidectomy. Seventeen conversions (1%) were necessary due to difficult dissection or large thyroid volume. Final histology showed a malignant tumour in 86 patients (74, papillary thyroid cancer; 6, follicular thyroid cancer; 5, medullary thyroid cancer; 1, metastasis

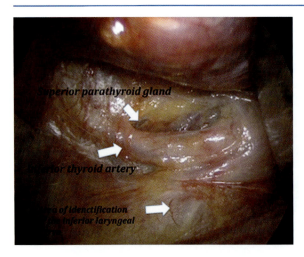

Fig. 10.5 Endoscopic view dorsally to the thyroid lobe (*right side*)

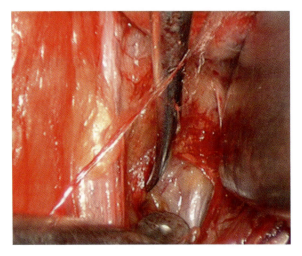

Fig. 10.6 Endoscopic view of the left inferior laryngeal nerve

Table 10.3 MIVAT: personal experience on 1,637 patients

Preoperative diagnosis	N°
Suspicious nodule	548
Multinodular goitre	772
Multinodular toxic goitre	54
Toxic adenoma	43
Papillary cancer	23
Graves' disease	189
Hashimoto-thyroiditis	5
RET-oncogene mutation	3

Table 10.4 MIVAT: 1,659 surgical procedures by 1,637 patients

Type of surgery	N°
Thyroid lobectomy	753
Subtotal thyroidectomy	311
Total thyroidectomy	499
Total thyroidectomy and central neck dissection	15
Completion thyroidectomy	22
Subtotal lobectomy/nodule resection	59

from renal cell carcinoma). Postoperative complications included 76 (8.9%; calculated on 847 bilateral operations) cases of symptomatic hypocalcaemia requiring in 26 patients vitamin D substitution, 19 transient recurrent laryngeal nerve palsy (1.1%; calculated on 1,637 patients) and bleeding or haematoma requiring reoperation in 30 cases (1.8%; calculated on 1,659 surgical procedures). A wound infection occurred in four cases (0.2%).

10.5 Conclusions

Many studies have demonstrated safety and feasibility of MIVAT (Fan et al. 2010; Lai et al. 2008; Lombardi et al. 2009; Miccoli et al. 2004; Samy et al. 2010; Schabram et al. 2004; Snissarenko et al. 2009) according to the indicated selections' criteria. It can be considered an appropriate treatment for benign thyroid diseases (Alesina et al. 2011; Miccoli et al. 2008) and for low-risk papillary thyroid cancer (Miccoli et al. 2009). Nevertheless, the advocated advantage in terms of postoperative pain and improved cosmetic outcome needs better clarification in the setting of prospective and long-term analysis (Alesina et al. 2010; Sahm et al. 2011).

References

Alesina PF, Rolfs T, Rühland K et al (2010) Evaluation of postoperative pain after minimally invasive video-assisted and conventional thyroidectomy: results of a prospective study. Langenbecks Arch Surg 395:845–849

Alesina PF, Singaporewalla RM, Eckstein A et al (2011) Is minimally invasive, video-assisted thyroidectomy feasible in Graves' disease? Surgery 149:556–560

Bellantone R, Lombardi CP, Raffaelli M et al (1999) Minimally invasive, totally gasless video-assisted thyroid lobectomy. Am J Surg 177:342–343

Bellantone R, Lombardi CP, Bossola M et al (2002) Video-assisted vs conventional thyroid lobectomy. Arch Surg 137. 301–304

Fan Y, Guo B, Guo S et al (2010) Minimally invasive video-assisted thyroidectomy: experience of 300 cases. Surg Endosc 24:2393–2400

Gagner M (1996) Endoscopic parathyroidectomy. Br J Surg 83:875

Huscher CS, Chiodini S, Napolitano C et al (1997) Endoscopic right thyroid lobectomy. Surg Endosc 11:877

Lai SY, Walvekar RR, Ferris RL (2008) Minimally invasive video-assisted thyroidectomy: expanded indications and oncologic completeness. Head Neck 30:1403–1407

Lombardi CP, Raffaelli M, De Crea C et al (2009) Video-assisted thyroidectomy: lessons learned after more than one decade. Acta Otorhinolaryngol Ital 29:317–320

Miccoli P, Pinchera A, Cecchini G et al (1997) Minimally invasive, video-assisted parathyroid surgery for primary hyperparathyroidism. J Endocrinol Invest 20:429–430

Miccoli P, Berti P, Conte M et al (1999) Minimally invasive surgery for thyroid small nodules: preliminary report. J Endocrinol Invest 22:849–851

Miccoli P, Berti P, Raffaelli M et al (2001) Comparison between minimally invasive video-assisted thyroidectomy and conventional thyroidectomy: a prospective randomized study. Surgery 130:1039–1043

Miccoli P, Bellantone R, Mourad M et al (2002) Minimally invasive video-assisted thyroidectomy: multiinstitutional experience. World J Surg 26:972–975

Miccoli P, Berti P, Materazzi G et al (2004) Results of video-assisted parathyroidectomy: single institution's six-year experience. World J Surg 28:1216–1218

Miccoli P, Minuto MN, Ugolini C et al (2008) Minimally invasive video-assisted thyroidectomy for benign thyroid disease: an evidence-based review. World J Surg 32:1333–1340

Miccoli P, Pinchera A, Materazzi G et al (2009) Surgical treatment of low- and intermediate-risk papillary thyroid cancer with minimally invasive video-assisted thyroidectomy. J Clin Endocrinol Metab 94:1618–1622

Sahm M, Schwarz B, Schmidt S et al (2011) Long-term cosmetic results after minimally invasive video-assisted thyroidectomy. Surg Endosc 2011. doi:10.1007/s00464-011-1693-2

Samy AK, Ridgway D, Orabi A et al (2010) Minimally invasive, video-assisted thyroidectomy: first experience from the United Kingdom. Ann R Coll Surg Engl 92:379–384

Schabram J, Vorländer C, Wahl RA (2004) Differentiated operative strategy in minimally invasive, video-assisted thyroid surgery results in 196 patients. World J Surg 28:1282–1286

Snissarenko EP, Kim GH, Simental AA Jr et al (2009) Minimally invasive video-assisted thyroidectomy: a retrospective study over two years of experience. Otolaryngol Head Neck Surg 141:29–33

Walz MK, Lederbogen S, Limmer JC et al (2001) Video-assisted hemithyroidectomy: surgical technique and early results. Chirurg 72:1054–1057

Minimally Invasive Non-Endoscopic Thyroidectomy: The MINET Approach

11

Dimitrios Linos

11.1 Introduction

The main advantage of minimally invasive thyroidectomy (MIT) appears to be the smaller incision in the neck compared to the traditional Kocher incision (Linos 2011). The most established MIT procedure in the neck appears to be the minimally invasive video-assisted thyroidectomy (MIVAT) in which a 1.5- to 3-cm incision is necessary to complete the thyroidectomy (Bellantone et al. 2002; Lombardi et al. 2007; Miccoli et al. 2001; Terris and Chin 2006; Wu et al. 2010). We describe a minimally invasive non-endoscopic thyroidectomy (MINET) technique where through a similar in length (1 in.) skin incision, we obtain similar (if not better) results without the need of endoscopic assistance. The smaller incision in the neck approach has been gradually accepted by several thyroid surgeons in response to the "pressure" for better outcomes (including patients' satisfaction) promoted extensively in the MIVAT literature (Brunaud et al. 2003; Cavicchi et al. 2006; Ferzli et al. 2001; Miccoli et al. 2002; Rafferty et al. 2006; Terris et al. 2005).

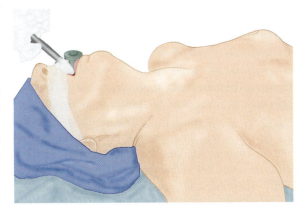

Fig. 11.1 Patient position

11.2 Patient Position

The patient is positioned supine with both arms tucked at the patient's side. A soft roll is placed underneath the shoulders in order to have a slight extension of the neck (Fig. 11.1). Pressure sites are protected with foam. Elastic stockings are placed in all patients and a sequential compression system to avoid intraoperative deep venous thrombosis. The surgical field is prepared with chlorhexidine solution, and four sterile drapes cover the patient exposing only the neck. Two additional small drapes placed laterally protect further the sterile operative filed.

D. Linos, M.D., Ph.D.
Professor of Surgery, St. George's University of London Medical School at the University of Nicosia,
Nicosia, Cyprus

Department of Surgery, Hygeia Hospital,
7 Fragoklisias St., Marousi, Athens 15125, Greece
e-mail: dlinos@hms.harvard.edu

11.3 Incision

The secret of a successful minimally invasive non-endoscopic thyroidectomy (MINET) is to place the skin incision much higher than the traditional Kocher

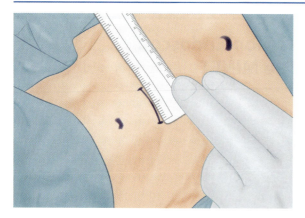

Fig. 11.2 The length of the incision is 1 in. (2.5 cm) for the minimally invasive non-endoscopic thyroidectomy (MINET) technique

11.4 Flaps

The skin incision is continued through the subcutaneous space and the platysma using electrocautery. Using skin hooks, the superior and inferior subplatysmal flaps are developed using electrocautery and blunt dissection with the finger, the back of the toothed pick up or the pressure of a peanut (Fig. 11.4). It is important to extend the superior flap to the superior edge of the thyroid cartilage and the inferior flap to the sternal notch. Freeing the flaps laterally with the electrocautery provides the final initial exposure for the thyroidectomy.

11.5 Lateral Retraction of the Strap Muscles

The midline "yellowish" connection of the sternohyoid muscles is divided by electrocautery, exposing the thyroid cartilage, the pyramidal lobe, the isthmus, and the trachea above the sternal notch (Fig. 11.5).

The sternothyroid muscle covering each thyroid lobe is separated by using electrocautery initially and blunt dissection of the areolar tissue between the thyroid lobe and the common carotid artery (Fig. 11.6).

This dissection is facilitated by dividing the middle thyroid vein with the Focus Harmonic scalpel (Ultracision®, Ethicon Endosurgery Cincinnati, OH, USA) (Fig. 11.7). A Kocher clamp is positioned on the stump retracting the lobe anteromedially. The appropriate countertraction of the sternohyoid muscle using

incision. There are, in most people, one or two natural skin creases at the level of thyroid and cricoid cartilages. We decide which of the two to use based on the anticipated level of the superior poles of the thyroid and the isthmus. Marking the skin crease by applying pressure with a silk suture facilitates the incision especially when the skin crease is not clearly seen. The length of the incision is 1 in. (2.5 cm) symmetrically measured from the midline (Fig. 11.2).

It is always amazing how from such a small incision a total thyroidectomy is so easily done (Fig. 11.3). So, the incision should not be extended unless later in the thyroidectomy if the surgeon feels the need for better exposure.

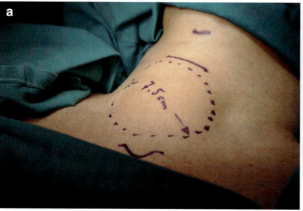
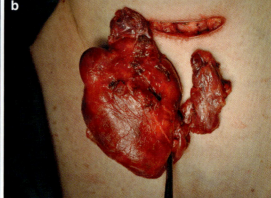

Fig. 11.3 MINET: (**a**) a thyroid nodule with a diameter of 7.5 cm can be extracted from a 1-in. incision, (**b**) the surgical specimen

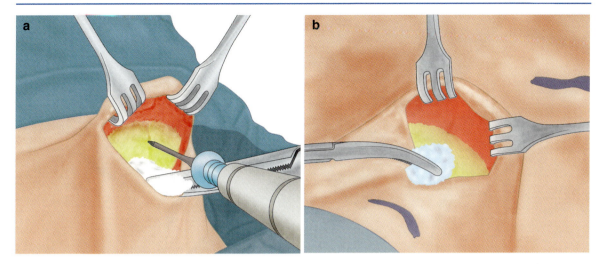

Fig. 11.4 (**a**) Superior and (**b**) inferior subplatysmal flaps developed using electrocautery and the pressure of a peanut

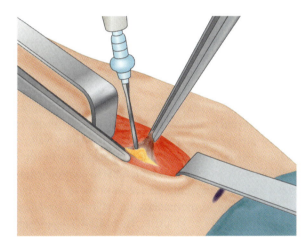

Fig. 11.5 The midline "*yellowish*" connection of the sternohyoid muscles is divided by electrocautery

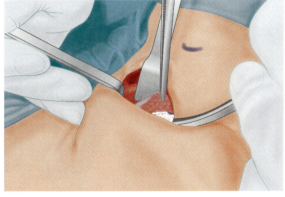

Fig. 11.6 Blunt dissection of the space between the sternothyroid muscle and the thyroid lobe

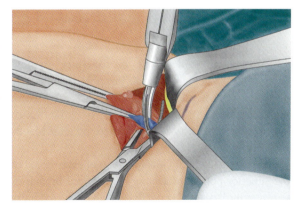

Fig. 11.7 Dividing the middle thyroid vein with the Focus Harmonic scalpel (Ultracision®, Ethicon Endosurgery Cincinnati, OH, USA)

two retractors allows the almost full exposure of the thyroid lobe.

11.6 Mobilization of the Superior Pole

Another Kocher clamp is positioned on the superior pole of the thyroid lobe applying anterior and lateral traction. Blunt dissection with a "peanut" further sweeps the fibers of the sternothyroid muscle in order to clearly visualize the superior pole vessels. Usually, the Kocher clamp is repositioned further upward for better traction and exposure of the vessels (Fig. 11.8).

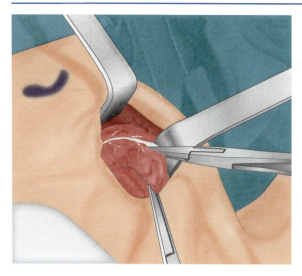

Fig. 11.8 Mobilization of the superior pole; the Kocher clamp facilitates with the exposure of the vessels

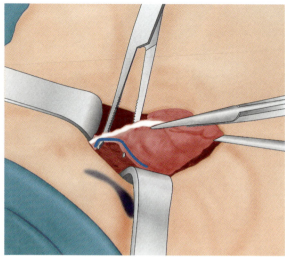

Fig. 11.10 Individual ligation of each superior pole thyroid vessel

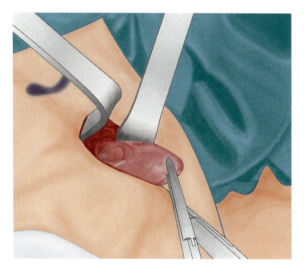

Fig. 11.9 The cricothyroid space is opened carefully

The cricothyroid space is carefully opened (Fig. 11.9). The larger superior pole vessels are now clearly seen and individually divided by using both Harmonic scalpel and 3- or 4-0 silk ties to avoid any possibility for immediate or later bleeding (Fig. 11.10).

The careful and individual ligation of each vessel of the superior pole is protecting the external branch of the superior laryngeal nerve that usually goes medially to the vessels as it enters the cricothyroid muscle. Occasionally, this nerve might loop around the superior vessels.

11.7 Identification of the Superior Parathyroid Gland

At the very tip of the superior pole of the thyroid lobe, and posteriorly, the superior parathyroid gland is almost always there (Fig. 11.11a). Its darker yellow color is easily recognized and separated from the thyroid tissue. A 4-0 silk tie is preferable to control hemostasis than the harmonic device in order to avoid the thermal spread to the underlying recurrent laryngeal nerve (RLN) (Fig. 11.11b). The MINET approach allows direct vision and control of the crucial laryngeal entry point of the RLN as it enters the larynx posteromedial to the lower margin of the cricothyroid muscle at the cricoid cartilage.

11.8 Mobilization of the Inferior Pole

The mobilization of the inferior pole starts medially below the isthmus by dividing the inferior thyroid veins (Fig. 11.12). Blunt sweeping of the trachea with a peanut allows the exposure of the anterior and "safe" area of the trachea as well as the vessels. The superomedial traction of the inferior pole and the countertraction with the retractors facilitates the full mobilization of large goiters. At this point, attention is paid to discover the inferior parathyroid gland (Fig. 11.13). Often, it is covered within the thyroid capsule or well attached to the

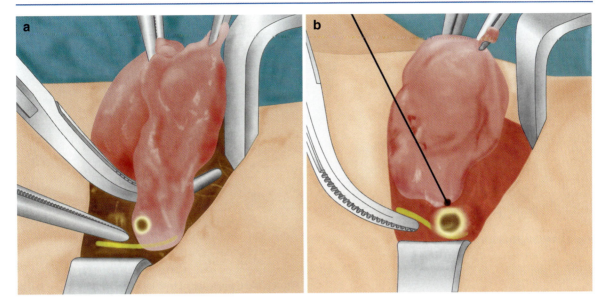

Fig. 11.11 (**a**) Identification of the superior parathyroid gland, (**b**) use of tie for hemostasis

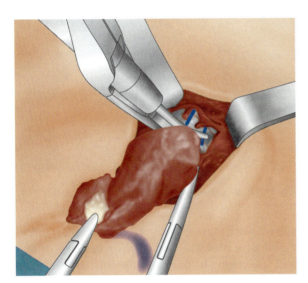

Fig. 11.12 Mobilization of the inferior pole

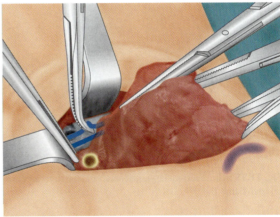

Fig. 11.13 Identification of the inferior parathyroid gland

thyroid, making its separation and protection more difficult than the superior parathyroid gland.

11.9 Mobilization of the Lobe

The lobe that had been freed from its attachments to the superior and inferior poles is pulled medially in order to complete its full mobilization (Fig. 11.14). At this point, all our attention is given to see and protect the recurrent laryngeal nerve which comes very close to the thyroid and the ligament of Berry before entering the larynx. A very constant landmark is the tubercle of Zuckerkandl. This is a lateral nodular projection of the thyroid of different sizes. Underneath the tubercle of Zuckerkandl, the RLN is almost always recognized both visually and confirmed with the intraoperative nerval monitoring devices (Fig. 11.15). Lifting the tubercle of Zuckerkandl anteromedially provides a more complete and safer lobectomy. The ligament of Berry which is a condensation of the

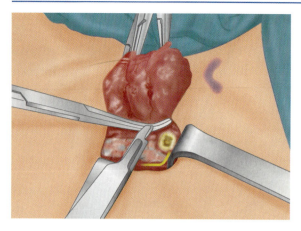

Fig. 11.14 Mobilization of the lobe

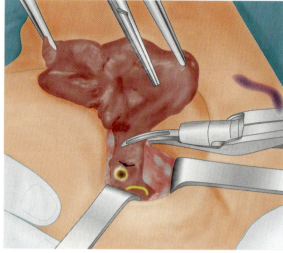

Fig. 11.16 Completion of hemithyroidectomy

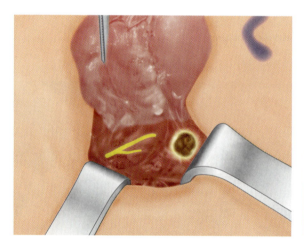

Fig. 11.15 The recurrent laryngeal nerve and the superior parathyroid gland

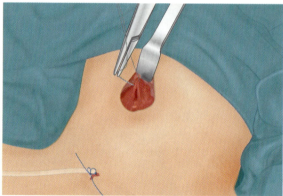

Fig. 11.17 Reapproximation of the sternohyoid muscles

thyroid capsule with or without thyroid tissue is the last step before the lobectomy is completed. This should be done having the course of the RLN visible at all times.

11.10 Mobilization of Isthmus and Pyramidal Lobe

The high entrance to the thyroid field in the MINET approach allows an easy mobilization of the pyramidal lobe and its complete extirpation. The full mobilization of isthmus is safely done using the electrocautery. The different steps described above are repeated on the opposite lobe to complete a total thyroidectomy unless the surgical plan was for hemithyroidectomy or thyroid lobectomy. In this case, the isthmus is divided using Ultracision energy, and the operation is completed (Fig. 11.16).

11.11 Closure

The operative field is irrigated with sterile water, and careful inspection for bleeding sites is meticulously done.

Hemostasis is obtained with pressure and careful use of electrocautery. Manual pressure of oozing areas close to the recurrent laryngeal nerves, as well as the occasional use of antithrombin agents, will provide a

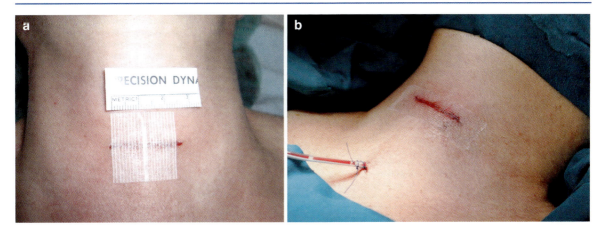

Fig. 11.18 Final outcome using either (**a**) steri-strips or (**b**) silicone sheets

bloodless field before each closure. A Valsalva maneuver by the anesthesiologist will further reveal potential bleeders.

Although a drain is not used routinely, there is no problem to leave a small (closed wound) drain exiting from above the sternal notch and remove it the following morning before discharging the patient.

The sternohyoid muscles are reapproximated in the midline using a 3-0 absorbable suture (Fig. 11.17). The platysma muscle is reapproximated using the 4-0 absorbable suture, and the skin is closed using a subcuticular 5-0 Monocryl suture. Steri-strips or special adhesive silicone gel sheets protect the skin from the development of hypertrophic neck scar (Fig. 11.18).

11.12 Advantages of the MINET Approach

1. *More safety*
   The small incision placed high at the level of the superior pole of the thyroid provides the surgeon with direct vision and ability to protect the recurrent laryngeal nerve as it enters the larynx, the external branch of the superior laryngeal nerve as it enters the cricothyroid muscle and the superior parathyroid gland.
2. *No limitations*
   The technique can be applied to the majority of thyroidectomies for benign and malignant diseases without lateral lymphadenopathy. The small 2.5- to 3-cm-high places in the natural skin crease incision can always be extended to accommodate larger goiters.
3. *More "radical"*
   The option for avoiding the use of the energy devices very close to the recurrent laryngeal nerve (RLN) provides a more "radical" thyroidectomy (as proven by the very low iodine uptake postoperatively). In the other endoscopic MIT techniques where the use of energy devices is obligatory, there is a need to avoid thermal spread to the RLN by leaving some thyroid tissue behind.
4. *Less expensive*
   The MINET approach is less costly because there is no need for additional endoscopic technology and disposable instruments.
5. *Easy to learn*
   The learning curve for the MINET procedure is easy because the same principles are followed as in the traditional open thyroidectomy. The only difficulty is to overcome the initial hesitancy for a small incision placed high in the neck.

11.13 Summary

The minimally invasive non-endoscopic thyroidectomy (MINET) technique followed the "pressure" of the minimally invasive video-assisted thyroidectomy (MIVAT) offering better esthetics and other advantages via a small incision in the neck. In the MINET approach, a similarly small incision (1 in.) is used but placed very high in the neck along the nearly always existing skin crease(s). The direct approach to the superior pole provides better and safer management of the recurrent laryngeal nerve as it enters into the larynx, the preservation of the external branch of the superior laryngeal nerve and the preservation of the superior parathyroid glands. The possibility of avoiding the thermal spread of the energy devices in this sensitive area provides "more" total thyroidectomy and potentially less complications, although the remaining steps of the MINET procedure can be expedited with the use of energy devices with less blood loss. Finally, the MINET procedure is less expensive and easy to learn by the thyroid surgeon.

References

Bellantone R, Lombardi CP, Bossola M, Boscherini M, De Crea C, Alesina PF, Traini E (2002) Video-assisted vs conventional thyroid lobectomy: a randomized trial. Arch Surg 137(3):301–304; discussion 305

Brunaud L, Zarnegar R, Wada N, Ituarte P, Clark OH, Duh QY (2003) Incision length for standard thyroidectomy and parathyroidectomy: when is it minimally invasive? Arch Surg 138(10):1140–1143

Cavicchi O, Piccin O, Ceroni AR, Caliceti U (2006) Minimally invasive nonendoscopic thyroidectomy. Otolaryngol Head Neck Surg 135(5):744–747

Ferzli GS, Sayad P, Abdo Z, Cacchione RN (2001) Minimally invasive, nonendoscopic thyroid surgery. J Am Coll Surg 192(5):665–668

Linos D (2011) Minimally invasive thyroidectomy: a comprehensive appraisal of existing techniques. Surgery 150(1):17–24

Lombardi CP, Raffaelli M, de Crea C, Princi P, Castaldi P, Spaventa A, Salvatori M, Bellantone R (2007) Report on 8 years of experience with video-assisted thyroidectomy for papillary thyroid carcinoma. Surgery 142(6):944–951; discussion 944–951

Miccoli P, Berti P, Raffaelli M, Materazzi G, Baldacci S, Rossi G (2001) Comparison between minimally invasive video-assisted thyroidectomy and conventional thyroidectomy: a prospective randomized study. Surgery 130(6):1039–1043

Miccoli P, Elisei R, Materazzi G, Capezzone M, Galleri D, Pacini F, Berti P, Pinchera A (2002) Minimally invasive video-assisted thyroidectomy for papillary carcinoma: a prospective study of its completeness. Surgery 132(6):1070–1073; discussion 1073–1074

Rafferty M, Miller I, Timon C (2006) Minimal incision for open thyroidectomy. Otolaryngol Head Neck Surg 135(2):295–298

Terris DJ, Chin E (2006) Clinical implementation of endoscopic thyroidectomy in selected patients. Laryngoscope 116(10): 1745–1748

Terris DJ, Bonnett A, Gourin CG, Chin E (2005) Minimally invasive thyroidectomy using the Sofferman technique. Laryngoscope 115(6):1104–1108

Wu CT, Yang LH, Kuo SJ (2010) Comparison of video-assisted thyroidectomy and traditional thyroidectomy for the treatment of papillary thyroid carcinoma. Surg Endosc 24(7): 1658–1662

Endoscopic Transaxillary Thyroidectomy

12

Simon K. Wright

12.1 Introduction

Until the past decade, there have been no significant advances in the surgical technique of thyroidectomy established early in the last century. The advent of energized dissecting and cutting instruments, most notably the Harmonic scalpel, relieved the surgeon of the necessity of clamping and tying vessels. This facilitated the contemplation of minimization and relocation of incisions distant from the neck. Combined with advances in laparoscopic surgical instrumentation and techniques, which occurred in the 1990s, the stage was set for the field of minimally invasive surgery (MIS) of the thyroid gland to develop.

Thyroid surgery is intrinsically well suited for minimally invasive surgery. Many patients undergoing thyroid surgery are young or middle-aged women. Frequently, thyroidectomy is performed as an "excisional biopsy" to determine the character of a lesion with the foreknowledge that it is likely benign; in selected cases, extirpative surgery provides all the treatment necessary. While accuracy of thyroid fine needle aspiration biopsy (FNAB) generally correlates with the experience of the procedurist (Ghorfrani et al. 2006), the rate of benign final histology for indeterminate FNAB remains 70% even at leading cancer centers (Scalabs et al. 2003). It is commonplace for patients to be more concerned with the potential for visible scarring than with the underlying disease itself, particularly in young women. This can contribute to a delay in treatment. While the recovery from conventional thyroid surgery is not difficult, the surgical approach is a major contributor to recovery compared to the actual surgical maneuvers required to excise the gland itself. As such, the potential to reduce the recovery period through MIS represents an opportunity to significantly reduce the overall morbidity of the procedure as a whole.

The world was introduced to MIS for thyroid and parathyroid surgery when Gagner performed an endoscopic parathyroidectomy (Gagner 1996). A flourish of MIS activity followed, most notably, the development of the minimally invasive video-assisted technique (MIVAT) which has become the workhorse of contemporary MIS of the thyroid and parathyroid surgical fields (Miccoli 2000; Gagner and Inabnet 2001). Among others, Miccoli was an early champion of this technique who generated a large experience and published widely (Miccoli et al. 2002, 2011).

While clearly beneficial from an aesthetic standpoint, MIVAT still results in a visible incision. The demand for remote incision placement led to a variety of surgical approaches involving the chest, the breast, and the axilla. Chief advantages have been the relocation and minimization of incisions through the use of trocars and CO_2 insufflation. Initial experience by Ikeda demonstrated a transaxillary approach. Subsequent authors have demonstrated safe and effective approaches including transaxillary, bilateral breast approaches, and others (Ikeda et al. 2000; Ohgami et al. 2000). This chapter will describe the technique of transaxillary totally endoscopic (TATE) thyroid lobectomy.

S.K. Wright, M.D.
Minimally Invasive and Robotic Head
and Neck Surgery, ENT Clinic of Iowa,
1455 29th Street, West Des Moines, IA 50323, USA
e-mail: swright@entclinicofiowa.com

This approach offers advantages of excellent visualization of key structures including parathyroid glands, recurrent laryngeal nerve (RLN), and vascular structures. It avoids visible incisions and is performed through trocar incisions, maintaining status as a true minimally invasive procedure.

12.2 CO$_2$ Insufflation

Carbon dioxide insufflation is a key component of the TATE technique, and brief synopsis of the world experience with CO$_2$ insufflation of the neck deserves review. Initial application of CO$_2$ insufflation to the neck occurred in the late 1990s and resulted in hypercarbia and extensive subcutaneous emphysema (Gottlieb et al. 1997). In this case, insufflation pressures of 20 mmHg then 42 mmHg were utilized. Later, the pressure level was reduced to 15 mmHg for a prolonged surgery. Extensive subcutaneous emphysema occurred. Subsequently, a series of studies were conducted. Using a large animal model, Rubino et al. indicated no change in intracranial pressure with CO$_2$ insufflation pressures less than 10 mmHg (Rubino et al. 2000). Bellantone measured arterial PCO$_2$ and cardiovascular function in a porcine model and determined that at 10 mmHg, no significant PaCO$_2$ changes occur; furthermore, neither acidosis nor adverse hemodynamic changes were observed (Bellantone et al. 2001). Minor changes were seen in both studies at 15 mmHg, and explicit adverse changes were observed at 20 mmHg. Ochiai determined that at pressure of 6 mmHg, pCO$_2$ level remained normal when performing endoscopic thyroid surgery under CO$_2$ insufflation (Ochiai et al. 2000). This author has performed over 100 transaxillary endoscopic approaches without complications related to CO$_2$ and knows of no reported complication related to CO$_2$ at pressures less than 10 mmHg.

12.3 Indications

Indications for transaxillary totally endoscopic thyroidectomy include follicular neoplasms, hemorrhagic cysts, microcarcinomas, hyperfunctional nodules, and oxyphilic cell tumors. In general, lesions should be less than 4 cm in size. Relative contraindications include Hashimoto's thyroiditis, obesity, Graves disease, and age greater than 50. We have found that CO$_2$ tends to become more diffuse in older patients. Absolute contraindications include substernal thyroid, morbid obesity, prior neck surgery, shoulder pathology, and known advanced malignancy.

12.4 Preoperative Evaluation

Preoperative evaluation is the same as for a conventional thyroidectomy including application of ultrasonography and FNAB according to standard indications. TATE-specific evaluation includes assessment of the general body habitus. This includes BMI, neck size, neck length, thyroid and laryngeal position in neck, shoulder mobility, and flexibility in general. Thyroid tumor characteristics including size, mobility, firmness/compressibility, and position all factor into candidacy. A woman with a high BMI but a long neck with a small compressible lateral tumor would be a good candidate, while a thin patient with a low, medially based firm tumor in a short neck with poor flexibility would be a less-favorable candidate. Because the arm may be positioned in a "salute" position, recreating this position in the office to assess for patient mobility and comfort is useful to determine whether the patient is suited to this positioning option.

12.5 Operative Procedure

12.5.1 Operative Room Setup

The operating room is set up as it would be for conventional thyroidectomy. The table is maintained orientated to anesthesia without turning. The video tower is placed contralateral to the operative axilla, and surgeon typically sits during the procedure. Camera holder assistant is cranial to the surgeon (Fig. 12.1). The patient is prepped from chin to border of abdomen, including axilla.

12.5.2 Patient Positioning

Arm positioning is an important consideration for transaxillary thyroid surgery. Two options exist. The first option simply involves having the operative arm allowed tucked in a neutral position with conventional

Fig. 12.1 The operative table is *left straight*, and the surgeon typically sits at the bedside. To optimize continuous orientation, the *line* of sight of the surgeon should cross the incision, thyroid, and align with the video tower

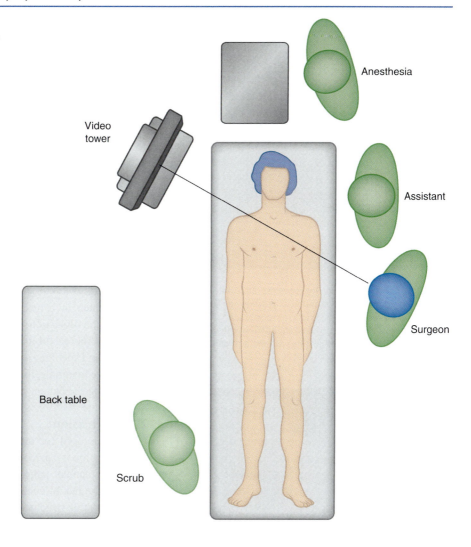

padding to prevent ulnar nerve injury. Depending on body type, the arm may be slightly lowered to expose superior-lateral axilla. Slight shoulder roll placement may be useful. Rotation of head opposite may be useful (Fig. 12.2). The advantage of this is safety, as there is no risk to the shoulder girdle; however, exposure is more difficult, and access more limited. Incisions will typically have to be placed slightly more anteriorly, potentially making them visible.

The second option is preferable from the standpoint of exposure and incision placement. This is a "salute" position with the forearm suspended over the face. Prior to the induction of anesthesia, having the patient self-position her arm in the most comfortable position allows for optimal arm positioning specific to that individuals innate anatomy and flexibility profile. This position is reproduced for the procedure. In general, important principles include avoidance of raising the upper arm, bending elbow no more than 90°, and no IV in the suspended arm. Extensive padding is recommended (Figs. 12.3 and 12.4).

12.5.3 Instrumentation

Laparoscopic instruments are utilized for TATE procedures. We use a combination of laparoscopic Maryland forceps, blunt grasping forceps, and a 10-mm camera. Energy is used with a hook cautery and Harmonic Ace scalpel (Ethicon Endosurgery, Cincinnati, OH). Laparoscopic suction should be available, though use may not be necessary. We use two 5-mm trocars and one extra-long 10-mm camera trocar. Our protocol does include intraoperative nerve monitoring.

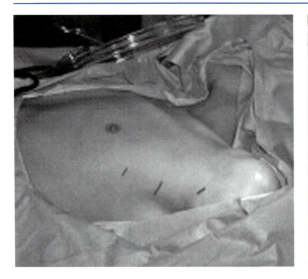

Fig. 12.2 For patients with longer necks and more cranially located thyroid glands, an "arm-down" position can be utilized. This requires a somewhat more anterior positioning of the incisions. The arm should be at a plane slightly lower than the back to prevent collisions of instruments with the arm and facilitate instrument range of motion

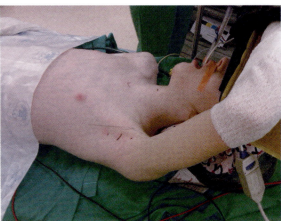

Fig. 12.4 Extensive padding is recommended in this position. No intravenous line in the suspended arm

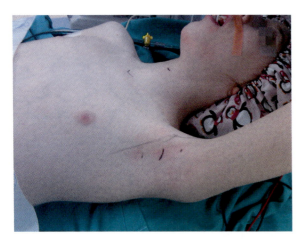

Fig. 12.3 The arm suspended or "salute position" greatly improves access to the thyroid compartment and is the preferred position. Awake positioning is recommended to account for anatomic variation and minimize traction

12.5.4 Operative Sequence

12.5.4.1 Initial Access

Incision Placement. Three incisions are utilized – one central 15-mm camera trocar incision and two 5-mm instrument trocar incisions, one superior and one inferior. The more medial the incisions, the easier the access; the more widely spaced the superior and inferior instrument incisions, the better the triangulation and easier the dissection. Proper incision placement is critical to a successful dissection. Generally, cheating anteriorly and medially with widely spaced incisions will be more favorable, though aesthetically less pleasing. Marking the patient preoperatively is desirable.

12.5.4.2 Incision

#15 blade is used for the incision just through skin. Next, dissection is carried to lateral border of pectoralis muscle. Bimanual palpation of the lateral margin (pinching the lateral border of pectoralis muscle) will help identify this structure and guide initial dissection.

12.5.4.3 Initial Pocket Creation

Using finger dissection only through central camera trocar, blunt dissection is used to separate the pectoralis fascia from the underlying muscle. Working lateral to medial, aggressive blunt dissection can be freely utilized to create a large working space. Aggressive blunt dissection to the level of the clavicle is desired (Fig. 12.5).

"Reverse dissection" to region of instrument trocars is done by retroflexing finger toward dissection. A segment of intact subcutaneous tissue adjacent to instrument incisions is desirable, as this facilitates a "cuff" around instrument trocar once placed.

12.5.4.4 Trocar Placement

Three trocars are used: one 10-mm central camera trocar and two 5-mm instrument trocars. We recommend using blunt instrument trocars. Learn to use trocars in

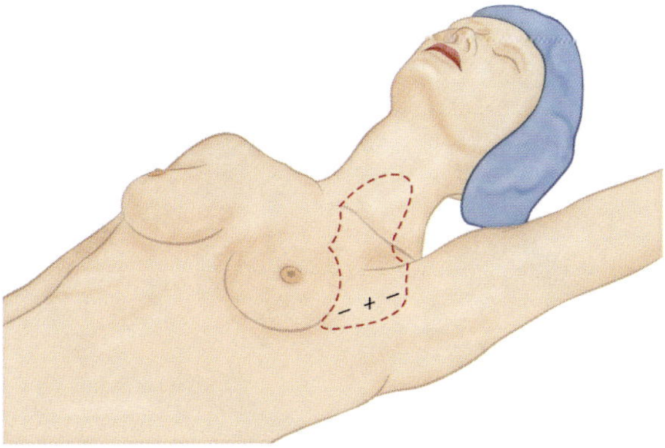

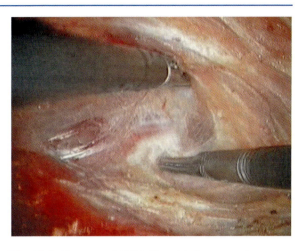

Fig. 12.5 Ideal exposure involves more cranial rotation of the upper arm, which is limited by patient's awake comfort report. The distal extremity is placed over the region of the eyes or forehead and padded

Fig. 12.6 Exposure of SCM. The *right* instrument is running roughly parallel to the fibers of the pectoralis muscle and crosses over the clavicle. It is pointing to the posterior border of the clavicular insertion of the SCM. The *left* instrument is directed parallel to the clavicular head of the SCM, whose shiny tendonous fibers can be seen running roughly horizontally. The lateral aspect of the SCM should be dissected cranially as far as possible to expose at least the lower one-half to one-third of the SCM

cadavers. Trocars have blades and can cause injury. It is conceivable that one could enter the thorax or subclavian vasculature with careless trocar handling. I generally try to use "blunt" or bladeless trocars, as there is no advantage to using sharp trocars. Instrument trocars are placed first under direct forefinger palpation through the camera trocar incision. Central camera trocar (10 mm) is then placed and secured with 0 silk purse string suture. Leave long tails to the purse string so that they can be tied around barrel of trocar to secure this and prevent inadvertent removal.

12.5.4.5 Insufflation and Endoscopy

Once trocars are secure, CO_2 insufflation is initiated. As per protocol, maximum insufflation pressure is 8 mmHg. Flow should be set as "high flow." You must double check insufflation pressure, as most general surgery laparoscopy procedures are done at much higher pressures. The surgical scrub nurse will not automatically perceive a problem with a higher pressure. If the tower turned off, it may reset to a default pressure that is much higher. Use a 10-mm scope – 0°. Use scope warmer to prevent fogging; slightly vent one of the trocars to continuously vent smoke.

12.5.4.6 Initial Dissection

Dissection is carried out across the pectoralis toward the clavicle and sternocleidomastoid muscle (SCM). Once the clavicle is identified, dissection medially toward the clavicular insertion of the SCM is carried out, watching for the decussating fibers of the SCM with characteristic shiny white tendonous insertion. This process is aided by bimanual palpation externally and internally with instruments to aid in orientation and landmark definition. It is important to maintain a wide cranio-caudal pocket of dissection and to avoid tunneling into a hole where visualization is limited. The key landmark is the lower SCM (Fig. 12.6). The middle and anterior supraclavicular nerves are occasionally encountered at the level of the clavicle. Traction of these nerves can result in transient postoperative clavicular cutaneous numbness which normally resolves over a period of weeks to months.

12.5.4.7 Entry to Neck

For the thyroid gland, entry to the neck is carried out between the sternal and clavicular heads of the SCM. In most cases, a natural split is present; if not, it can be developed between the two heads. At this point, it is important to develop a plane of dissection along the lateral border of the SCM at least to the cranial level of the cricoid cartilage; this facilitates adequate access to the upper pole vessels. Once this superior level of dissection has been achieved, the triangle bordered by the posterior margin of the sternal head of the SCM, clavicle, and anterior margin of the clavicular head of the SCM can be entered. The SCM will split superior with blunt retraction. In some cases, the Harmonic scalpel

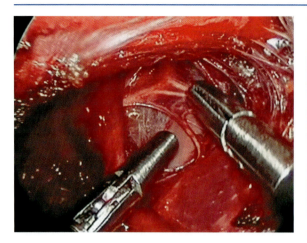

Fig. 12.7 View of ansa cervicalis/omohyoid muscle/jugular vein relation. The posterior border of the SCM can be seen coursing horizontally across the superior view of the field. The *left* instrument is pointing at the jugular vein while simultaneously retracting the omohyoid inferiorly at its central tendon. The *right* instrument is pointing at the inferior root of the ansa cervicalis, which can be seen coursing deep to the central tendon of the omohyoid and superficial to the jugular vein. The ansa cervicalis is an excellent landmark to alert the vicinity of the jugular vein

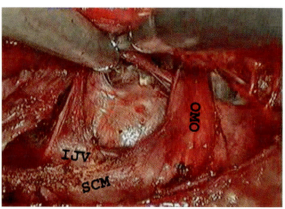

Fig. 12.8 Ansa cervicalis/omohyoid muscle/jugular vein relations. Note that the jugular vein can tent forward and up into view where it can be at risk of injury. *OMO* omohyoid, *SCM* sternocleidomastoid muscle, *IJV* internal jugular vein

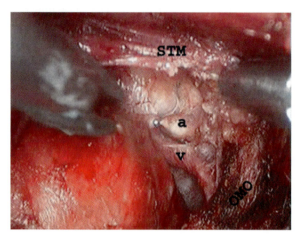

Fig. 12.9 The superior pedicle is well demonstrated in this view which demonstrates the artery (with hema-clip) and vein. The omohyoid muscle (*OMO*) and sternothyroid muscle (*STM*) can be seen as they relate to the superior pedicle

can be used to release muscle attachments to the SCM to improve exposure.

12.5.4.8 Dissection of Gland

The next landmark is the lateral border of the strap muscles. This is heralded by the ansa cervicalis nerve, which runs just deep to the omohyoid, also an important landmark. Understanding of the neural, muscular, and vascular anatomy of the lateral aspect of the thyroid gland is essential (Fig. 12.7). The omohyoid will run transversely and under the strap muscles. Directly deep to the strap muscles and omohyoid is the jugular vein. These structures are intimately associated with one another, and careful dissection is essential in this area. The jugular vein is at risk of tenting forward with retraction and may be hard to recognize if compressed of venous blood (Fig. 12.8). Injury to the jugular vein represents a serious risk and must be avoided by explicit dissection. The lateral margin of the strap muscles is elevated superiorly to the omohyoid. The anterior-inferior surface of the omohyoid is the best location to dissect to the jugular vein and thyroid gland. The thyroid is invested with fascia, and this must be carefully peeled back to the true surface of the gland. Bimanual instrument blunt dissection and judicious harmonic use is best, taking care to avoid injury to the jugular vein.

At this point, the lateral aspect of the gland can be identified. Working along the anterolateral aspect of the gland, the entire lateral gland is dissected. This can be aided by lifting the strap muscles off the gland to release the anterior surface of the gland. The superior pole vessels are dissected by maintaining inferior retraction (Fig. 12.9). These are released with the Harmonic scalpel's help close to the gland to avoid injury to the superior laryngeal nerve (SLN) (Fig. 12.10). Next, attention is turned inferiorly where the lower border of the gland is released with a target

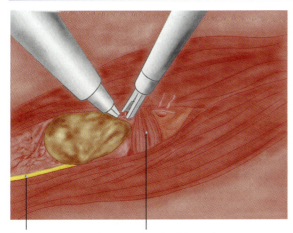

Recurrent laryngeal nerve | Omohyoid muscle

Fig. 12.10 Sketch demonstrating relation of sternothyroid muscle, omohyoid muscle (*OMO*), and recurrent laryngeal nerve (*RLN*)

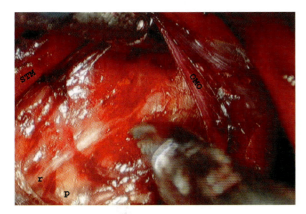

Fig. 12.11 Endoscopic view of lower pole of thyroid gland, which is retracted superiorly with the left instrument. The recurrent laryngeal nerve (*r*) is seen in the trachea-esophageal groove. Just lateral to this is the parathyroid gland (*p*). Sternothyroid muscle (*STM*) and omohyoid muscle (*OMO*) relationship can be appreciated

of tracheal identification. The strap muscles are retracted anteriorly, and the lower border of the gland is released. Blunt dissection and external/internal bimanual palpation aid in the process.

Once the trachea is identified, the lower border of the gland is reflected cranially. Now, the RLN is identified. Careful probing with a curved Maryland dissection is useful. The parathyroid glands are identified (Fig. 12.11). The nerve is dissected superiorly; it tends to fall posteriorly as it approaches Berry's ligament. Once the ligament is released, the isthmus can be divided, and the gland is fully mobilized. It is delivered through the camera trocar after placing in a bag or finger of a sterile glove. The area is inspected, and a ten French suction drain is placed, taken out through the axilla. Wounds are closed in layers, and skin glue is applied. Local anesthetic can be injected to the trocar sites for postoperative analgesia. The drain is removed 24–48 h after surgery.

12.6 Clinical Results

Literature review for transaxillary thyroid surgery has been favorable with no increase in complication rates compared to conventional open surgery (Lobe et al. 2005; Lobe and Wright 2011; Udomsawaengsup et al. 2004; Miyano et al. 2008; Chang et al. 2009; Duncan et al. 2006, 2007). Because of the variation in trocar placement, it is difficult to draw conclusions about differences in operative time, pain levels, and other factors; however, it is clear that rates of major morbidity such as death, recurrent laryngeal nerve injury, parathyroid gland injury, bleeding, and hematoma formation are not increased through the transaxillary approach (Rao and Duncan 2009; Enoz et al. 2011; Ryu et al. 2010; Kang et al. 2010; Kuppersmith and Holsinger 2011). The whole point of incision relocation is to avoid morbidity related to visible incisions. Every study involving transaxillary surgical approaches for thyroid surgery has clearly demonstrated convincing patient satisfaction with the aesthetic result. Over time, we can expect indications for transaxillary surgery to change as equipment, such as retractors, and experience evolve. In most cases, the learning curve for adoption includes approximately 10–20 cases, making this an accessible method for an experienced thyroid surgeon. We must emphasize the importance of mastery of the Harmonic scalpel as a precondition for minimally invasive surgery engagement.

12.7 Conclusion

A decade ago, the gold standard for thyroid surgery clearly would have been a conventional technique. In the past decade, the proliferation of MIVAT has challenged the concept of one-size-fits-all surgery for the thyroid. Given the immensely pleomorphic spectrum of disease that the thyroid represents, it is only logical that a variety of surgical options should be possible for treatment. The TATE surgical approach is particularly well suited for unilateral benign or very early stage disease. It is also excellent for parathyroid excision under strict indications. The main advantage of this approach is that it remains a true minimally invasive surgery which not only relocates incisions but also incurs only minimal disruption to accomplish the basic surgical goal. For this reason, it should be contemplated as an option for selected patients.

References

Bellantone R, Lombardi CP, Rubino F, Perilli V, Sollazzi L, Mastroianni G, Gagner M (2001) Arterial PCO_2 and cardiovascular function during endoscopic neck surgery with carbon dioxide insufflation. Arch Surg 136(7):822–827

Chang EH, Lobe TE, Wright SK (2009) Our initial experience of the transaxillary totally endoscopic approach for hemithyroidectomy. Otolaryngol Head Neck Surg 141(3):335–339

Duncan TD, Ejeh IA, Speights F, Rashid QN, Ideis M (2006) Endoscopic transaxillary near total thyroidectomy. JSLS 10(2):206–211

Duncan TD, Rashid Q, Speights F, Ejeh I (2007) Endoscopic transaxillary approach to the thyroid gland: our early experience. Surg Endosc 21(12):2166–2171

Enoz M, Inancli HM, Hafiz G (2011) Robotic thyroidectomy using a transaxillary approach can be performed by experienced surgeons in selected surgical clinics. Surg Endosc 25(3):977

Gagner M (1996) Endoscopic subtotal parathyroidectomy in patients with primary hyperparathyroidism. Br J Surg 83(6):875

Gagner M, Inabnet WB 3rd (2001) Endoscopic thyroidectomy for solitary thyroid nodules. Thyroid 11(2):161–163

Ghorfrani M, Beckman D, Rimm D (2006) The value of onsite adequacy assessment of thyroid fine-needle aspirations is a function of operator experience. Cancer 108:110–113

Gottlieb A, Sprung J, Zheng XM, Gagner M (1997) Massive subcutaneous emphysema and severe hypercarbia in a patient during endoscopic transcervical parathyroidectomy using carbon dioxide insufflation. Anesth Analg 84(5):1154–1156

Ikeda Y, Takami H, Sasaki Y, Kan S, Niimi M (2000) Endoscopic neck surgery by the axillary approach. J Am Coll Surg 191(3):336–340

Kang SW, Lee SH, Ryu HR, Lee KY, Jeong JJ, Nam KH, Chung WY, Park CS (2010) Initial experience with robot-assisted modified radical neck dissection for the management of thyroid carcinoma with lateral neck node metastasis. Surgery 148(6):1214–1221

Kuppersmith RB, Holsinger FC (2011) Robotic thyroid surgery: an initial experience with North American patients. Laryngoscope 121(3):521–526

Lobe TE, Wright SK (2011) The transaxillary, totally endoscopic approach for head and neck endocrine surgery in children. J Laparoendosc Adv Surg Tech A 21(1):97–100

Lobe TE, Wright SK, Irish MS (2005) Novel uses of surgical robotics in head and neck surgery. J Laparoendosc Adv Surg Tech A 15(6):647–652

Miccoli P, Berti P, Bendinelli C, Conte M, Fasolini F, Martino E (2000) Minimally invasive video-assisted surgery of the thyroid: a preliminary report. Langenbecks Arch Surg 385(4):261–264

Miccoli P, Berti P, Raffaelli M, Materazzi G, Baldacci S, Rossi G (2001) Comparison between minimally invasive video-assisted thyroidectomy and conventional thyroidectomy: a prospective randomized study. Surgery 130(6):1039–1043

Miccoli P, Bellantone R, Mourad M, Walz M, Raffaelli M, Berti P (2002) Minimally invasive video-assisted thyroidectomy: multiinstitutional experience. World J Surg 26(8):972–975

Miccoli P, Materazzi G, Baggiani A, Miccoli M (2011) Mini-invasive video assisted surgery of the thyroid and parathyroid glands: A 2011 update. J Endocrinol Invest 34(6):473–480. Epub 2011 Mar 22

Miyano G, Lobe TE, Wright SK (2008) Bilateral transaxillary endoscopic total thyroidectomy. J Pediatr Surg 43(2):299–303

Ochiai R, Takeda J, Noguchi J, Ohgami M, Ishii S (2000) Subcutaneous carbon dioxide insufflation does not cause hypercarbia during endoscopic thyroidectomy. Anesth Analg 90(3):760–762

Ohgami M, Ishii S, Arisawa Y, Ohmori T, Noga K, Furukawa T, Kitajima M (2000) Scarless endoscopic thyroidectomy: breast approach for better cosmesis. Surg Laparosc Endosc Percutan Tech 10(1):1–4

Rao RS, Duncan TD (2009) Endoscopic total thyroidectomy. JSLS 13(4):522–527

Rubino F, Pamoukian VN, Zhu JF, Deutsch H, Inabnet WB, Gagner M (2000) Endoscopic endocrine neck surgery with carbon dioxide insufflation: the effect on intracranial pressure in a large animal model. Surgery 128(6):1035–1042

Ryu HR, Kang SW, Lee SH, Rhee KY, Jeong JJ, Nam KH, Chung WY, Park CS (2010) Feasibility and safety of a new robotic thyroidectomy through a gasless, transaxillary single-incision approach. J Am Coll Surg 211(3):e13–e19

Scalabs G, Staerkel G, Shapioro S et al (2003) Fine-needle aspiration of the thyroid and correlation with histopathology in a contemporary series of 240 patients. Am J Surg 186:702–709

Udomsawaengsup S, Navicharern P, Tharavej C, Pungpapong SU (2004) Endoscopic transaxillary thyroid lobectomy: flexible vs rigid laparoscope. J Med Assoc Thai 87(Suppl 2):S10–S14

Endoscopic Thyroidectomy Using the Gasless Transaxillary Approach

13

Dimitrios Linos

13.1 Introduction

The scarless in the neck thyroidectomy has been widely practiced in South Korea in the last few years. The surgeons at Yonsei University under the leadership of Prof. Chung have proven that this approach is as safe and as effective as the traditional thyroidectomy (Lee et al. 2011).

The transaxillary robot-assisted thyroidectomy appears to be their standard approach in the management of most surgical thyroid pathology; thus, an extensive experience has been accumulated in this group. While in Europe and America, this approach has not been accepted favorably for several reasons (Linos 2011; Duh 2011), I believe there are few and specific indications that this approach should be offered to the patient. The most important indication is the young female patient with a known predisposition to keloids. As seen in Fig. 13.1, even the smallest incision in the neck will leave a catastrophy for the psychology of this patient's esthetic outcome. A keloid in the axilla, though (Fig. 13.2), will have no serious effect on the patient since it is easily covered.

The main limitation for the average thyroid surgeon is the lack of experience in robotic surgery and, more

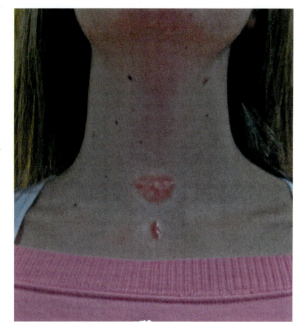

Fig. 13.1 Keloid scar in the neck after minimally invasive thyroidectomy

often, the lack of the expensive robot system in his/her hospital. Thus, we believe that the endoscopically assisted transaxillary approach is a valid and easily reproduced technique for the experienced thyroid surgeon that requires minimal learning curve.

We decided to present our approach based on relatively limited experience mainly to encourage the non-Korean thyroid surgeon that this is an easy, reproducible technique that provides no scar in the neck or other daily visible aspects of the body.

D. Linos, M.D., Ph.D.
Professor of Surgery, St.George's University of London Medical School at the University of Nicosia, Nicosia, Cyprus

Department of Surgery, Hygeia Hospital,
7 Fragoklisias St., Marousi, Athens 15125, Greece
e-mail: dlinos@hms.harvard.edu

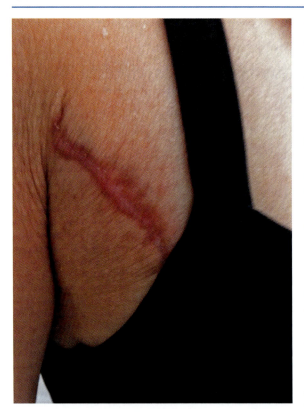

Fig. 13.2 Keloid scar in the axilla after endoscopically assisted transaxillary thyroidectomy

13.2 Patient Position

The patient is placed in a supine position with the neck slightly extended. Homolateral to the thyroid largest lesion arm is raised and comfortably fixed, providing the shortest distance from the axilla to the thyroid (Fig. 13.3).

13.3 Incision

A 6-cm skin incision in the axilla, along the lateral border of the pectoralis major muscle, is made (Fig.13.4). Using the cautery, we start developing the flap that will lead us to the thyroid. The anterior surface of the pectoralis major muscle is our inferior landmark, continuing to the upper surface of the clavicle all the way to the manubrium.

Exposing the loose triangle of the sternocleidomastoid muscle is our next target. We search the yellowish, loose triangle with fat between the sternal and clavicular attachments (heads) of the sternocleidomastoid muscle (SCM) (Fig. 13.5). This avascular space is extended upward allowing the insertion of the special Chung retractor to lift the strap muscles (Fig. 13.6).

13.4 Establishing the Working Tunnel

Once we have in view the thyroid lobe and usually the trachea above and below the isthmus, we stabilize the lifting system on the opposite side of the operating table. On the same side of the incision, we stabilize a flat metallic platform with several holes, allowing the insertion of the endoscopic camera and the different endoscopic instruments. We found that

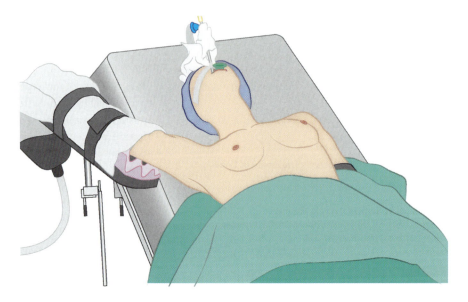

Fig. 13.3 Patient position

13 Endoscopic Thyroidectomy Using the Gasless Transaxillary Approach

13.5 Lobectomy and Isthmusectomy

The first step is to recognize the upper pole of the thyroid and its vessels. Using the appropriate traction, each vessel is identified and individually ligated using the Harmonic scalpel (Johnson & Johnson Medical, Cincinnati, OH, USA) (Fig. 13.8). We continue moving down until the superior parathyroid gland is clearly seen and protected (Fig. 13.9). Similarly, the external branch of the superior laryngeal nerve (Fig. 13.10) is protected by remaining close to thyroid lobe and protecting the cricothyroid muscle from inadvertent thermal injury.

At this point, the upward course of the recurrent laryngeal nerve (Fig. 13.11) is clearly seen with magnification of the endoscopic view.

The second step is to mobilize the inferior pole of the thyroid, trying to recognize and protect the inferior parathyroid gland (Fig. 13.11).

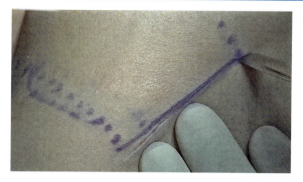

Fig. 13.4 Skin incision in the axilla, along the lateral border of the pectoralis major muscle

this simple device facilitates and stabilizes the operating maneuvers of the surgeon and assistants (Fig. 13.7).

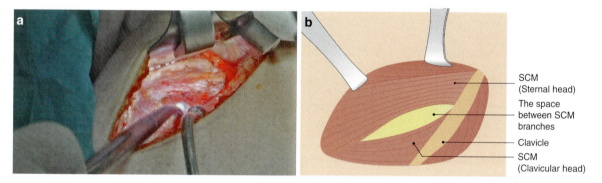

Fig. 13.5 Loose triangle with fat between the sternal and clavicular heads of the sternocleidomastoid muscle, (**a**) operative view, (**b**) illustration image

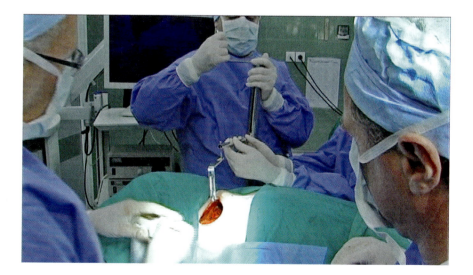

Fig. 13.6 Insertion of Chung retractor

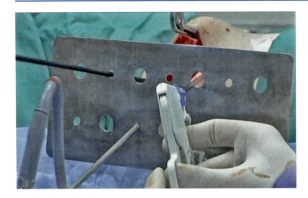

Fig. 13.7 Flat metallic platform with several holes, allowing the insertion of the endoscopic camera and the different endoscopic instruments

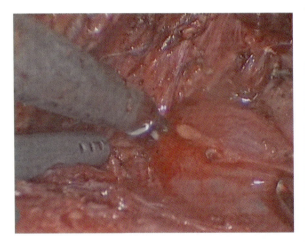

Fig. 13.8 The Harmonic scalpel (Johnson & Johnson Medical, Cincinnati, OH, USA)

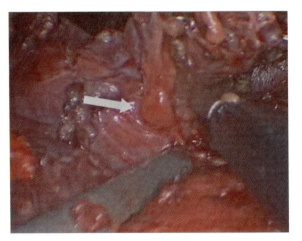

Fig. 13.9 Superior parathyroid gland (*white arrow*)

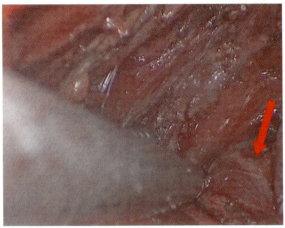

Fig. 13.10 External branch of the superior laryngeal nerve (*red arrow*)

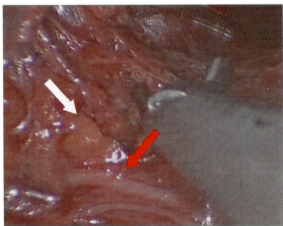

Fig. 13.11 Recurrent laryngeal nerve (*red arrow*) and inferior parathyroid gland (*white arrow*)

The third step is to mobilize the homolateral lobe superiorly and medially. The RLN is protected at all times, and each brand of the inferior thyroid artery is clearly seen before using the Harmonic scalpel for complete hemostasis. At this stage, the isthmusectomy will complete the lobectomy. The contralateral lobectomy can be performed by applying similar steps with the anteromedial traction of the remaining lobe.

When indicated, central compartment lymph node dissection can be easily done, taking advantage of the excellent endoscopic view of the lymph nodes and the direct vision of their relationship to the recurrent

Fig. 13.12 The surgical specimen is removed through the tunnel

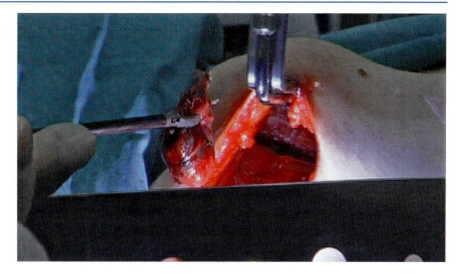

laryngeal nerve. Finally, the surgical specimen is removed through the tunnel (Fig. 13.12).

13.6 Closure

Closing the relatively large space used to perform the transaxillary thyroidectomy requires special attention and patience. Absolute hemostasis is required. In addition to the harmonic sealing, thrombin hemostatic material is used. Also antiadhesive membranes are applied on top of the exposed pectoralis major muscle. Finally, a closed suction drain is always left in the operative field exciting by a separate skin incision. The initial axillary skin incision is closed in layers using absorbable sutures (Fig. 13.13).

13.7 Comments

The endoscopically assisted gasless transaxillary thyroidectomy is using the Chung robotically assisted approach, as presented in the next chapter. Obviously, there is no need for the robot and no extra skin incision on the anterior chest wall. The Yonsei Group (Kang et al. 2009; Yoon et al. 2006) have published large numbers of thyroidectomies (581 patients) using this

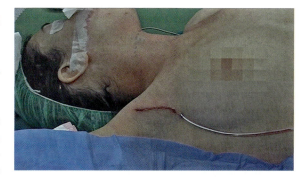

Fig. 13.13 Closed axillary skin incision with the suction drain

approach prior to embarking to the robotically assisted transaxillary thyroidectomy. The reported results using this approach have been excellent with complication rates and outcomes similar to the open thyroidectomy ones (Kang et al. 2009).

Again, the main advantage of this technique is the complete absence of a scar in the neck (Fig. 13.14). I have to repeat that even the smallest skin incision in the neck on a patient who has a keloid formation tendency (Fig. 13.1) can be catastrophic esthetically and psychologically, especially to a young woman (Bayat et al. 2003; Brown et al. 2008). Thus, the alternative approach of the transaxillary thyroidectomy should be available in the hands of the thyroid surgeon.

Fig. 13.14 A 27-year-old woman treated with endoscopic thyroidectomy using gasless transaxillary approach. There is no incision in the neck

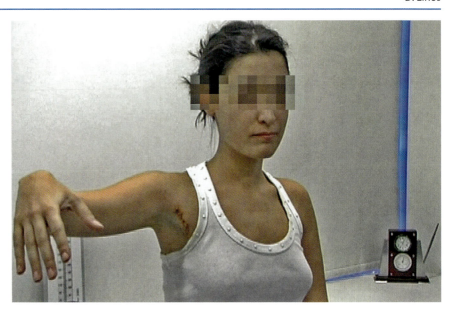

References

Bayat A, McGrouther DA, Ferguson MW (2003) Skin scarring. BMJ 326(7380):88–92

Brown BC, McKenna SP, Siddhi K, McGrouther DA, Bayat A (2008) The hidden cost of skin scars: quality of life after skin scarring. J Plast Reconstr Aesthet Surg 61(9):1049–1058

Duh QY (2011) Robot-assisted endoscopic thyroidectomy: has the time come to abandon neck incisions? Ann Surg 253(6):1067–1068

Kang SW, Jeong JJ, Yun JS, Sung TY, Lee SC, Lee YS, Nam KH, Chang HS, Chung WY, Park CS (2009) Gasless endoscopic thyroidectomy using trans-axillary approach; surgical outcome of 581 patients. Endocr J 56(3):361–369

Lee S, Ryu HR, Park JH, Kim KH, Kang SW, Jeong JJ, Nam KH, Chung WY, Park CS (2011) Excellence in robotic thyroid surgery: a comparative study of robot-assisted versus conventional endoscopic thyroidectomy in papillary thyroid microcarcinoma patients. Ann Surg 253(6):1060–1066

Linos D (2011) Minimally invasive thyroidectomy: a comprehensive appraisal of existing techniques. Surgery 150(1): 17–24

Yoon JH, Park CH, Chung WY (2006) Gasless endoscopic thyroidectomy via an axillary approach: experience of 30 cases. Surg Laparosc Endosc Percutan Tech 16(4):226–231

Robotic Gasless Transaxillary Thyroidectomy

Woong Youn Chung

14.1 Introduction

The application of innovative surgical technology to thyroid surgery has yielded new approaches that are less invasive, reducing the size of neck incisions required to remove the thyroid gland (Kuppersmith et al. 2009; Miccoli et al. 2001a; Inabnet et al. 2003; Yoon et al. 2006; Miyano et al. 2008; Terris et al. 2006; Ikeda et al. 2002a; Sasaki et al. 2008).

The minimally invasive thyroidectomy technique includes mini-open-incision thyroidectomy, video-assisted thyroidectomy, and pure endoscopic thyroidectomy (Yoon et al. 2006; Hüscher et al. 1997; Ohgami et al. 2000; Miccoli et al. 2001b; Ikeda et al. 2000; Gagner and Inabnet 2001; Shimazu et al. 2003; Choe et al. 2007; Tae et al. 2007; Koh et al. 2009). Endoscopic thyroidectomy was first performed by Hüscher et al. in 1997 via a cervical approach (Hüscher et al. 1997). Endoscopic thyroidectomy has several advantages over conventional thyroidectomy (Ikeda et al. 2003; Ikeda et al. 2004; Chung et al. 2007; Jeong et al. 2009; Koh et al. 2010). However, endoscopic thyroidectomy is a difficult technique for surgeons because of difficulties with adequate visualization and precise manipulation of the surgical field. Therefore, endoscopic thyroidectomy remains limited in application and practiced in a relatively small number of specialist centers worldwide (Hüscher et al. 1997; Gagner 1996; Ikeda et al. 2002b).

Recently, robotic technology using the da Vinci Surgical System robot has been applied to minimally invasive thyroid surgery to overcome the limitations of endoscopic thyroidectomy (Miyano et al. 2008; Tanna et al. 2006; Kang et al. 2009a; Lee et al. 2009). The da Vinci Surgical System robot (Intuitive Surgical Inc., Sunnyvale, CA, USA) provides a three-dimensional magnified view of the surgical area. It also provides hand-tremor filtration, fine-motion scaling, and precise and multiarticulated hand-like motions.

Several different approaches have been developed with respect to the location of the incisions and whether or not CO_2 insufflation is required to keep the operative space open (Kuppersmith et al. 2009). The limitations of CO_2 insufflation in the head and neck have been documented including the lack of a natural space, potential complications, difficulty with visualization when smoke plume is created, and difficulty maintaining the space when suction is required to control bleeding (Kuppersmith et al. 2009; Miyano et al. 2008; Duncan et al. 2009; Gottlieb et al. 1997).

Robotic gasless transaxillary thyroidectomy has been used clinically in Korea since late 2007 (Kang et al. 2009a, b, c). It also has been validated for surgical management of the thyroid gland (Kang et al. 2009a, b, c; Lewis et al. 2010).

14.2 Advance of Robotic Gasless Transaxillary Thyroidectomy

Based on the feasibility and the safety of endoscopic thyroidectomy on papillary thyroid microcarcinoma, (Jeong et al. 2009) the initial cases of robotic thyroidectomy was limited to the well-differentiated thyroid carcinoma with

W.Y. Chung, M.D., Ph.D.
Department of Surgery, Yonsei University College of Medicine, 50 Yonsei-ro, Seodaemun-gu, Seoul 120-752, South Korea
e-mail: woungyounc@yuhs.ac

a tumor size of ≤2 cm without definite extrathyroidal tumor invasion (T1 lesion) or follicular neoplasm with a tumor size of ≤5 cm (Kang et al. 2009a). A lesion located in the thyroid dorsal area, especially adjacent to the tracheoesophageal groove, was considered ineligible due to the possibility of injuring the trachea, esophagus, or RLN during robotic thyroidectomy. As robotic experience accumulated, it was able to successfully manage unexpectedly encountered advanced cases such as definite adjacent muscle invasion or multiple-nodal metastasis without open conversion. Currently, the indication of robotic thyroidectomy to include those patients with T3 or larger size lesions has been expanded. The initial robotic thyroidectomy resembled the endoscopic thyroidectomy using two separate incisions, both axilla and anterior chest wall. With sufficient experience, the anterior chest wall incision was removed and developed a less invasive transaxillary single-incision robotic thyroidectomy. This procedure have reduced the dissection and the surgical invasiveness with similar surgical outcomes (Ryu et al. 2010).

Additionally, robotic thyroidectomy for Graves' disease or multinodular goiter which was difficult to manage with endoscopic method alone due to the tumors' large sizes has been performed, and the robotic extraction of the large thyroid gland can successfully be achieved with excellent cosmesis and without increasing the complications. Recently, more than 60 cases of compartment-oriented MRND with acceptable postoperative outcomes and excellent cosmesis had been also performed with da Vinci robotic system (Kang et al. 2010).

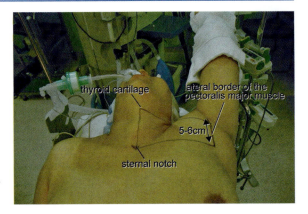

Fig. 14.1 Patient's position for the robotic thyroidectomy

14.3 Surgical Techniques

14.3.1 Double-Incision Robotic Thyroidectomy

With the patient placed in the supine position under general anesthesia, the neck was slightly extended, and the lesion-side arm was raised and fixed for the shortest distance from the axilla to the anterior neck (Fig. 14.1). A 5- to 6-cm vertical skin incision was made along the lateral border of the pectoralis major muscle in the axilla. The subplatysmal skin flap from the axilla to the anterior neck area was dissected over the anterior surface of the pectoralis major muscle and clavicle using an electrical cautery under direct vision. After exposing the medial border of the sternocleidomastoid (SCM) muscle, the dissection was approached through the avascular space between the sternal and the clavicular heads of the SCM muscle and beneath the strap muscle until the contralateral lobe of the thyroid was exposed. Next, an external retractor was inserted through the skin incision in the axilla and raised to maintain the working field. A second skin incision (0.8 cm in length) was made on the medial side of the anterior chest wall, 2 cm superior and 6–8 cm medial to the nipple, for insertion of the fourth robot arm. The camera (Intuitive Inc.), Harmonic curved shears (Intuitive Inc.), and Maryland dissector (Intuitive Inc.) were inserted through the axillary incision. The Harmonic curved shears together with the Maryland dissector was placed on both lateral sides of the camera. A ProGrasp forceps (Intuitive Inc.) was placed on the anterior chest arm (Fig. 14.2). The Harmonic curved shears were used for all the dissections and ligations of vessels. After the upper pole of the thyroid was drawn downward and medially by the ProGrasp forceps, the superior thyroid vessels were identified and divided. The lower pole was dissected from the adipose and cervical thymic tissue and then the inferior thyroid artery was divided close to the thyroid gland. Then, after the thyroid gland was retracted medially with the ProGrasp forceps, the perithyroidal fascia was divided and sharply dissected. Careful dissection proceeded to identify the inferior thyroid artery and the recurrent laryngeal nerve in their usual anatomic relationship. After tracing the entire running course of RLN and identification of the superior parathyroid gland, the thyroid gland was dissected from the trachea. The

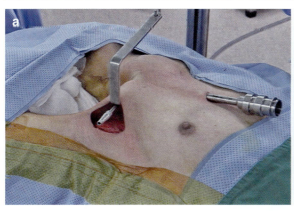 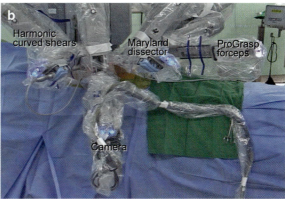

Fig. 14.2 Double-incision robotic thyroidectomy. (**a**) Insertion of the external retractor (Chung's retractor) and anterior chest wall trocar. (**b**) External view of robotic arms

contralateral thyroidectomy was performed using the same method applied for medial traction of the thyroid. The resected specimen was extracted through the axillary skin incision. A 3-mm closed suction drain was inserted through a separate skin incision under the axillary skin incision. The wound then was closed.

14.3.2 Single-Incision Robotic Thyroidectomy

The patient positioning and the working space creation are same as with the double-incision robotic thyroidectomy except for an anterior chest incision. After making the working space, the robot arms are docked. Unlike the previously described double-incision method, in this method, robotic arms are inserted through a single incision in the axilla. To prevent interference between robotic arms, the placement of the ProGrasp forceps and the angle and inter-arm distances of the robotic arms are extremely important. The actual locations of the robotic arms are the same with the double-incision method except the ProGrasp forceps. For the right side approach, a 12-mm trocar for the camera and a 30° dual channel endoscope are located in the center of the axillary incision. The camera should be placed in the lowest part of the incision and its tip directed upward. An 8-mm trocar for the ProGrasp forceps is then positioned on the right of the camera parallel with the suction tube of the retractor blade. At this point, the ProGrasp forceps must be located as close as possible to the retractor blade. The 5-mm trocar of a Maryland dissector is then positioned on the left of the camera, and the 5-mm trocar for the Harmonic curved shears on the right side of the camera. The Maryland dissector and Harmonic curved shears should be as far apart as possible (Fig. 14.3). The procedure used is same as that of the double-incision robotic thyroidectomy, except for the use of the ProGrasp forceps. Previously, we used the movements of the endowrist and the external joint of the ProGrasp forceps to achieve tissue traction. However, during the single-incision approach, tissue should be drawn using only endowrist motion of the forceps, and its external joint should be articulated as little as possible. Because all four robotic arms are inserted through the same incision, it is best to avoid large movements of the external joints of the robotic arms to prevent collisions.

14.4 Future of Robotic Gasless Transaxillary Thyroidectomy

Despite its excellence, robotic thyroidectomy still has some limitations to overcome. Robotic gasless transaxillary thyroidectomy is more invasive because of the wide dissection from the axilla to the anterior neck and more time consuming than the conventional open method. Also, it is difficult to approach the contralateral upper pole of the thyroid with this method (Yoon et al. 2006; Ikeda et al. 2000). Some reports, pointing out the limitations of bilateral total thyroidectomy using a one-sided axillary approach, have introduced a bilateral axillary approach (Miyano et al. 2008; Lobe

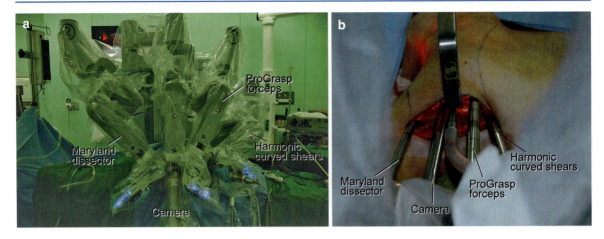

Fig. 14.3 Single-incision robotic thyroidectomy. (**a**) External view of robotic arm. (**b**) All robotic instruments are inserted through the axillary skin incision

et al. 2005). Furthermore, the use of the nonarticulating Harmonic curved shears resulted in some inaccessible areas in the deep and narrow working spaces during robotic thyroidectomy. Although the Harmonic curved shears results in minimal thermal spread compared to the various other energy sources, some limitations exist in applying it to taxing cases such as RLN nerve invasion or trachea invasion. To overcome such limitations, many instrumental experiments have been tried. Also, development of image-guided surgery such as fusion of various preoperative imaging studies with the high-definition three-dimensional image of the surgical field may guide beginner surgeons to preserve important structure like RLN and parathyroid glands with ease (Garg et al. 2010).

This surgical procedure requires multiple steps including positioning and preparation of the patient, creating the surgical working space, docking the robot, using the robot to remove the thyroid, and wound closure. In addition to mastering the technical aspects of the robotic surgical system, a team approach and consistency of the team members including operating room staff and anesthesia personnel are more important than in a conventional open and endoscopic thyroid surgery (Kuppersmith and Holsinger 2011).

Although early operative outcomes have been satisfactory as compared with conventional, open, (Kang et al. 2009b) and endoscopic cases (Shimizu et al. 1999) in terms of postoperative hospital stay, pain degree, complications, and degree of complete resection, as determined by postoperative serum thyroglobulin levels, a prospective, controlled study with long-term follow-up is needed to determine the operative outcomes and oncologic safety of the described procedure.

14.5 Conclusion

Robotic gasless transaxillary thyroidectomy has several advantages over conventional endoscopic thyroid surgery (Kang et al. 2009a, b, c; Lewis et al. 2010). These advantages include a three-dimensional working field, a magnified view, and a tremor-filtering system, all of which enable a surgeon to preserve the parathyroid gland and RLN more easily and safely. In addition, multiarticulated instruments provide easy access to deep and narrow corner spaces and allow complete central node dissection (Kang et al. 2009c; Lewis et al. 2010). Compared with endoscopic thyroidectomy, use of the robot in an endoscopic approach provides a broader view of the thyroid bed, albeit from a lateral rather than the conventional anterior perspective. The use of "wristed" instruments and the elimination of operator tremor by use of the robot have made the device easier to handle, significantly expanding the applications of this procedure (Lewis et al. 2010). These findings suggest that robotic assistance may revolutionize the field of thyroid surgery.

Additionally, it has been suggested that experience with robotic gasless transaxillary thyroidectomy may ultimately lead to the ability to perform more complicated procedures including neck dissection (Holsinger et al. 2010). The instrumentation currently used for robotic thyroid surgery was not originally designed for this purpose. It is likely that specially designed instrumentation and upgrades to the technology will facilitate further innovation within the neck.

References

Choe JH, Kim SW, Chung KW, Park KS, Han W, Noh DY, Oh SK, Youn YK (2007) Endoscopic thyroidectomy using a new bilateral axillo-breast approach. World J Surg 31:601–606

Chung YS, Choe JH, Kang KH, Kim SW, Chung KW, Park KS, Han W, Noh DY, Oh SK, Youn YK (2007) Endoscopic thyroidectomy for thyroid malignancies: comparison with conventional open thyroidectomy. World J Surg 31:2302–2308

Duncan TD, Rashid Q, Speights F, Ejeh I (2009) Transaxillary thryoidectomy: an alternative to traditional open thyroidectomy. J Natl Med Assoc 101:783–787

Gagner M (1996) Endoscopic subtotal parathyroidectomy in patients with primary hyperparathyroidism. Br J Surg 83:875

Gagner M, Inabnet WB III (2001) Endoscopic thyroidectomy for solitary thyroid nodules. Thyroid 11:161–163

Garg A, Dwivedi RC, Sayed S et al (2010) Robotic surgery in head and neck cancer: a review. Oral Oncol 46(8):571–576

Gottlieb A, Sprung J, Zheng XM, Gagner M (1997) Massive subcutaneous emphysema and severe hypercarbia in a patient during endoscopic transcervical parathyroidectomy using carbon dioxide insufflations. Anesth Analg 84:1154–1156

Holsinger FC, Sweeney AD, Jantharapattana K et al (2010) The emergence of endoscopic head and neck surgery. Curr Oncol Rep 12:216–222

Hüscher CS, Chiodini S, Napolitano C, Recher A (1997) Endoscopic right thyroid lobectomy. Surg Endosc 11:877

Ikeda Y, Takami H, Sasaki Y, Kan S, Niimi M (2000) Endoscopic neck surgery by the axillary approach. J Am Coll Surg 191: 336–340

Ikeda Y, Takami H, Niimi M, Kan S, Sasaki Y, Takayama J (2002a) Endoscopic thyroidectomy and parathyroidectomy by the axillary approach. Surg Endosc 16:92–95

Ikeda Y, Takami H, Sasaki Y, Takayama J, Niimi M, Kan S (2002b) Comparative study of thyroidectomies: endoscopic surgery versus conventional open surgery. Surg Endosc 16:1741–1745

Ikeda Y, Takami H, Sasaki Y, Takayama J, Niimi M, Kan S (2003) Clinical benefits in endoscopic thyroidectomy by the axillary approach. J Am Coll Surg 196:189–195

Ikeda Y, Takami H, Sasaki Y, Takayama J, Kurihara H (2004) Are there significant benefits of minimally invasive endoscopic thyroidectomy? World J Surg 28:1075–1078

Inabnet WB 3rd, Jacob BP, Gagner M (2003) Minimally invasive endoscopic thyroidectomy by a cervical approach. Surg Endosc 17:1808–1811

Jeong JJ, Kang SW, Yun JS, Sung TY, Lee SC, Lee YS, Nam KH, Chang HS, Chung WY, Park CS (2009) Comparative study of endoscopic thyroidectomy versus conventional open thyroidectomy in papillary thyroid microcarcinoma (PTMC) patients. J Surg Oncol 100:477–480

Kang SW, Lee SC, Lee SH, Lee KY, Jeong JJ, Lee YS, Nam KH, Chang HS, Chung WY, Park CS (2009a) Robotic thyroid surgery using a gasless, transaxillary approach and the da Vinci S system: the operative outcomes of 338 consecutive patients. Surgery 146:1048–1055

Kang SW, Jeong JJ, Yun JS, Sung TY, Lee SC, Lee YS, Nam KH, Chang HS, Chung WY, Park CS (2009b) Robot-assisted endoscopic surgery for thyroid cancer: experience with the 100 patients. Surg Endosc 23:2399–2406

Kang SW, Jeong JJ, Nam KH, Chang HS, Chung WY, Park CS (2009c) Robot-assisted endoscopic thyroidectomy for thyroid malignancies using a gasless transaxillary approach. J Am Coll Surg 209:e1–e7

Kang SW, Lee SH, Ryu HR, Lee KY, Jeong JJ, Nam KH, Chung WY, Park CS (2010) Initial experiences of robot-assisted modified radical neck dissection for the management of thyroid carcinoma with lateral neck node metastasis. Surgery 148(6):1214–1221

Koh YW, Kim JW, Lee SW, Choi EC (2009) Endoscopic thyroidectomy via a unilateral axillo-breast approach without gas insufflation for unilateral benign thyroid lesions. Surg Endosc 23:2053–2060

Koh YW, Park JH, Kim JW, Lee SW, Choi EC (2010) Endoscopic hemithyroidectomy with prophylactic ipsilateral central neck dissection via an unilateral axillo-breast approach without gas insufflation for unilateral micropapillary thyroid carcinoma: preliminary report. Surg Endosc 24:188–197

Kuppersmith RB, Holsinger FC (2011) Robotic thyroid surgery: an initial experience with North American patients. Laryngoscope 121(3):521–6

Kuppersmith RB, Salem A, Holsinger FC (2009) Advanced approaches for thyroid surgery. Otolaryngol Head Neck Surg 141:340–342

Lee KE, Rao J, Youn YK (2009) Endoscopic thyroidectomy with the da Vinci robot system using the bilateral axillary breast approach (BABA) technique; our initial experience. Surg Laparosc Endosc Percutan Tech 19(3):e71–e75

Lewis CM, Chung WY, Holsinger FC (2010) Feasibility and surgical approach of transaxillary approach robotic thyroidectomy without CO2 insufflation. Head Neck 32:121–126

Lobe TE, Wright SK, Irish MS (2005) Novel uses of surgical robotics in head and neck surgery. J Laparoendosc Adv Surg Tech A 15:647–652

Miccoli P, Berti P, Raffaelli M et al (2001a) Minimally invasive video-assisted thyroidectomy. Am J Surg 181:567–570

Miccoli P, Berti P, Raffaelli M, Materazzi G, Baldacci S, Rossi G (2001b) Comparison between minimally invasive video-assisted thyroidectomy and conventional thyroidectomy: a prospective randomized study. Surgery 130:1039–1043

Miyano G, Lobe TE, Wright SK (2008) Bilateral transaxillary endoscopic total thyroidectomy. J Pediatr Surg 43:299–303

Ohgami M, Ishii S, Arisawa Y, Ohmori T, Noga K, Furukawa T, Kitajima M (2000) Scarless endoscopic thyroidectomy: breast approach for better cosmesis. Surg Laparosc Endosc Percutan Tech 10:1–4

Ryu HR, Kang SW, Lee SH, Lee KY, Jeong JJ, Nam KH, Chung WY, Park CS (2010) Feasibility and safety of a new robot-assisted thyroidectomy technique based on a gasless, transaxillary approach; transaxillary single incision surgery. J Am Coll Surg 211(3):e13–e19

Sasaki A, Nakajima J, Ikeda K, Otsuka K, Koeda K, Wakabayashi G (2008) Endoscopic thyroidectomy by the breast approach: a single institutions 9-year experience. World J Surg 32:381–385

Shimazu K, Shiba E, Tamaki Y, Takiguchi S, Taniguchi E, Ohashi S, Noguchi S (2003) Endoscopic thyroid surgery through the axillo-bilateral breast approach. Surg Laparosc Endosc 13:196–201

Shimizu K, Akira S, Jasmi AY et al (1999) Video-assisted neck surgery: endoscopic resection of thyroid tumors with a very minimal neck wound. J Am Coll Surg 188:697–703

Tae K, Kim SY, Lee YS, Lee HS (2007) Gasless endoscopic thyroidectomy by an axillary approach: preliminary report. Korean J Otolaryngol 50:252–256

Tanna N, Joshi AS, Glade RS, Zalkind D, Sadeghi N (2006) Da Vinci robot-assisted endocrine surgery: novel application in otolaryngology. Otolaryngol Head Neck Surg 135:633–635

Terris DJ, Gourin CG, Chin E (2006) Minimally invasive thyroidectomy: basic and advanced techniques. Laryngoscope 116:350–356

Yoon JH, Park CH, Chung WY (2006) Gasless endoscopic thyroidectomy via an axillary approach: experience of 30 cases. Surg Laparosc Endosc Percutan Tech 16:226–231

Robotic Lateral Neck Node Dissection for the Thyroid Cancer via the Transaxillary Approach

15

Sang-Wook Kang and Woong Youn Chung

15.1 Introduction

Since the era of Crile, the conventional open neck dissection had been the gold standard of surgery for the management of lateral neck nodes metastasis (Crile 1905). Hereafter, many head and neck surgeons have made some modifications of this original technique, and the extent of surgical dissection has been diminished for the less surgical morbidity within the same oncologic safety (Martin et al. 1951; Jesse et al. 1978). In recent years, profound comprehensions of the pathophysiology in head and neck cancers and intensive treatment experiences have drawn the alternative surgical options for the cervical lymph node metastasis, such as selective or hyperselective neck dissection in accordance with the primary tumor biology (Lim et al. 2006, 2009; Caron and Clark 2005).

Lately, to correspond with this concepts, modified radical neck dissection (MRND) type III (actually selective neck dissection (levels II–VI)) has been the treatment of choice for the management of well-differentiated thyroid carcinoma (WDTC) with lateral neck node metastasis (LNM) based on its lymphatic drainage pattern (Caron and Clark 2005).

With the recent advances of surgical instruments and techniques, the trials to adopt the endoscopic or minimally invasive techniques to the thyroid surgery have continuously run for avoiding the prominent cervical scars, and many of early satisfactory results for these techniques have been reported (Shimizu et al. 1999; Miccoli et al. 2000; Ikeda et al. 2000; Park et al. 2003; Shimazu et al. 2003; Choe et al. 2007; Koh et al. 2009; Kang et al. 2009a). Furthermore, the incorporation of dexterous robotic technology to neck surgery has facilitated to perform more precise and meticulous endoscopic movement in the complex procedure. Accordingly, robotic MRND technique for thyroid cancer with LNM have been introduced with the excellent cosmetic result, and the technical feasibility and safety of robotic MRND have been reported showing the capability of complete compartment-oriented dissection using robotics (Kang et al. 2010).

In this chapter, the detailed method of robotic MRND for the management of well-differentiated thyroid cancer with LMN will be described.

15.2 Surgical Indications

The eligibility criteria for robotic MRND are as follows: 1) well-differentiated thyroid carcinoma with clinical LNM (cases with one or two minimal metastatic lymph nodes (LNs) in the lateral neck), 2) the primary tumor size of ≤4 cm, and 3) minimal invasion of primary tumor into the anterior thyroid capsule and strap muscle.

All patients should be diagnosed to have WDTC by preoperative fine needle aspiration biopsy (FNAB). High-resolution staging ultrasonography (US) and computed tomography (CT) of the neck can be performed for the evaluation of preoperative disease staging (Choi et al. 2009).

S.-W. Kang, M.D. (✉) • W.Y. Chung, M.D., Ph.D.
Department of Surgery, Yonsei University College of Medicine, 50 Yonsei-ro, C.P.O. Box 8044, Seodaemun-gu, Seoul 120-752, South Korea
e-mail: oralvanco@yuhs.ac; woungyounc@yuhs.ac

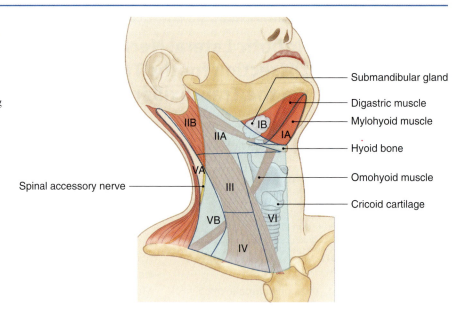

Fig. 15.1 The anatomic landmarks used to divide the lateral and central lymph node compartments into levels I–VI; the area with a deviant *crease line* is where LN dissection is made during MRND

The presence of lateral neck node metastasis can be determined by US-guided FNAB histology or by thyroglobulin (Tg) levels in FNAB washout fluid (FNA-Tg > 10 ng/mL, > mean +2SD of FNA-Tg measured in node negative patients, or > serum-Tg) from lateral neck lymph nodes (Kim et al. 2009).

The role of robotic procedure for the management of thyroid cancer with LMN is still controversial. For experienced surgeons, this approach may be well suited for cases with limited LNM from the WDTC, but its role for more locally advanced disease is uncertain. So, there are clear contraindicated cases for the robotic MRND.

The exclusion criteria that should be applied are: 1) definite tumor invasion to an adjacent organ (recurrent laryngeal nerve (RLN), esophagus, major vessels, or trachea) 2) multilevel LN metastases in the lateral neck, or 3) perinodal infiltration at a metastatic lymph node.

15.3 Extent of Dissection for MRND

Most commonly used surgical approaches to the cases with LNM from WDTC are bilateral total thyroidectomy with central compartment neck dissection and concurrent MRND (type III, sparing sternocleidomastoid muscle, spinal accessory nerve, and the internal jugular vein). In terms of dissection extent, the submental, submandibular, parotid, and retroauricular nodes are virtually never dissected (Caron and Clark 2005), and level IIb and VA lymph nodes are not routinely dissected either in thyroid cancer with LNM due to its rare metastatic pattern to levels I, IIb, and VA (Lee et al. 2008; Caron et al. 2006). However, if an enlarged or suspicious node is encountered by palpation or by preoperative US at the I or IIb levels or among VA lymph nodes, these compartments are included in en bloc dissection. So, the actual extents of surgical dissection for MRND in WDTC with LNM are usually levels IIa, III, IV, Vb, and VI, and this surgical extent is the same in the robotic and the open MRND procedure (Fig. 15.1).

15.4 Special Equipment or Considerations

For the patient position, arm board (lesion side) which can be attached to the operative table and soft pillow (for neck extension) should be prepared (Fig. 15.2). During the development of working space, electrocautery with regular and extended-sized tip, vascular Debakey or Russian forceps (extended length), two army-navy retractors, right-angled retractors, and breast lighted retractors are used. Laparoscopic clip appliers can be used for the ligation of external jugular vein during this procedure. After placing the wide and long blade of external retractor (special set of Chung's retractor for

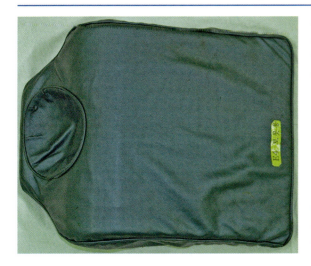

Fig. 15.2 Soft pillow for patient neck extension

MRND, Fig. 15.3) for maintenance of the working space, actual robotic procedures are started. For the robotic MRND, da Vinci S or Si system (Intuitive, Inc., Sunnyvale, CA, USA) can be used. Three robotic instruments (5-mm Maryland dissector, 8-mm ProGrasp forceps, and 5-mm Harmonic curved shears) and dual-channel camera (30-degree, used in the rotated down position) are needed. For the energy device, Harmonic curved shears is preferred (Table 15.1).

15.5 Operative Techniques

15.5.1 Patient Preparation

With a patient in a supine position under general anesthesia, the neck is slightly extended by inserting a soft pillow under the shoulder, and the face is turned to the opposite direction of the lesion. The lesion-side arm is stretched out laterally and abducted about 80° from the body (for the optimal exposure of the axillary and lateral neck area) (Fig. 15.4). The landmarks for dissection are demarcated by the sternal notch and the midline of anterior neck medially, anterior border of trapezius muscle laterally, and submandibular gland superiorly (Fig. 15.5).

15.5.2 Development of Working Space

A 7–8-cm vertical skin incision is placed in the axilla along the anterior axillary fold and the lateral border of the pectoralis major muscle. A subcutaneous skin flap is made over the anterior surface of the pectoralis muscle from axilla to the clavicle and the sternal notch. After crossing the clavicle, a subplatysmal skin flap is made. The flap is dissected medially over the sternocleidomastoid (SCM) muscle toward the midline of anterior neck. Laterally, the trapezius muscle is identified and dissected upward along its anterior border. The spinal accessory nerve is preserved by careful skeletonization of the trapezius muscle and is traced along its course until it passes on the undersurface of the SCM muscle. The subplatysmal skin flap is elevated upward over the anterior surface of the SCM muscle until the submandibular gland superiorly and upper third of SCM muscle is exposed laterally. After subplatysmal flap dissection, the posterior branch (clavicular head) of SCM is transected at the level of clavicle-attached point (for the complete exposure of junction area between internal jugular vein (IJV) and subclavian vein). The dissection of the SCM muscle fascia begins at the posterior edge of the muscle and proceeds in a medial direction beneath the two heads of SCM muscle. The external jugular vein is ligated at the crossing point of the SCM muscle, and the dissection proceeds upward until the submandibular gland and the posterior belly of digastric muscle are exposed. The superior belly of omohyoid muscle is divided at

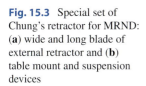

Fig. 15.3 Special set of Chung's retractor for MRND: (**a**) wide and long blade of external retractor and (**b**) table mount and suspension devices

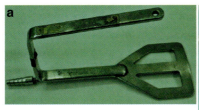
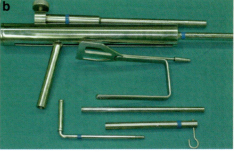

Table 15.1 Special equipments for the robotic MRND

Patient position
Arm board
Soft pillow
Development of working space
Electrocautery with regular and extended-sized tip
Vascular Debakey or Russian forceps (extended length)
Army-navy retractor × 2
Right-angled retractors × 2
Breast lighted retractor × 2
Laparoscopic clip appliers for hemostasis
Maintenance of working space
Chung's retractor (special set of retractor for MRND, Fig. 15.3a)
Table mount and suspension device (BioRobotics Seoul, Korea, or Marina Medical, Sunrise, FL) (Fig. 15.3b)
Robotic procedure
5-mm Maryland dissector
8-mm ProGrasp forceps
5-mm Harmonic curved shears
Dual-channel 30-degree endoscope (used in the rotated down position)
Ethicon Endopath graspers and forceps
Ethicon Endopath suction irrigator

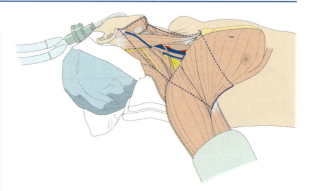

Fig. 15.5 Actual surgical extent of flap dissection from the axilla to the anterior neck (margined by the *dotted line*; *unbroken line* is skin incision line)

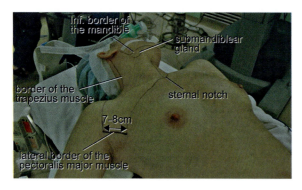

Fig. 15.4 Patient position and superficial landmark for flap dissection

the level of thyroid cartilage. The thyroid gland is detached from the strap muscles.

After flap dissection, the patient's face is turned back to the front. A long and wide retractor blade (Chung's retractor) designed for the modified radical neck dissection is inserted through the axillary incision and placed between thyroid and the strap muscle. The entire thyroid gland and level IIa, III, IV, Vb, and VI area are fully exposed by elevating the two heads of the SCM muscle and the strap muscles. A second skin incision for the fourth robotic arm is made on the anterior chest wall, 6–8 cm medially, 2–4 cm superiorly from the nipple (Fig. 15.6).

15.5.3 Docking and Instrumentation

The patient cart is placed to the lateral side of the patient (opposite to the main lesion). The operative table should be positioned slightly oblique with respect to the direction of the robotic column to allow direct alignment between the axis of the robotic camera arm and the surgical approach route (from axilla to anterior neck, usually the direction of retractor blade insertion).

Four robotic arms are used for the operation. Three arms are inserted through the axillary incision: the 30-degree dual-channel endoscope is placed on the central camera arm through a 12-mm trocar; the Harmonic curved shears is placed on the right arm of the scope through a 5-mm trocar; and the 5-mm Maryland dissector (Intuitive Inc.) is placed on the left side arm of the scope. The ProGrasp forceps (Intuitive Inc.) is placed on the fourth arm and inserted through the 8-mm anterior chest trocar. To prevent collisions between the robotic arms, the introduction angle is important. In particular, the camera arm should be placed in the center of the axillary skin incision. The camera is inserted upward direction (the external third joint should be placed in the lowest part (floor) of the incision entrance, and the camera tip should be directed upwardly). The Harmonic curved shears and 5-mm Maryland dissector arms should be inserted through the opposite angle (downward direction). Finally, the

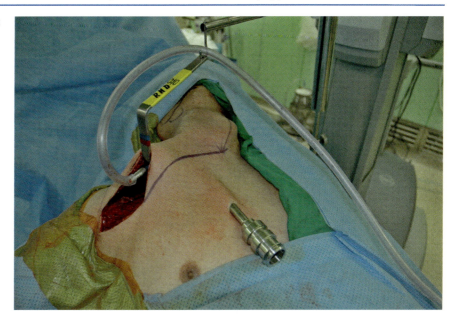

Fig. 15.6 After development of working space

external three joints of the robotic arms should form an inverted triangle.

15.5.4 Robotic Total Thyroidectomy with Central Compartment Neck Dissection

The robotic total thyroidectomy with central compartment node dissection is well described in the previous chapter, so the detailed description of the procedure would be omitted. The procedure goes along with the same manner as the double-incision robotic thyroidectomy (Kang et al. 2009b).

15.5.5 Robotic MRND

After total thyroidectomy with central compartment neck dissection, lateral neck dissection is started at the level III/IV area around IJV. The IJV is hauled medially using the ProGrasp forceps; soft tissues and lymph nodes are pulled lateral direction by Maryland dissector and detached from the anterior surface of the IJV to the posterior aspect of IJV until the common carotid artery and vagus nerve are identified. The smooth, sweeping lateral movements of Harmonic curved shears can establish proper plane and delineate the vascular structures from the specimen tissues. The skeletonization of IJV progresses upwardly from level IV to upper level III area. During this procedure, superior belly of omohyoid muscle is cut at the level of thyroid cartilage. After then, the packets of lymph nodes are drawn superiorly using ProGrasp forceps, and the LNs are meticulously detached from the junction of IJV and subclavian vein. Careful dissection is performed to avoid injury to the thoracic duct. There can be some difficulty in reaching the straight Harmonic curved shears to this point due to obstruction from clavicle. In these cases, heightening of external third joint of the robotic arm equipped with Harmonic curved shears and making steeper introduction angle of the shears can resolve these problems, and the instrument can reach the target point. In general, the transverse cervical artery (a branch of the thyrocervical trunk) courses laterally across the anterior scalene muscle, anterior to the phrenic nerve. Using this anatomic landmark, the phrenic nerve and transverse cervical artery may be preserved without injury or ligation. Further dissection is followed along with the subclavian vein to lateral direction. After clearing level IV area, the inferior belly of omohyoid muscle is cut at the point which trapezius muscle meets. The distal external jugular vein (which can join IJV or subclavian vein) is ligated with Hemolock clip at the inlet to the subclavian vein. Then the dissection proceeds upward along the anterior border of trapezius muscle while preserving the spinal accessory nerve. After finishing the level III, IV, and Vb node dissections, redocking was needed for better

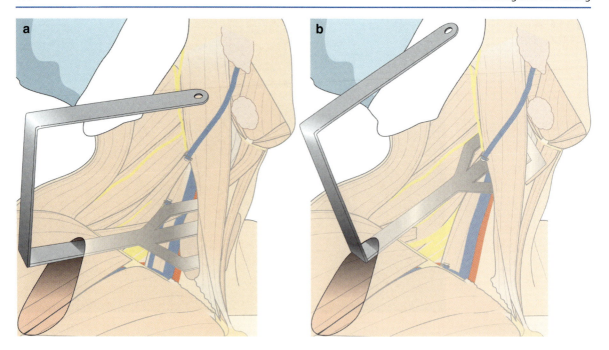

Fig. 15.7 External retractor insertion: (**a**) Initial position of retractor for thyroidectomy and neck dissection of levels III, IV, and Vb. (**b**) Repositioned external retractor for level II dissection

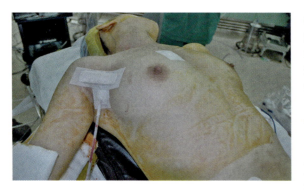

Fig. 15.8 After the robotic MRND

operation view to dissect the level II lymph node. The external retractor was removed and reinserted through the axillary incision toward the submandibular gland (Fig. 15.7a, b). The second docking procedure is done in the same manner as the first docking, and thus the operative table should be repositioned more obliquely with respect to the direction of the robotic column to allow same alignment between the axis of the robotic camera arm and the direction of retractor blade insertion. Drawing the specimen tissue inferiolaterally, the soft tissues and lymph nodes are detached from the lateral border of sternohyoid muscle, submandibular gland, anterior surface of carotid arteries, and IJV. The level IIa dissection proceeds to the posterior belly of digastric muscle and the submandibular gland superiorly. After the specimen is delivered, 3-mm closed suction drain is inserted as described for the previous robotic thyroidectomy. The wound is closed cosmetically (Fig. 15.8).

15.6 Conclusion

In head and neck area, neck dissection is one of the most complex and precision-needed procedure. The long cervical scar and postoperative neck discomfort have been also inevitable brands after this procedure. Heretofore, nobody dares to try the minimally invasive surgical technique to the neck dissection mainly due to its complexity and jeopardy of complication. Although, there have been several reports about the endoscopic approaches for functional neck dissection or MRND (Kang et al. 2009a; Lombardi et al. 2007), they had so many technical and instrumental limitations.

The dexterities of the cutting-edge robotics have far advanced the techniques of endoscopic and minimally invasive surgery. With this technology, the most exacting procedure in head and neck area could be managed by endoscopic approach with excellent cosmesis. The technical feasibility and early surgical outcomes of robotic

MRND for the management of WDTC with LNM have already been reported as satisfactory (Kang et al. 2010). Robotic MRND using the transaxillary approach can allow complete compartment-oriented lymph node dissection without any injuries to major vessels or nerves, or compromising surgical oncologic principles.

With instrumental advance and more experiences, the robotic MRND would be emerged as an acceptable alternative method in low-risk WDTC patients with LNM.

Sources of Financial Support The authors have no conflict of interest to declare.

References

Caron NR, Clark OH (2005) Papillary thyroid cancer: surgical management of lymph node metastases. Curr Treat Options Oncol 6(4):311–322

Caron NR, Tan YY, Ogilvie JB et al (2006) Selective modified radical neck dissection for papillary thyroid cancer-is level I, II and V dissection always necessary? World J Surg 30(5):833–840

Choe JH, Kim SW, Chung KW, Park KS, Han W, Noh DY, Oh SK, Youn YK (2007) Endoscopic thyroidectomy using a new bilateral axillo-breast approach. World J Surg 31(3):601–606

Choi JS, Kim J, Kwak JY et al (2009) Preoperative staging of papillary thyroid carcinoma: comparison of ultrasound imaging and CT. AJR Am J Roentgenol 193:871–878

Crile GW (1905) On the surgical treatment of cancer of the head and neck. With a summary of one hundred and five patients. Trans South Surg Gynecol Assoc 18:109–127

Ikeda Y, Takami H, Sasaki Y, Kan S, Niimi M (2000) Endoscopic neck surgery by the axillary approach. J Am Coll Surg 191:336–340

Jesse RH, Ballantyne AJ, Larson D (1978) Radical or modified neck dissection: a therapeutic dilemma. Am J Surg 136:516–519

Kang SW, Jeong JJ, Yun JS, Sung TY, Lee SC, Lee YS, Nam KH, Chang HS, Chun WY, Park CS (2009a) Gasless endoscopic thyroidectomy using trans-axillary approach; surgical outcome of 581 patients. Endocr J 56(3):361–369

Kang SW, Jeong JJ, Nam KH, Chang HS, Chung WY, Park CS (2009b) Robot-assisted endoscopic thyroidectomy for thyroid malignancies using a gasless transaxillary approach. J Am Coll Surg 209(2):e1–e7

Kang SW, Lee SH, Ryu HR et al (2010) Initial experience with robot-assisted modified radical neck dissection for the management of thyroid carcinoma with lateral neck node metastasis. Surgery 148(6):1214–1221

Kim MJ, Kim EK, Kim BM et al (2009) Thyroglobulin measurement in fine-needle aspirate washouts: the criteria for neck node dissection for patients with thyroid cancer. Clin Endocrinol (Oxf) 70(1):145–151

Koh YW, Kim JW, Lee SW, Choi EC (2009) Endoscopic thyroidectomy via a unilateral axillo-breast approach without gas insufflation for unilateral benign thyroid lesions. Surg Endosc 23(9):2053–2060

Lee J, Sung TY, Nam KH, Chung WY, Soh EY, Park CS (2008) Is level IIb lymph node dissection always necessary in N1b papillary thyroid carcinoma patients? World J Surg 32(5):716–721

Lim YC, Koo BS, Lee JS, Lim JY, Choi EC (2006) Distributions of cervical lymph node metastases in oropharyngeal carcinoma: therapeutic implications for the N0 neck. Laryngoscope 116:1148–1152

Lim YC, Lee JS, Choi EC (2009) Therapeutic selective neck dissection (level II-V) for node-positive hypopharyngeal carcinoma: is it oncologically safe? Acta Otolaryngol 129:57–61

Lombardi CP, Raffaelli M, Princi P, De Crea C, Bellantone R (2007) Minimally invasive video-assisted functional lateral neck dissection for metastatic papillary thyroid carcinoma. Am J Surg 193:114–118

Martin H, Del Valle B, Ehrlich H, Cahan WG (1951) Neck dissection. Cancer 4:441–499

Miccoli P, Berti P, Bendinelli C, Conte M, Fasolini F, Martino E (2000) Minimally invasive video-assisted surgery of the thyroid: a preliminary report. Langenbecks Arch Surg 385:261–364

Park YL, Han WK, Bae WG (2003) 100 cases of endoscopic thyroidectomy: breast approach. Surg Laparosc Endosc Percutan Tech 13(1):20–25

Shimazu K, Shiba E, Tamaki Y, Takiguchi S, Taniguchi E, Ohashi S et al (2003) Endoscopic thyroid surgery through the axillo-bilateral breast approach. Surg Laparosc Endosc 13:196–201

Shimizu K, Akira S, Jasmi AY, Kitamura Y, Kitagawa W, Akasu H et al (1999) Video-assisted neck surgery: endoscopic resection of thyroid tumors with a very minimal neck wound. J Am Coll Surg 188:697–703

16
Bilateral Axillo-Breast Approach (BABA) Endoscopic and Robotic Thyroid Surgery

June Young Choi, Kyu Eun Lee, and Yeo-Kyu Youn

16.1 Terminology

The term "bilateral axillo-breast approach" (BABA) endoscopic thyroid surgery describes the endoscopic thyroid surgery which is using a closed endoscopic technique with four-port methods, and the ports come through the small incisions of both axillae and breasts. Bilateral axillo-breast approach robotic thyroid surgery is the endoscopic surgery using a robot system performing thyroidectomy with bilateral axillo-breast approach. BABA endoscopic thyroid surgery is an abbreviation of bilateral axillo-breast approach endoscopic thyroid surgery.

16.2 Introduction

As endoscopic thyroid surgery has been developed in late 1990s, various techniques have been introduced by many surgeons including cervical, axillary, breast, and anterior chest approaches. The major advantage of endoscopic thyroid surgery over conventional open surgery is the cosmetic results. In performing thyroid surgery with endoscopic approach, the surgeon should pursue the completeness and safety of the operation as well as the cosmetic results because thyroid nodules, including well-differentiated thyroid cancer, have good prognosis and most of the patients are young females.

As BABA endoscopic thyroid surgery was developed in 2004, it has been applied to various operations for thyroid diseases such as well-differentiated thyroid cancer, thyroid goiter, Graves' disease, and reoperation for completion lobectomy. The advantages of BABA endoscopic thyroidectomy are as follows: (1) the procedures use the midline approach like the conventional open thyroidectomy, which gives the surgeon familiarity and comfort, (2) BABA gives symmetric view of bilateral thyroid lobes and gives an optimal visualization of major structures such as recurrent laryngeal nerves and parathyroid glands during the operation, (3) there is no interference between instruments because the ports are remote from each other and as mentioned above, (4) good cosmetic results with no visible scar.

After the introduction of da Vinci Robotic Surgical System to BABA endoscopic surgery, the operator can perform the operation with a three-dimensional high-definition vision and the endowrist function that allows doing complex tasks in the limited working space.

16.3 BABA Endoscopic Thyroidectomy

16.3.1 Basic Equipment and Instruments

- Endoscope: flexible 5-mm endoscope (Olympus, Center Valley, PA, USA)
- Vascular tunneler (Gore-Tex, Flagstaff, AZ, USA)
- Suction-irrigator
- Harmonic® (Ethicon Endo-Surgery, Cincinnati, OH, USA)
- Trocars: one 12-mm and three 5-mm trocars
- Endobag
- Endosuture and endoneedle holder

Fig. 16.1 Snake retractors (*left* and *right*)

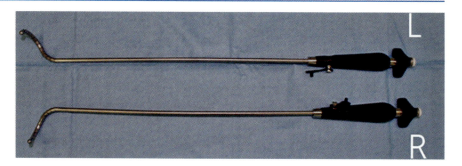

- Basic instruments: 1 endoclinch, 1 endo-Maryland, 1 endo-right angle
- 10-mL syringes with 22-gauge spinal needle: 200 mL normal saline with 1 mL epinephrine (1:200,000)
- Snake retractor (Fig. 16.1)

16.3.2 Patient Selection: Indications and Contraindications

BABA endoscopic thyroidectomy has been used in patients with the following indications:
- Benign thyroid nodules that need to be excised. The size of nodule is not considered to be important, but for beginners, the nodule less than 3–4 cm in diameter is preferable.
- For diagnosis of the nodules that are suspicious for follicular neoplasm or Hurthle cell neoplasm.
- Completion thyroidectomy of the patient diagnosed with follicular carcinoma or Hurthle cell carcinoma of previous diagnostic lobectomy.

Absolute contraindications for BABA endoscopic thyroidectomy are as follows:
- The patient with previous open neck surgery
- Thyroid malignancy which expected to recur easily (i.e., advanced papillary thyroid cancer and poorly differentiated thyroid cancer)
- The patient with overt breast malignancy

Relatively not recommended patients for BABA endoscopic thyroidectomy:
- With large-size thyroid nodules over 5 cm in diameter
- Male patient (due to the prominent clavicle and no breast mound which cause immovability of the instruments)
- Graves' disease
- With well-differentiated thyroid carcinoma over 1 cm in diameter

16.3.3 Surgical Technique

16.3.3.1 Patient Positioning and Preparation
The patient is placed in supine position on the operating table with a pillow under her shoulders. Extend the patient's neck to expose the neck. Arms should be fixed in the abducted position in order to expose the axillae.

Antiseptic solution is applied to the patient's skin from the patient's chin to the xiphoid process. Axillae and proximal regions of arms are also prepared with antiseptic solution. Cover the patient with sterile universal drapes, except the anterior neck and both axillae and breasts.

16.3.3.2 Operating Room Setup
When performing right lobectomy of the patient, the operator stands on the left side of the patient. The assistant and the camera operator stand on the right side of the patient. And for left lobectomy, the operator stands on the right side of the patient; the assistant and the camera operator stand on the left side of the patient (Fig. 16.2).

16.3.3.3 Drawing Guidelines
Draw marking lines along the landmarks of the chest and the neck – midline, thyroid cartilage (V), cricoids cartilage (+), anterior border of the SCM muscle, superior border of the clavicles, suprasternal notch (U), incisions, trajectory lines from the port site to the thyroid gland, and the working spaces (Fig. 16.3).

16.3.3.4 Saline Injection
Diluted epinephrine solution (1:200,000) is injected in the working area under the platysma in the neck and subcutaneously in the anterior chest. In the neck area, a "pinch and raise" maneuver of the skin facilitates the injection of saline into the subplatysmal area (Fig. 16.4).

16 Bilateral Axillo-Breast Approach (BABA) Endoscopic and Robotic Thyroid Surgery

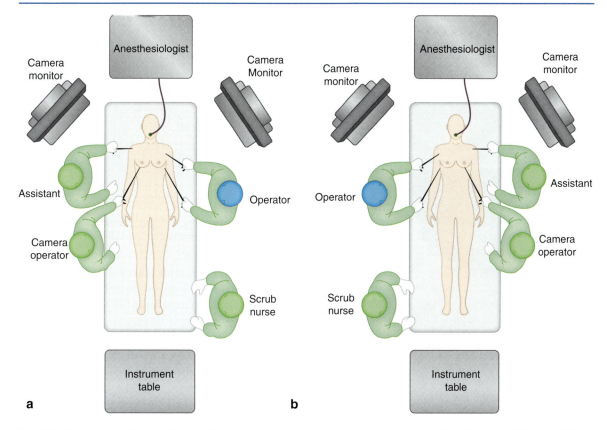

Fig. 16.2 Schematic depiction of the aerial view of the operating room setting for endoscopic thyroidectomy: (**a**) for right lobectomy and (**b**) for left lobectomy

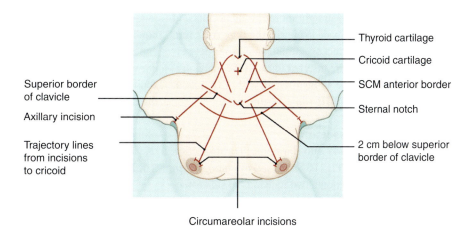

Fig. 16.3 Guidelines for BABA endoscopic thyroidectomy

This "hydrodissection" technique results in the formation of a saline pocket in the subplatysmal layer, which decreases the bleeding in the flap area and makes the subsequent dissection easier.

Note that drawing the plunger backward before making the injection will prevent intravenous injection of the solution which may cause spiking blood pressure and tachycardia.

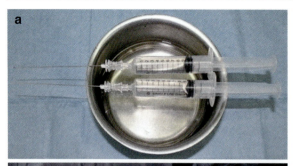

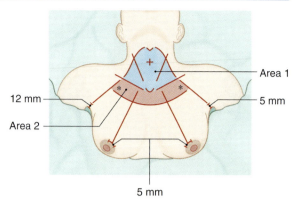

Fig. 16.5 Skin incisions and flap elevation: The dissections should start in red area (marked by*) and elongate to blue area

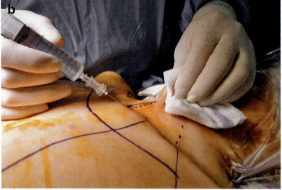

Fig. 16.4 (a) Preparation for saline injection. (b) "Pinch and raise" maneuver

16.3.3.5 Skin Incision, Blunt Dissection, and Port Insertion

After two incisions are made in both axillae (a 12-mm incision on right side and a 5-mm incision on left side), a blunt dissection with straight mosquito hemostats and a vascular tunneler is made to elevate the flap. A 12-mm incision is used to extract specimen later. After dissecting bluntly, the ports are inserted through the incisions.

The working space is insufflated with CO_2 gas at the pressure of 5–6 mmHg via a 12-mm port.

16.3.3.6 Sharp Dissection

Sharp dissection is made with Harmonic. The dissection should start in area 2 (Fig. 16.5, marked by stars). When dissection of area 2 is done, two incisions in superomedial margins of the areolar of the breasts are made. And the flap is extended to area 1, up to the thyroid cartilage in the cephalad direction and towards the anterior border of the SCM muscle, laterally (Fig. 16.5).

16.3.3.7 Division in the Midline and Isthmectomy

To identify the midline, first, externally palpate the thyroid cartilage. Make an incision through the cervical fascia in the midline with a hook electrocautery and extend the incision from the thyroid cartilage to the suprasternal notch to expose the full length of the strap muscle. After making a midline incision, divide the isthmus in the midline using the ultrasonic shears or a hook electrocautery. Prior to isthmectomy, make certain that there are no isthmus lesions on any of the preoperative workups such as the ultrasonography.

Due to its close proximity to the trachea, isthmectomy should be done with great care (Fig. 16.6).

16.3.3.8 Lateral Dissection

Medially retract the thyroid gland with an endoclinch; then, the right side of the strap muscles should be retracted laterally with the forceps. It is then dissected down to the deep aspect of the gland to expose the lateral side of the thyroid gland. With a snake retractor drawing the upper portion of the strap muscles in a cephalad direction, use the ultrasonic shears to dissect the upper pole of the thyroid gland. In order to expose the lateral part of the thyroid gland, the medial traction of the gland is made with switching motion (Fig. 16.7).

16.3.3.9 Preservation of the Inferior Parathyroid Gland and Recurrent Laryngeal Nerve

Before the inferior thyroid artery enters the thyroid glands, it passes directly underneath or above the recurrent laryngeal nerve. Therefore, the inferior thyroid artery can be used as a guide to finding the recurrent laryngeal nerve. If the nerve cannot be exposed immediately, further dissection of the loose fibrous tissue is needed at the inferior point of the artery near the tracheal esophageal groove.

16 Bilateral Axillo-Breast Approach (BABA) Endoscopic and Robotic Thyroid Surgery

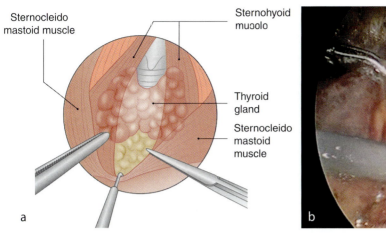
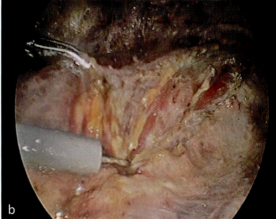

Fig. 16.6 (a–b) Division of strap muscles in the midline

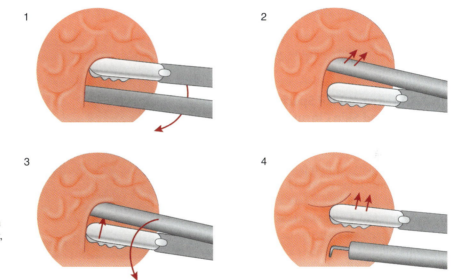

Fig. 16.7 Switching motion in endoscopic thyroidectomy, which allows retracting the thyroid gland medially

Then, identify the inferior parathyroid gland. It is generally located near the branching point of the inferior thyroid artery. When preserving the inferior parathyroid glands, avoid any damage to the feeding vessels in order to maintain the blood supply to the parathyroid is the most critical factors.

If the parathyroid glands could not be saved, reimplantation of the parathyroid gland could be an option. Pectoralis major muscle is often used as a reimplantation site in endoscopic thyroidectomy.

Once the nerve is identified, delineate the plane just superficial to the nerve with a dissecting tool. Continue following this plane of dissection in a cephalad direction up to the inferior cornu of the thyroid cartilage that is near the nerve entrance point to the larynx (Fig. 16.8).

16.3.3.10 Dissection of the Thyroid Upper Pole

It is important to preserve the fascia of the cricothyroid muscle because the external branch of the superior laryngeal nerve is closely associated with the cricothyroid muscle.

One or two small veins may be entering the posterior portion of the upper pole. Identifying and ligating these branches requires much attention. Then, identify the terminal branches of the superior thyroidal artery

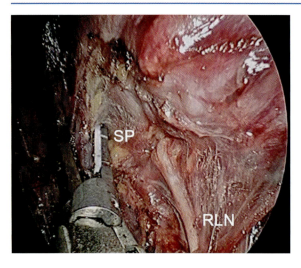

Fig. 16.8 Delineation of the recurrent laryngeal nerve; *SP* superior parathyroid gland, *RLN* recurrent laryngeal nerve

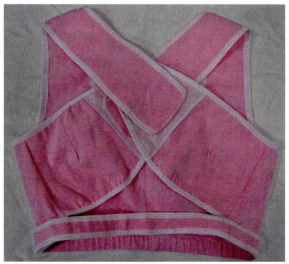

Fig. 16.9 Surgi-Bra®

and vein and carefully separate these vessels with the ultrasonic shears.

16.3.3.11 Removal of Specimen and Skin Closure

After dissecting the thyroid gland away from the trachea, encase the specimen in a plastic bag and remove it via right axillary 12-mm port.

The specimen is inspected with care to find out the parathyroid gland, and the nodules are sent for an intraoperative frozen section to determine the extent of the operation.

After the meticulous hemostasis with electrocautery, the right and left strap muscles are reapproximated. A Jackson-Pratt (JP) drain is placed into the thyroid pockets through the midline incision, via left axillary ports. The skin of the breasts and axillae are sutured with knot-buried stitching by absorbable sutures.

Finally, the anterior chest is compressed with a Surgi-Bra® (Fig. 16.9).

16.4 Bilateral Axillo-Breast Approach (BABA) Robotic Thyroidectomy

16.4.1 Basic Equipment and Instrument

- da Vinci Si HD robot system (intuitive) (Fig. 16.10)
- Endowrist instruments: 1 Maryland bipolar forceps, 1 electrocautery hook, 1 ProGrasp™ forceps, 1 Harmonic
- Vascular tunneler (Gore-Tex, Flagstaff, AZ, USA)
- Harmonic® (Ethicon Endo-Surgery, Cincinnati, OH, USA)

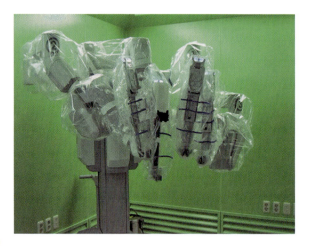

Fig. 16.10 da Vinci robot system is ready for the operation

- Trocars: one 12-mm and three 8-mm trocars
- Endobag
- 10-mL syringes with 22-gauge spinal needle: 200 mL normal saline with 1 mL epinephrine (1:200,000)
- Suction-irrigator (Fig. 16.11)

16.4.2 Patient Selection: Indications and Contraindications

Indications for BABA robotic thyroidectomy are as follows:
- Cytological diagnosed well-differentiated thyroid carcinoma such as papillary thyroid carcinoma and follicular thyroid carcinoma. The size of the cancer less than 2–3 cm is recommended.

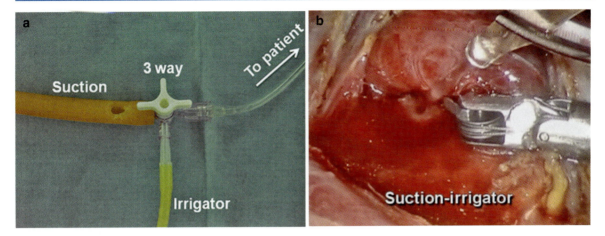

Fig. 16.11 (**a–b**) Suction-irrigator for robotic surgery. A small hole of suction is for intermittent air vent

- The patient with Graves' disease.
- Male patient with thyroid nodules that are needed to be excised.
- Large size of the thyroid nodule, more than 5 cm.

Absolute contraindications for BABA robotic thyroidectomy are the patient with:

- Previous open neck surgery
- Thyroid malignancy which expected to be recurred easily (i.e., advanced papillary thyroid cancer and poorly differentiated thyroid cancer)
- Overt breast malignancy

Relatively not recommended patients for BABA robotic thyroidectomy are with:

- Large-size thyroid nodules over 8 cm in diameter
- Thyroid malignancy with suspicious for lateral neck lymph node metastases

Previous breast operation due to breast carcinoma or breast augmentation is not to be considered as contraindication, and we experienced scores of patients with breast augmentation. Moreover, with BABA robotic thyroidectomy, lateral neck dissection can be effectively performed; patient with suspicion for lateral neck metastases are not considered as relative contraindication recently.

16.4.3 Advantages of Robotic System

- Endowrist function: this allows the surgeon to perform sophisticated and complex maneuvers.
- High-definition three-dimensional imaging: a good operative view with excellent depth perception.
- Suitable for deep narrow operative fields of thyroid surgery.
- Reduction of hand tremor.
- No muscle tension or strain of operator.

16.4.4 Disadvantages of Robotic System

- No touch sensation
- Unawareness of possible damages of the patient
- Impossibility to react immediately against unexpected accident
- High cost, even in developed countries

16.4.5 Surgical Technique

16.4.5.1 Patient Positioning and Preparation

The patient should be placed in the supine position on the operating table, with the arms tucked close to the side.

A folded sheet or a pillow is placed vertically under the patient's shoulders to extend the head and neck.

The operative field is prepared with a routine surgical maneuver. And a large sterile drape is covered over the patient's shoulder, anterior chest wall, and the lower body.

16.4.5.2 Operating Room Setup

While making the flap, the operating room setting is same as BABA endoscopic thyroidectomy. After the flap elevation is done, the robot is docked from left shoulder of the patient. The anesthesiologist and the ventilator can be placed at the patient's feet or right side of the patient (Fig. 16.12.).

16.4.5.3 Drawing Guidelines and Saline Injection

Guidelines and saline injection for BABA robotic surgery are same as BABA endoscopic thyroid surgery.

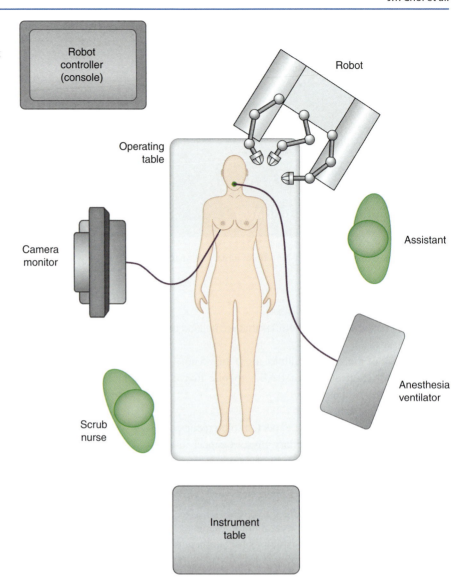

Fig. 16.12 Schematic depiction of the aerial view of the operating room setting for BABA robotic thyroidectomy

One thing that is different from BABA endoscopic thyroid surgery is the length of incision of the right breast. da Vinci robot system uses scope of 12 mm in diameter; right breast incision is always 12 mm in BABA robotic thyroid surgery.

16.4.5.4 Skin Incision and Flap Elevation

Circumareolar incisions are made bilaterally along the superomedial margin of each areola. Each incision is further deepened by electrocautery.

Blunt dissections are held with a straight mosquito hemostat and a vascular tunneler to elevate the flap. The ports are inserted through the breast incision, and sharp dissections with ultrasonic shears are performed. In robotic surgery, it is very important to have the ultrasonic shears always in the field of camera view to compensate for loss of touch sensation with visualization.

After making the working space on the anterior chest, two 8-mm axillary incisions are made. Two 8-mm ports are inserted through the axillary incisions (Fig. 16.13).

16.4.5.5 Docking of Robot System

The patient's head is positioned toward the robot system, and the center column of the robot system is aligned with the camera port of right breast. After the robot system is in place, the robotic arms are docked to each port.

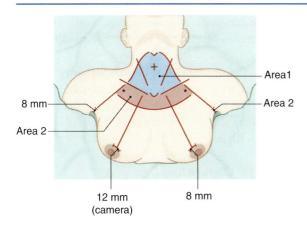

Fig. 16.13 Guidelines and incisions. Dissection should start at "area 2" (marked by *) and elongate to "area 1"

16.4.5.6 Division in the Midline and Isthmectomy

To identify the midline, the first assistant should palpate externally the prominence of the thyroid cartilage, while the operator marks the midline with the hooked electrocautery. After dividing in the midline, the isthmus is divided with a hook or a Harmonic scalpel. Isthmectomy should be carefully performed to avoid giving injury to the trachea.

16.4.5.7 Lateral Dissection

The thyroid gland is retracted in medial direction with a ProGrasp™ forceps, and the right side of the strap muscles is retracted laterally using a Maryland forceps.

The strap muscles are separated from the capsule of the thyroid gland, and this dissection is continued down to the deep aspect of the gland to expose the lateral side of the thyroid gland. To facilitate the medial traction of the thyroid lobe, the surgeon can gradually grasp the thyroid gland on its medial portion by manipulating both robot arms with switching motion (Fig. 16.14).

16.4.5.8 Preservation of the Inferior Parathyroid Gland and Recurrent Laryngeal Nerve

The inferior parathyroid gland and recurrent laryngeal nerve are identified with the Maryland forceps. The inferior parathyroid gland is usually just over the recurrent laryngeal nerve, so one can make each one as a guide to the other. The operator does not cut any structures before recurrent laryngeal nerve is identified. The tubercle of Zuckerkandl can also be used as a guide to the recurrent laryngeal nerve, so the area under the tubercle of Zuckerkandl should be dissected with the Maryland forceps with great care. The ultrasonic shears are used to retract the strap muscles at this moment.

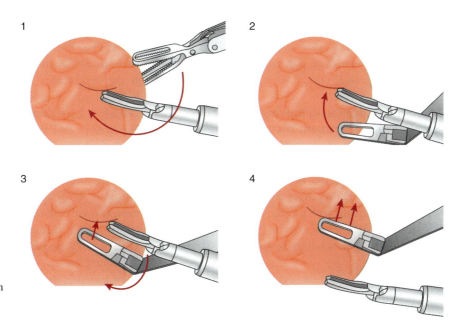

Fig. 16.14 Switching motion in BABA robotic thyroid surgery

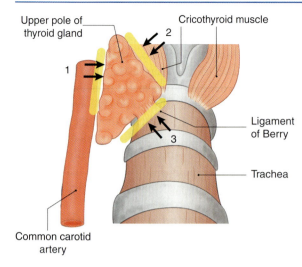

Fig. 16.15 Three ways to dissect the thyroid upper pole

The dissection is continued in the cephalad direction near the point of the nerve entering the larynx. Nerve may divide into two or more branches along its course from the level of the inferior thyroid artery to that of the larynx.

16.4.5.9 Dissection of the Thyroid Upper Pole

With the retractor drawing the upper portion of the strap muscles in a cephalad direction, the ultrasonic shears is used to dissect the upper pole of the thyroid gland. The medial and lateral sides are dissected alternately to free the upper pole of the thyroid gland. There are three ways to dissect the upper thyroid pole. These are (1) lateral approach, (2) anteromedial approach, and (3) posteromedial approach, and in BABA robotic thyroidectomy, lateral or posteromedial approach is preferable (Fig. 16.15).

16.4.5.10 Specimen Removal and Central Compartment Dissection

After dissecting the thyroid gland away from the trachea, the specimen is wrapped with the plastic bag and taken out via left axillary port. If the incision of left axilla is not enough to extract the specimen, the incision may be widened with a knife.

Once the specimen is extracted, an intraoperative frozen section is obtained to determine the extent of the operation.

When the frozen section is proved to be malignant, central compartment dissection and contralateral lobectomy are performed. Lesion-side central compartment dissection is performed with care to ensure that the recurrent laryngeal nerve is not damaged.

16.4.5.11 Contralateral Thyroidectomy

The contralateral lobe is dissected in the same fashion. As shown in Fig. 16.16, the operator has the comfortable and symmetric view of each side of the operative field with BABA.

16.4.5.12 Closure and Dressing

After achieving hemostasis, right and left strap muscles are sutured together with continuous running sutures. Two Jackson-Pratt (JP) drains are placed into both thyroid pockets via both axillary incisions. The skin incisions are closed with knot-buried stitches by an absorbable suture. Finally, the anterior chest is compressed with a Surgi-Bra®.

16.5 Special Considerations of BABA Oncoplastic Surgery

16.5.1 Surgical Outcomes of BABA: Comparison with Open Thyroidectomy

Surgical outcomes of BABA endoscopic thyroid surgery were evaluated in the study of comparing 198 patients with open total thyroidectomy and 103 patients with BABA endoscopic total thyroidectomy for papillary thyroid microcarcinoma in Seoul National University Hospital between 2003 and 2006. Thyroglobulin (Tg) level 3 months after the operation was used to assess the completeness of the two methods, and the percentages of Tg level < 1.0 ng/mL were 90.4% in open thyroidectomy and 88.9% in BABA endoscopic thyroidectomy. Complications including hypocalcemia and vocal cord palsy were evaluated, and transient hypocalcemia occurred in 17.7% in open thyroidectomy and 25.2% in BABA endoscopic thyroidectomy, respectively. Permanent hypocalcemia occurred in 4.5% and 1.0% of patients, respectively. Transient vocal cord palsy occurred in 2.5% and 25.2% ($p < 0.0001$), but permanent vocal cord palsy occurred in 0.5% and 0%, respectively (Chung et al. 2007).

The completeness of BABA robotic thyroid surgery was evaluated in the study of comparing 327 patients with open total thyroidectomy and 423 patients with BABA robotic total thyroidectomy for papillary

Fig. 16.16 After total thyroidectomy; (**a**) right and (**b**) left

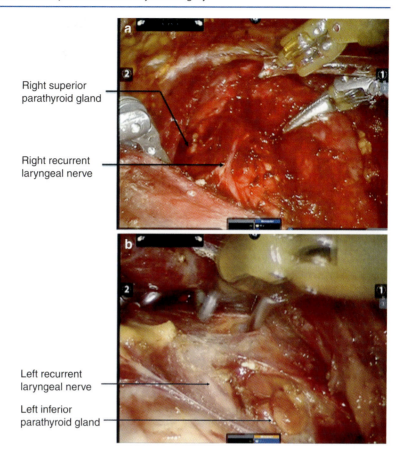

thyroid carcinoma in Seoul National University Hospital between 2008 and 2010. Of them, 174 robotic and 237 open thyroidectomy patients who received radioactive iodine (RAI) ablation were selected. Propensity score matching using 3 demographic and 5 pathological factors was used to generate 2 matched cohorts, each composed of 108 patients. The radioactive iodine (RAI) uptake ratio and stimulated thyroglobulin (Tg) levels on the first RAI scan were measured to assess surgical completeness, and the matched BABA robotic thyroidectomy and open thyroidectomy cohorts (108 patient sets) were not different in terms of the RAI uptake ratio ($p=0.319$), stimulated Tg levels ($p=0.564$), or proportion of patients with stimulated Tg levels below 1.0 ng/mL ($p=0.593$) on the first ablation. The number of RAI ablation sessions and RAI doses needed to achieve a complete ablation also did not differ significantly ($p=0.774$ and 0.468, respectively).

In these studies, BABA oncoplastic thyroid surgery is safe and effective method for the patient with papillary thyroid carcinoma, and furthermore it may be suitable for any thyroid diseases that come up to the current indications.

16.5.2 Issue of Gas Insufflation of BABA

It has been reported that subcutaneous emphysema and hypercarbia may be experienced when endoscopic surgery is performed using very high pressure (over 30 mmHg) CO_2 insufflation (Gottlieb et al. 1997). However, no adverse effects have been noted when the pressure of gas is low enough (<6 mmHg) (Brunt et al. 1997). The study evaluating the hemodynamic changes according to the pressure of gas insufflation showed that the hemodynamics of the patient including peripheral CO_2 concentration, pH, cardiac output, heart rate, and maximum airway pressure were stable under

6 mmHg pressure of gas insufflation. But it was dangerous to infuse over 12 mmHg pressure of gas (unpublished data).

16.5.3 Issue of Breast Sensory Change of BABA

As the remote approach, BABA endoscopic and robotic thyroidectomy tends to be more invasive than conventional operation due to the created wide skin flaps at the anterior chest and neck. According to our recent studies with Semmes-Weinstein monofilament test, the numbness of the neck and anterior chest including both breasts was resolved in 90.5% within 3 months after the operation ($p=0.019$) (unpublished data).

And as Yeung has pointed out before, there is a concern about the scars around the nipple, especially in Western women (Yeung 2002). Though this issue that the breast incision is inevitable in BABA oncoplastic thyroid surgery can be an insoluble problem for us, the circumareolar wound can heal very well and be invisible at some distance. And it is promising that the recently developed areolar repigmentation techniques can camouflage the circumareolar wound more satisfactorily.

16.5.4 BABA Endoscopic Lateral Neck Dissection

The patients with suspicious metastatic lateral lymph node of papillary thyroid carcinoma were treated with BABA endoscopic and robotic thyroid surgery in Seoul National University since 2004. In the study of comparing 27 BABA endoscopic lateral neck dissection and 34 BABA robotic lateral neck dissection in Seoul National University Hospital between 2004 and 2009, the yields of lymph node were 3.26 ± 1.95 in central and 4.52 ± 3.65 in lateral compartment in endoscopic cases and 6.59 ± 4.55 and 5.82 ± 4.19 in robotic cases ($p=0.075, p=0.289$). Nine patients (33.3%) had central node metastases, and 5 patients (18.5%) had lateral node metastases in endoscopic cases; 12 patients (35.3%) and 6 patients (17.6%) in robotic cases, respectively ($p=0.517$, $p=0.808$). Mean operative time was 181.3 ± 45.4 min in endoscopic cases and 177.0 ± 33.7 min in robotic cases ($p=0.249$). During and after the operations, no significant blood loss or postoperative complications occurred, and no evidences of residual disease were found at follow-up (unpublished data).

16.5.5 External Branch of Superior Laryngeal Nerve

External branch of superior laryngeal nerve (EBSLN) is essential for maintaining good voice quality. In BABA endoscopic and robotic thyroid surgery with intraoperative neuromonitoring (IONM), 61% of EBSLN could be visualized and identified, and 29% of EBSLN could be identified with twitching of the cricothyroid muscles. The quality of voice of the patients was measured by using the voice handicap index-10 (VHI-10), and the results were statistically significant compared to the group without IONM of the EBSLN (unpublished data).

16.5.6 BABA Endoscopic Completion Thyroidectomy

Patients with a confirmed thyroid malignancy on permanent pathology after prior endoscopic thyroid lobectomy require completion thyroidectomy. The safety and feasibility of BABA endoscopic completion thyroidectomy were evaluated in the study of 13 patients after diagnosed with follicular or papillary carcinoma on permanent pathology in Seoul National University Hospital between 2006 and 2009 (Kim et al. 2010). The median interval between thyroid lobectomy and completion thyroidectomy was 5.6 months (range, 4.2–28.2 month). The mean operation time was 109.3 ± 23.3 min. There were no cases of converting to open surgery. There were six (46.2%) cases of transient hypocalcemia and restored within 2 postoperative weeks and there were no cases of vocal cord palsy. The flap elevation was not difficult in all cases because the flap adhesion was minimal. Preoperative CT scan or ultrasound is absolutely necessary to perform BABA endoscopic completion thyroidectomy, and the possibility of conversion to open surgery should be informed to the patient.

References

Brunt LM, Jones DB, Wu JS, Quasebarth MA, Meininger T, Soper NJ (1997) Experimental development of an endoscopic approach to neck exploration and parathyroidectomy. Surgery 122:893–901

Chung YS, Choe JH, Kang KH, Kim SW et al (2007) Endoscopic thyroidectomy for thyroid malignancies: comparison with conventional open thyroidectomy. World J Surg 31:2302–2306; discussion 7–8

Gottlieb A, Sprung J, Zheng XM, Gagner M (1997) Massive subcutaneous emphysema and severe hypercarbia in a patient during endoscopic transcervical parathyroidectomy using carbon dioxide insufflation. Anesth Analg 84: 1154–1156

Kim SJ, Lee KE, Choe JH, Lee J et al (2010) Endoscopic completion thyroidectomy by the bilateral axillo breast approach. Surg Laparosc Endosc Percutan Tech 20:312–316

Yeung GH (2002) Endoscopic thyroid surgery today: a diversity of surgical strategies. Thyroid 12:703–706

Other Minimally Invasive Thyroidectomy Techniques Using Remote Skin Incision Outside of the Neck

Sang-Wook Kang and Woong Youn Chung

17.1 Introduction

From the beginning of twenty-first century, with the raised socioeconomic status of the global people, they can afford to think about the other things more than the struggling to survive. The "well-being" of life has been the main issues of present-day life, and these trends have greatly influenced on the medical area also. Many surgical therapeutic plans for the diseases had been changed as the risk stratification–matched treatment with consideration into the patient's quality of life without any confliction of their treatment outcomes.

Nowadays, the factors of postoperative pain or discomfort, cosmetic problems of operation scar, and time to the work after the operation have also been important considerations in surgical result, as well as treatment outcomes. With this concept, since the late twentieth century, the endoscopic and minimally invasive surgical techniques have been remarkably advanced with the development of surgical instruments.

In the thyroid and parathyroid surgeries, the endoscopic and minimally invasive techniques have been lately introduced mainly due to the anatomical limitations: no preformed working space, abundant blood supply to the target organ, and critical location of target organ which is surrounded by major vessels and nerves.

Just after the first report of endoscopic parathyroidectomy by Gagner (1996) in 1996 and video-assisted thyroid lobectomy by Hüscher et al. (1997) in 1997, various methods of endoscopic thyroidectomy have been serially introduced during the past decade (Shimazu et al. 2003; Shimizu et al. 1998, 1999; Kitagawa et al. 2003; Ikeda et al. 2000a, b, 2002; Ohgami et al. 2000; Gagner and Inabnet 2001; Inabnet et al. 2003; Miccoli et al. 2000, 2001; Kim et al. 2001; Park et al. 2003; Yoon et al. 2006; Kang et al. 2009; Bärlehner and Benhidjeb 2008; Miyano et al. 2008; Koh et al. 2009, 2010; Choe et al. 2007; Chung et al. 2007; Lee et al. 2009). Shimizu et al. (1998, 1999; Kitagawa et al. 2003) had introduced video-assisted neck surgery (VANS) using gasless technique in 1998, and Ikeda et al. (2000a, b, 2002) using axillary approach and Ohgami et al. (2000) using breast approach have introduced their own methods in 2000. For the better cosmetic results, each endoscopic thyroidectomy has used various approaching routes such as cervical (minimally invasive video-assisted thyroidectomy, MIVAT) (Gagner and Inabnet 2001; Inabnet et al. 2003; Miccoli et al. 2000, 2001), anterior chest wall (Shimizu et al. 1998, 1999; Kitagawa et al. 2003; Kim et al. 2001), breast (Ohgami et al. 2000; Park et al. 2003), axillary (Ikeda et al. 2000a, b, 2002; Yoon et al. 2006; Kang et al. 2009), axillo-bilateral-breast (ABBA) (Shimazu et al. 2003; Bärlehner and Benhidjeb 2008), bilateral axillary (Miyano et al. 2008), unilateral axillo-breast (Koh et al. 2009, 2010), bilateral axillo-breast (BABA) (Choe et al. 2007; Chung et al. 2007), and postauricular and axillary approaches (Lee et al. 2009). And for the creation of working space, continuous CO_2 gas insufflation method and gasless method using external retractor have been applied. These various approaching routes and methods for sustaining working space have each own advantages and pitfalls, so no one can confirmatively say yet which

S.-W. Kang, M.D. (✉) • W.Y. Chung, M.D. Ph.D.
Department of Surgery, Yonsei University College of Medicine,
C.P.O. Box 8044, 50 Yonsei-ro, Seodaemun-gu, Seoul
120-752, South Korea
e-mail: oralvanco@yuhs.ac; woungyounc@yuhs.ac

technique is better and optimal. However, with the relapse of time and experiences, more comfortable and efficient methods are favored and widely used by the beginner surgeons. These days, MIVAT, BABA, and axillary approaches have been the most commonly used method for endoscopic thyroidectomy (Ikeda et al. 2000a, b, 2002; Miccoli et al. 2000, 2001; Yoon et al. 2006; Kang et al. 2009; Koh et al. 2009, 2010; Choe et al. 2007; Chung et al. 2007), and the others remained as fringe methods of MIT.

In this chapter, the author would introduce the no-mainstream methods of MIT using outside of the neck incision and describe their benefits.

17.2 Anterior Approach

Anterior approach means that the incision is made in the anterior chest area, and main instruments are accessed through the anterior chest route. In 1998, the Japanese surgeon Shimizu et al. have firstly described the gasless method of MIT using the anterior chest wall area incision and termed the technique as video-assisted neck surgery (VANS) (Shimizu et al. 1998, 1999; Kitagawa et al. 2003). In terms of working space maintenance, this techniques is the first method of endoscopic thyroidectomy using gasless method (anterior neck skin lifting using two pieces of Kirschner wire which are inserted horizontally) (Fig. 17.1). In 2001, Kim et al. also reported similar MIT method using gasless, anterior chest wall approach. They used different types of external retractor for sustaining of working space, and all the incisions for trocar are made in the anterior chest area (Fig. 17.2) (Kim et al. 2001). These gasless endoscopic methods have no risk of complications such as hypercapnia, respiratory acidosis, tachycardia, subcutaneous emphysema, and air embolism that can occur in CO_2 gas insufflation method (Shimizu et al. 1998, 1999; Kitagawa et al. 2003). Furthermore, gasless method can avoid the camera view disturbance by the smoke or fume occurred in electrical cautery and ultrasonic shear uses and also prevent easy disruption of the working space by the suction for bleeding or smoke clearance (Shimizu et al. 1998, 1999; Kitagawa et al. 2003; Yoon et al. 2006; Kang et al. 2009). Gasless method also allows relatively larger working space to the gas insufflation method, and large tumor of thyroid gland can be managed by this method (Shimizu et al. 1998, 1999; Kitagawa et al. 2003).

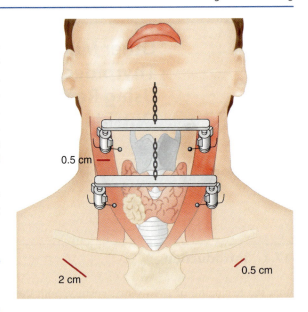

Fig. 17.1 The schematic illustration of the trochar accesses for the VANS methods

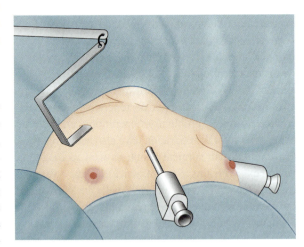

Fig. 17.2 The schematic illustration of the trochar accesses for anterior approach (Method of Kim et al. 2001)

The authors also emphasized on the merits of cosmetic effect as well. The main incision of this technique is made on the anterior chest area, so the scar is completely hidden even by widely open-neck clothes. Though VANS method uses 0.5-cm incision on the lateral side of the neck, it is almost inconspicuous within a few months (Shimizu et al. 1998, 1999; Kitagawa et al. 2003).

Because main incision is relatively close to the anterior neck area comparing to the other endoscopic methods, in the urgent situations which is difficult to be managed by endoscopic instruments, some parts of the procedure can be performed under the direct naked-eye view with instruments for open surgery.

17.2.1 Operative Technique (VANS Method) (Shimizu et al. 1998, 1999)

The main skin incision is made about 1.5 cm below the lesion-side clavicle, and it is normally covered by open-necked clothes. Through this incision, the main operative procedure is performed using Harmonic scalpel (Johnson & Johnson, Cincinnati, OH). Two other 0.5-cm incisions are made, one similarly placed as first incision but below the opposite clavicle and the other on the lateral part of the neck on the tumor side. A 5-mm grasper and an endoscope can be inserted through all the trochars depending on the stage of the operation. After a wide subplatysmal flap dissection, two pieces of Kirschner wire (1.2 mm in diameter) are inserted horizontally in the subcutaneous layer of the anterior neck. These are then lifted up and fixed to an L-shaped pole to create a tent-like working space. After making working space, both the sternohyoid muscle and the omohyoid muscle are divided on the inside of the sternocleidomastoid muscle (SCM). The ipsilateral sternohyoid and sternothyroid muscles are horizontally divided to create a wider operating field. With the grasper, the thyroid lobe can be gently mobilized cephalad, caudad, medially, and laterally. The superior and inferior thyroid vessels are ligated and cut. This permitted full mobilization of the lesion-side thyroid gland with the recurrent laryngeal nerve totally exposed. After dividing the isthmus, the one lobe of thyroid gland is completely resected and delivered out. The lymph node clearance is carried out in the central compartment from the prelaryngeal, pretracheal, and paratracheal area.

17.3 Breast Approach

In 2000, Ohgami et al. (2000) firstly introduced new endoscopic thyroidectomy method using breast approach. They had applied low-pressure CO_2 insufflation (6 mmHg) for the maintenance of working space and were able to obtain a satisfactory operative view. Through the low-pressure CO_2 insufflation methods, they could have the stable hemodynamics during the surgery and avoid massive subcutaneous emphysema, severe hypercarbia, and severe tachycardia. Through the application of a loose rubber bandage around the mandible during surgery, they just experienced only minimal emphysema around the neck without extension of subcutaneous emphysema to the face (Ohgami et al. 2000). Two years later, Park et al. also reported the same approach method with the large volume of experiences and showed the technical feasibility and satisfactory cosmetic effect (Park et al. 2003).

Comparing to the previous endoscopic thyroid surgery techniques such as cervical approach and VANS, breast approach method has sensational superiorities in terms of cosmesis. In the breast approach methods, the incision scars were minimal and completely hidden by the usual underwears. So, all the authors emphasized on the great benefit of esthetics using this method (Ohgami et al. 2000; Park et al. 2003).

The limitations of this method are as follows: (1) this method approaches from relatively remote accesses which is located lower part of the thyroid gland, so central neck node dissection for the thyroid cancer is not easy due to the disturbance of the clavicles; (2) the range of eligible instruments motion is narrow because the distances between each trocar accesses is short; (3) the scar in the parasternal area has much tendency to be changed to the hypertrophic scar; and (4) nipple deformities and hypesthesia could occur through the supra-circumareolar incision scar (Shimazu et al. 2003; Bärlehner and Benhidjeb 2008).

17.3.1 Operative Technique (Method of Park et al. 2003)

Patient is placed in the supine position with the neck extended with a shoulder pillow. A rubber bandage is applied loosely around the mandible to prevent subcutaneous emphysema from extending to the face during surgery. Diluted (1:200,000) epinephrine solution is injected into the subcutaneous space in the breast and subplatysmal space in the neck to reduce bleeding during the blunt dissection. Two incisions are made, on both upper circumareolar areas. Through these openings, subcutaneous and subplatysmal dissections are performed bluntly with use of a Rochester clamp and Dingman dissector. After the dissection is done to the designed area, the ports (12 and 15 mm) are inserted.

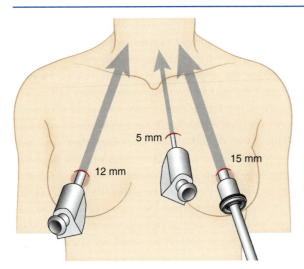

Fig. 17.3 The schematic illustration of the trochar accesses for the breast approach

The 15-mm port is put on the side of the thyroid mass, and the flexible endoscope is introduced through this port. The 12-mm port is used for the operational instruments. The working space is maintained with CO_2 insufflation at a pressure up to 6 mmHg. The remaining dissection is completed with the visual guidance of the endoscope. After the working space is set up, a 5-mm third port is inserted through the incision 3 cm below the clavicle on the side of the thyroid mass (Fig. 17.3). The dissection proceeds to the space between the anterior border of the SCM muscle and lateral border of strap muscle.

Dissection of the thyroid starts at the lower pole and proceeds to the posterior and lateral aspects of the gland. The authors used an ultrasonic shears for most of the dissections, without using endosurgical clips.

After lobectomy of thyroid gland, the resected specimen is inserted into a plastic bag and retrieved through the 15-mm port or 12-mm port. Closed suction drain is left in the operative place, and the skin is reapproximated cosmetically.

17.4 Axillo-Bilateral Breast Approach (ABBA)

Axillo-bilateral breast approach (ABBA) is the method of endoscopic thyroidectomy which uses lesion-side axillary skin incision and bilateral circumareolar incisions for the trocar accesses. This method is firstly introduced by Shimazu et al. in 2002 and is designed to overcome the limitations of breast approach with maintenance of the cosmetic excellences in the breast approach (Shimazu et al. 2003). In breast approach, the circumareolar incisions become inconspicuous several weeks after the surgery; however, the incision at the parasternal port site often becomes a hypertrophic scar. Furthermore, the range of instruments motion in breast approach is also narrow due to the short distances between each access. This pitfall can cause the limited viewing angle and the frequent interferences of the endoscope and surgical instruments during the surgery (Shimazu et al. 2003; Bärlehner and Benhidjeb 2008).

By converting the port site from the parasternal area to the axilla on the lesion side, the most promising cosmetic results can be obtained, because this method leaves no incision scars in the neck and upper anterior chest area. The lateral view from the axillary port makes it easy to observe the upper pole of the thyroid gland and identify the whole course of recurrent laryngeal nerve contrary to the breast approach (Shimazu et al. 2003; Bärlehner and Benhidjeb 2008). ABBA method also does some kind of bridge role to the development of the bilateral axillo-breast approach (BABA) for the bilateral total thyroidectomy.

However, this method also uses the circumareolar incisions, and there can be some other problems such as nipple deformity or hypesthesia. In the western countries, breast and nipples are regarded as important sexual organs, and they have some symbolic meanings more than just lactations. This is why many of western surgeons are reluctant to use the breast and nipples as the route for the surgery of thyroid disease even though excellent cosmesis.

Although some experiences about the breast approach and ABBA methods for MIT are still reported from China and some other Asian countries (Zhang et al. 2011; Irawati 2010), this approach needs careful modifications to gain the wide acceptances from the Western countries.

17.4.1 Operative Technique (Method of Shimazu et al. 2003)

Patient is placed in the supine position with the neck extended using a shoulder pillow, and the lesion-side arm is lifted up with a sterile cover to extend the axilla. A 2.5-cm incision is made along the upper margin of the areola on the tumor side. After blunt dissection of the subcutaneous tissue of the breast, a subplatysmal

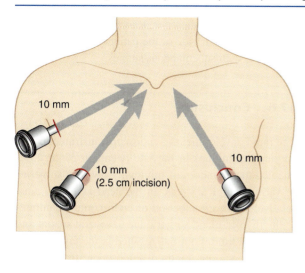

Fig. 17.4 The schematic illustration of the trochar accesses for the ABBA

working space is created with a balloon dissector. Following insertion of a 10-mm trocar through the incision, the working space is inflated with CO_2 gas at a pressure of 4–6 mmHg, and a 10-mm telescope is inserted through the trochar. Two additional 10-mm trochars are inserted through the incision at the lesion-side axilla and through the supra-circumareolar incision of the opposite breast, respectively (Fig. 17.4). The working space is made widely to the level of thyroid cartilage in the upper side and to the medial border of each of the SCM muscles in the lateral sides. Then, the strap muscles and SCM muscle are separated, and the strap muscles on the tumor side are transected using an ultrasonic shears.

After exposure of the thyroid gland, actual thyroidectomy is performed by the similar manners to the other methods.

The resected specimen is removed outside in a plastic bag, and no drainage tube is inserted. The divided strap muscles are sutured with absorbable suture materials, and the skin incisions are closed by subcutaneous sutures.

17.5 Bilateral Transaxillary Endoscopic Approach (BAEA)

Endoscopic thyroidectomy using transaxillary approach is firstly introduced by Ikeda et al. in 2000 (Ikeda et al. 2000a, b, 2002). This transaxillary approach for endoscopic thyroidectomy is the method that all the three trochars are inserted through the unilateral axillary area with CO_2 gas insufflation. This approach had been the cornerstones of the other transaxillary endoscopic thyroidectomies: bilateral transaxillary endoscopic approach (BAEA), unilateral axillo-breast approach without gas insufflations, and gasless transaxillary approach (Yoon et al. 2006; Kang et al. 2009; Miyano et al. 2008; Koh et al. 2009, 2010). In this transaxillary approach, the surgeon can approach the lateral aspect of the thyroid gland, and he can easily manipulate the superior and inferior pole of thyroid gland and identify the parathyroid and recurrent laryngeal nerve with ease (Ikeda et al. 2000a, b, 2002; Yoon et al. 2006; Kang et al. 2009). The surgeon also can perform complete central compartment neck dissection (from the carotid artery to the substernal notch and prelaryngeal area) in malignant tumor patients without any difficulty. In addition, the cosmetic result of this method is better than that of cervical or anterior chest wall approach because the operation scar remains in the axillary area which is covered with the arm in natural position (Ikeda et al. 2000a, b, 2002). However, this transaxillary approach has some technical limitations. Because all the trochars are introduced through the narrow axillary entrance, the discordance of each surgical instruments in the operation field (so-called sword fighting) is a considerable problem (Ikeda et al. 2000a, b, 2002). This problem can be resolved by second small incision (medial side of the anterior chest wall (similar area of VANS initial incision) 5-mm trocar) which enables multiangular approach and comfortable manipulation of endoscopic instruments (Yoon et al. 2006; Kang et al. 2009). Another major pitfall is the difficulty in contralateral lobectomy (Ikeda et al. 2000a, b, 2002; Miyano et al. 2008). Using unilateral transaxillary approach, bilateral total thyroidectomy is possible, but it is demanding and needs much skillful techniques (needs steep learning curve). To overcome these limitations, BAEA was developed by Miyano et al. in 2007 (Miyano et al. 2008). This method could conserve all the advantages of unilateral transaxillary approach, and furthermore enables even the beginner surgeons to perform bilateral total thyroidectomy without difficulty. The main problem of this method is it is a too time-consuming procedure. For the bilateral total thyroidectomy, BAEA needs separate two axillary approaching routes, and it takes too much time comparing to that of unilateral approach. The factor that two experienced surgeons and two independent endoscopic units are necessary is also an especially challenging barrier to the adoption of BAEA (Miyano et al. 2008).

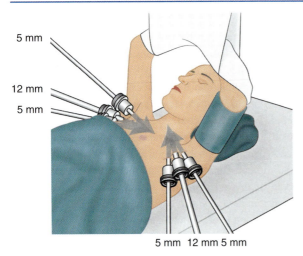

Fig. 17.5 The schematic illustration of the trochar accesses for the BAEA

17.5.1 Operative Technique (Method of Miyano et al. 2008)

The patient is positioned supine with a small roll placed beneath the shoulders to extend the neck slightly. After the patient is prepared and draped, two teams started simultaneously, one from each axilla.

Incisions for two lateral 5-mm operating trochars and one centrally placed 12-mm trocar for the camera are made in each bilateral anterior axillary fold (Fig. 17.5). Using finger dissection, a subcutaneous plane is developed anterior to the pectoralis fascia. Once the space is sufficiently large, all the trochars are inserted on each side, and the dissection proceeds under CO_2 insufflation to 10 mmHg with a Harmonic scalpel dissecting from lateral to medial toward the thyroid. A 0° or 30° telescope is used as the dissection progressed. Dissection is carried out to the SCM muscle and the thyroid gland on both sides. The clavicular head of the SCM muscles is partially divided to facilitate the inferior portion of the dissection. The deep cervical fascia is then identified, and dissection continues cephalad from the junction of the SCM to expose the omohyoid muscle. The space is further developed medially until the middle thyroid vein is encountered. This is divided with a Ligasure (Valleylab, Boulder, CO) for hemostasis. After exposure of the lateral aspect of the thyroid gland, the last thyroidectomy procedures are similar to the others. The specimen is extracted intact through one of the axillary port sites. A 7 F Petite Wound drainage system (Axiom Medical Inc, Rancho Dominguez, CA) is placed on either side of the patient, and the wounds are closed with subcutaneous sutures.

17.6 Conclusion

The rapid development of endoscopic instruments and surgical techniques in the late twentieth century has enabled the advances of minimally invasive surgeries in various surgical areas. In the head and neck area, relatively delayed adoption of endoscopic techniques to the thyroid gland surgery due to several spatial and anatomical limitations has resulted in the faster development of various kinds of endoscopic thyroidectomies based on the other organs experiences. All of these endoscopic methods have their own superiorities and pitfalls to the other methods according to the approach routes and ways to maintain working space.

Although the techniques described in this chapter are minor methods for the MIT, all of these procedures are technically feasible and safe and have definite their own merits. Furthermore, many surgeons still perform MIT using these techniques. If the complementary modifications are achieved based on each methods' pros and cons, the optimal minimally invasive surgical techniques not only for the thyroid but also for the other organs in the head and neck area can be developed in the near future.

Sources of Financial Support The authors have no conflict of interest to declare.

References

Bärlehner E, Benhidjeb T (2008) Cervical scarless endoscopic thyroidectomy: axillo-bilateral-breast approach (ABBA). Surg Endosc 22(1):154–157

Choe JH, Kim SW, Chung KW, Park KS, Han W, Noh DY, Oh SK, Youn YK (2007) Endoscopic thyroidectomy using a new bilateral axillo-breast approach. World J Surg 31(3):601–606

Chung YS, Choe JH, Kang KH, Kim SW, Chung KW, Park KS, Han W, Noh DY, Oh SK, Youn YK (2007) Endoscopic thyroidectomy for thyroid malignancies: comparison with conventional open thyroidectomy. World J Surg 31(12):2302–2306

Gagner M (1996) Endoscopic subtotal parathyroidectomy in patients with primary hyperparathyroidism. Br J Surg 83:875

Gagner M, Inabnet WB 3rd (2001) Endoscopic thyroidectomy for solitary thyroid nodules. Thyroid 11:161–164

Hüscher CSG, Chiodini S, Napolitano C, Recher A (1997) Endoscopic right thyroid lobectomy. Surg Endosc 11:877

Ikeda Y, Takami H, Sasaki Y, Kan S, Niimi M (2000a) Endoscopic resection of thyroid tumors by the axillary approach. J Cardiovasc Surg (Torino) 41:791–792

Ikeda Y, Takami H, Sasaki Y, Kan S, Niimi M (2000b) Endoscopic neck surgery by the axillary approach. J Am Coll Surg 191:336–340

Ikeda Y, Takami H, Sasaki Y, Takayama J, Niimi M, Kan S (2002) Comparative study of thyroidectomies. Endoscopic surgery versus conventional open surgery. Surg Endosc 16(112):1741–1745

Inabnet WB 3rd, Jacob BP, Gagner M (2003) Minimally invasive endoscopic thyroidectomy by a cervical approach. Surg Endosc 17:1808–1811

Irawati N (2010) Endoscopic right lobectomy axillary-breast approach: a report of two cases. Int J Otolaryngol 2010:958764

Kang SW, Jeong JJ, Yun JS, Sung TY, Lee SC, Lee YS, Nam KH, Chang HS, Chun WY, Park CS (2009) Gasless endoscopic thyroidectomy using trans-axillary approach; surgical outcome of 581 patients. Endocr J 56(3):361–369

Kim JS, Kim KH, Ahn CH, Jeon HM, Kim EG, Jeon CS (2001) A clinical analysis of gasless endoscopic thyroidectomy. Surg Laparosc Endosc Percutan Tech 11:268–272

Kitagawa W, Shimizu K, Akasu H, Tanaka S (2003) Endoscopic neck surgery with lymph node dissection for papillary carcinoma of the thyroid using a totally gasless anterior neck skin lifting method. J Am Coll Surg 196:990–994

Koh YW, Kim JW, Lee SW, Choi EC (2009) Endoscopic thyroidectomy via a unilateral axillo-breast approach without gas insufflation for unilateral benign thyroid lesions. Surg Endosc 23(9):2053–2060

Koh YW, Park JH, Kim JW, Lee SW, Choi EC (2010) Endoscopic hemithyroidectomy with prophylactic ipsilateral central neck dissection via an unilateral axillo-breast approach without gas insufflation for unilateral micropapillary thyroid carcinoma: preliminary report. Surg Endosc 24(1):188–197

Lee KE, Kim HY, Park WS, Choe JH, Kwon MR, Oh SK, Youn YK (2009) Postauricular and axillary approach endoscopic neck surgery: a new technique. World J Surg 33(4):767–772

Miccoli P, Berti P, Bendinelli C, Conte M, Fasolini F, Martino E (2000) Minimally invasive video-assisted surgery of the thyroid: a preliminary report. Langenbecks Arch Surg 385:261–364

Miccoli P, Berti P, Raffaelli M, Conte M, Materazzi G, Galleri D (2001) Minimally invasive video-assisted thyroidectomy. Am J Surg 181(6):567–570

Miyano G, Lobe TE, Wright SK (2008) Bilateral transaxillary endoscopic total thyroidectomy. J Pediatr Surg 43(2):299–303

Ohgami M, Ishii S, Arisawa Y, Ohmori T, Noga K, Furukawa T et al (2000) Scarless endoscopic thyroidectomy: breast approach for better cosmesis. Surg Laparosc Endosc Percutan Tech 10:1–4

Park YL, Han WK, Bae WG (2003) 100 cases of endoscopic thyroidectomy: breast approach. Surg Laparosc Endosc Percutan Tech 13(1):20–25

Shimazu K, Shiba E, Tamaki Y, Takiguchi S, Taniguchi E, Ohashi S et al (2003) Endoscopic thyroid surgery through the axillo-bilateral breast approach. Surg Laparosc Endosc 13:196–201

Shimizu K, Akira S, Tanaka S (1998) Video-assisted neck surgery: endoscopic resection of benign thyroid tumor aiming at scarless surgery on the neck. J Surg Oncol 69(3):178–180

Shimizu K, Akira S, Jasmi AY, Kitamura Y, Kitagawa W, Akasu H et al (1999) Video-assisted neck surgery: endoscopic resection of thyroid tumors with a very minimal neck wound. J Am Coll Surg 188:697–703

Yoon JH, Park CH, Chung WY (2006) Gasless endoscopic thyroidectomy via an axillary approach: experience of 30 cases. Surg Laparosc Endosc Percutan Tech 16:226–231

Zhang W, Jiang DZ, Liu S, Li LJ, Zheng XM, Shen HL, Shan CX, Qiu M (2011) Current status of endoscopic thyroid surgery in China. Surg Laparosc Endosc Percutan Tech 21(2):67–71

Robotic Facelift Thyroidectomy

David J. Terris and Michael C. Singer

18.1 Introduction

18.1.1 Evolution of Robotic Thyroidectomy

Thyroid surgery has evolved considerably over the last 10–15 years. After more than 100 years of doing a thyroidectomy essentially the way it was described by Theodore Kocher, a number of innovative techniques have emerged. Originally, these principally involved smaller incisions in a cervical location. Michel Gagner is credited with being the first to describe an endoscopic endocrine procedure in 1996 (Naitoh et al. 1998). However, Paolo Miccoli and his group in Pisa pioneered and then perfected a minimally invasive video-assisted cervical approach which has been embraced by high-volume centers throughout the world (Miccoli et al. 2004). At the same time as these techniques were being refined, surgeons located primarily in Asian countries explored the possibility of remote access endoscopic techniques. Ikeda at Teikyo University developed a totally endoscopic axillary insufflation-based approach (Ikeda et al. 2001). Others focused on access portals located in the anterior chest wall (Wang et al. 2009), the postauricular region (Lee et al. 2009), and in the breast and/or areolar location (Choe et al. 2007). While these numerous techniques were effective, they were tedious to perform and lengthy operations.

In 2009, Woong Youn Chung successfully married robotic technology with endoscopic remote access approaches to the thyroid compartment (Kang et al. 2009a). He very quickly demonstrated that these procedures could be done in a high-volume, safe, and efficient manner in a Korean population (Kang et al. 2009b). This generated tremendous enthusiasm in other parts of Asia and eventually in North America. However, the extrapolation of this technique to the United States was associated with the introduction of a substantial number of severe complications (Kuppersmith and Holsinger 2011; Landry et al. 2011).

18.1.2 Comparing American and Asian Patients

It became clear that application of the Chung robotic axillary thyroidectomy technique in American patients poses substantial challenges. This is likely because of the difference in the size of the patients, the size of their necks, and the size of the thyroid diseases being managed. The obesity epidemic in the United States is widely recognized. In addition, the average height of the patients is substantially greater than that in most Asian populations. Finally, because of the uniqueness of the Korean health system, many patients

D.J. Terris, M.D., FACS (✉)
Department of Otolaryngology, Georgia Health Thyroid/Parathyroid Center, Georgia Health Sciences University, 1120 Fifteenth Street, BP-4109, Augusta, GA 30912-4060, USA

Department of Otolaryngology – Head and Neck Surgery, Georgia Health Sciences University, Augusta, GA, USA
e-mail: dterris@georgiahealth.edu

M.C. Singer, M.D.
Department of Otolaryngology – Head and Neck Surgery, Georgia Health Sciences University, Augusta, GA, USA

have subclinical thyroid disease and even microcarcinomas that are being identified very early and managed surgically. By contrast, the American population has larger patients, larger overall surgical thyroid disease, and larger necks. Among the dramatic complications that have been witnessed in the United States included many instances of brachial plexopathy and arm paralysis. There were a number of esophageal perforations and even esophageal transection. There were patients where thyroid disease was inadvertently left behind, or was unable to be adequately exposed. Severe blood loss exceeding a liter has occurred in more than one case.

For these reasons, and others, the Chung thyroidectomy was abandoned in many centers in the United States. Nevertheless, there is clearly a demand for remote access techniques among the American population.

18.1.3 Emergence of Multiple Techniques and Principles

A number of important principles to consider when pursuing remote access surgery have been identified. A gasless technique is particularly important because there is no well-contained cavity within the thyroid compartment. A superior to inferior approach has been noted to be a suitable vector of dissection of the thyroid compartment (Terris et al. 2004). Robotic and endoscopic magnification and maneuverability have been demonstrated to be useful for any surgery in a confined space, such as the pelvis or the thyroid compartment (Terris and Amin 2008). Finally, we and subsequently others have reported the value of a facelift approach to the neck which results in a completely concealed incision (Terris et al. 1994).

We therefore set out to deliberately develop a hybrid surgical technique that draws from the benefits of each of these principles.

18.1.4 Procedure Development

A series of preclinical experiments has been undertaken in an animal and a cadaver model. In a porcine model, a variety of access points to the thyroid compartment were explored, including supraclavicular, axillary, and superior approaches. The superior to

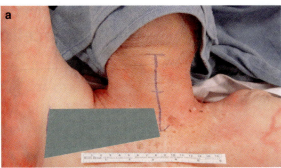
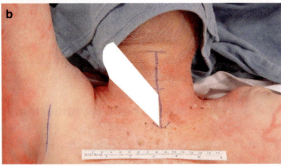

Fig. 18.1 The area of dissection required for a robotic axillary thyroidectomy (**a**) and a robotic facelift thyroidectomy (**b**) were calculated and found to be consistently greater with the axillary technique (by 38% on average) (Printed with permission from Singer et al. (2011))

inferior approach was determined to be the easiest and fastest for an endoscopic thyroidectomy (Terris et al. 2004).

Subsequent cadaveric experiments were undertaken to specifically explore a facelift access point (Singer et al. 2011). The optimal planes of dissection were explored, and the visualization of the thyroid compartment confirmed. A series of endoscopic and then robotic thyroidectomies was undertaken in a cadaver model successfully. A mannequin model was utilized to determine the precise and optimal location of the robot relative to the operating table and the positioning of the robotic arms.

Finally, a direct comparison of the area of dissection required for both a robotic axillary thyroidectomy (RAT) and the robotic facelift thyroidectomy (RFT) was undertaken (Singer et al. 2011). The RAT was found to require 38% greater area of dissection than the RFT (Fig. 18.1), representing important implications regarding time of surgery and rate of wound healing.

18.2 Selection Criteria

18.2.1 Patient Selection

The selection criteria for the robotic facelift thyroidectomy remain strict. There are both disease characteristics and patient characteristics that drive eligibility. Since the procedure is early in its development, we have been careful to reserve this procedure for patients with presumed benign disease who require unilateral surgery. The largest nodule should not exceed 30–35 mm in greatest dimension. The absence of thyroiditis is preferred, and there should be no substernal extension (Terris et al. 2011a).

The criteria that relate to the patient include non-morbidly obese individuals who can withstand a longer anesthetic than is required for conventional surgery. Perhaps the most important factor is that the patient should be motivated to completely eliminate a neck scar, as this represents the principal advantage of remote access surgery. The patient should be fully informed of the risks of the procedure, including the expectation of hypesthesia in the region of the greater auricular nerve.

18.2.2 Surgeon Selection

Because endoscopic and remote access surgery is more challenging than conventional techniques, surgeons wishing to pursue these procedures should have substantial experience in thyroid surgery with ongoing high surgical volumes. While there is no absolute cut-off, a thyroid practice in which more than 50 cases per year are performed is desirable.

18.2.3 Proper Training

In addition to possessing experience and advanced skills in thyroid surgery, surgeons who pursue robotic thyroidectomy should undergo considerable training in order to forge a short learning curve. At a minimum, this requires significant familiarity with robotic technology and the subtleties of both the surgeon console and the robotic arms. There should be exposure to both animate and inanimate simulation. Ideally, practice in a fresh cadaver model should be undertaken. Case observation and proctoring may also be helpful. After embarking upon a robotic thyroidectomy program, vigilance should be maintained regarding the outcomes.

18.3 Procedural Details

18.3.1 Anesthesia Considerations

The anesthesiologist is a fundamental member of the robotic thyroidectomy team and should be included in early planning of a robotic program. Several precautions can be taken to ensure safe and efficient procedures. These include use of anesthesia circuit extenders to facilitate maneuvering of the table. Laryngeal nerve monitoring is usually performed, and intubation using a Glidescope device helps to ensure proper positioning of the laryngeal EMG tube. The operating table should be rotated 180° away from the anesthesia cart after induction of anesthesia and intubation. We prefer a propofol drip and the absence of relaxation to facilitate nerve monitoring and to carefully titrate the depth of anesthesia.

Deep extubation at the completion of the procedure helps to minimize the likelihood of coughing and bucking on the tube which may prompt venous oozing. Liberal use of antiemetic agents is important to reduce the likelihood of emesis in the early postoperative period which may raise the intrathoracic pressures, further predisposing to the possibility of bleeding.

18.3.2 Positioning

Probably the most important advantage of robotic facelift thyroidectomy compared to other remote access techniques is the ease of positioning (Terris et al. 2011b). The patient is allowed to remain supine on the operating table, and the head is turned approximately 30° away from the side of the thyroidectomy (Fig. 18.2). A cushion placed next to the head on the side contralateral to the side of surgery helps to prevent excessive rotation of the neck during the procedure. Routine padding of the arms is accomplished. No urinary catheter is necessary.

18.3.3 Open Dissection

An incision is premarked in the holding area and begins just behind the ear lobule and runs in the postauricular

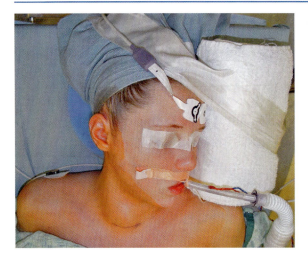

Fig. 18.2 The patient is positioned supine on the operating table, with the head turned 30° away from the side of the thyroidectomy with a cushion to prevent excessive rotation of the neck

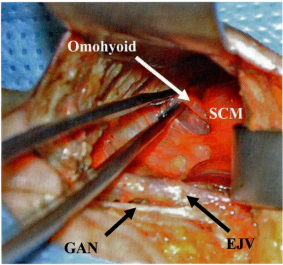

Fig. 18.4 A right-sided view of the open dissection necessary to expose the thyroid compartment. Easily seen are the greater auricular nerve (*GAN*), external jugular vein (*EJV*), sternocleidomastoid muscle (*SCM*), and the omohyoid muscle (Reprinted with permission from Terris et al. (2011a))

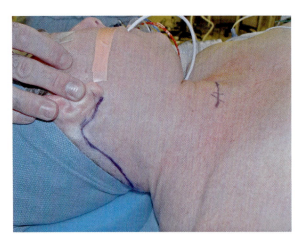

Fig. 18.3 The incision is made in the postauricular crease and extends into the occipital hairline so that it is completely hidden (Reprinted with permission from Terris et al. (2011b))

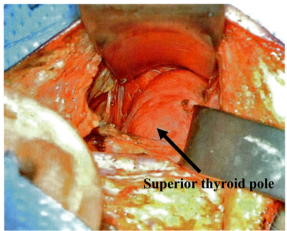

Fig. 18.5 Once the omohyoid, sternohyoid, and sternothyroid muscles are retracted ventrally, the superior pole of the right thyroid lobe becomes visible (Reprinted with permission from Terris et al. (2011a))

crease. It crosses into the occipital hairline at a point above where the incision will be hidden by the auricle and then extends down within the occipital hairline (Fig. 18.3). Once the patient is positioned at surgery, approximately 1 cm of hairline is clipped so that the incision may be completely hidden within the hair. The incision is infiltrated with quarter percent Marcaine with 1:200,000 of epinephrine. After sterile prepping and draping, the incision is made and carried down to the sternocleidomastoid muscle. A flap is elevated in the subcutaneous and then subplatysmal plane with care taken to stay ventral to the greater auricular nerve and then the external jugular vein (Fig. 18.4). The flap is extended along the length of the sternocleidomastoid muscle. The omohyoid muscle is identified and reflected ventrally. The sternohyoid and sternothyroid muscles are then reflected from lateral to medial exposing the upper pole of the thyroid gland (Fig. 18.5). These muscles are mobilized down to the sternum and

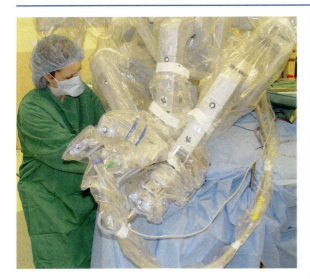

Fig. 18.6 The robot is deployed after a fixed retractor is properly placed. The camera is placed in the center of the field, a Maryland grasper is placed in the non-dominant hand, and the Harmonic is placed in the dominant hand (Reprinted with permission from Terris et al. (2011a))

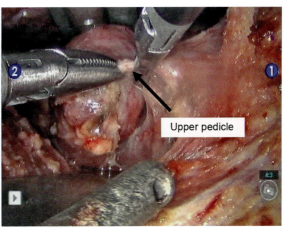

Fig. 18.7 Robotic view of the superior thyroid pedicle just prior to ligation (Reprinted with permission from Terris et al. (2011b))

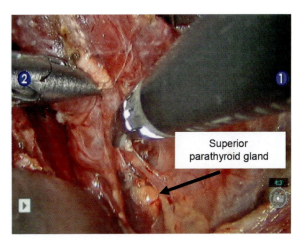

Fig. 18.8 The superior parathyroid gland is released posteriorly (Reprinted with permission from Terris et al. (2011b))

captured with a Chung retractor using a modified blade. The sternocleidomastoid muscle is retracted laterally using a Singer retractor fixed to the operating table.

18.3.4 Robotic Resection

The robot is deployed at this point. The pedestal of the patient side cart should be positioned opposite the side of the surgery and at an angle parallel to the long arm of the Chung retractor. The camera arm is positioned first utilizing a 30-degree down endoscope which is placed in the center just below the retractor and angled slightly upward. A Maryland dissector is placed in the non-dominant hand coming in laterally, and the Harmonic device is placed in the dominant hand also coming in from a lateral direction (Fig. 18.6).

Once these three arms are deployed, the procedure begins with mobilization of the superior pole and ligation of the upper pedicle as a single bundle (Fig. 18.7) using the Harmonic ACE device (Ethicon Endo-Surgery, Inc., Cincinnati, OH). The superior pole is reflected inferiorly exposing the inferior constrictor muscle. The superior parathyroid gland is seen at this point of the procedure and is dissected posterolaterally (Fig. 18.8). The superior pole is mobilized, and the superior laryngeal nerve is identified medially crossing on the inferior constrictor muscle (Fig. 18.9). When the inferior border of this muscle is reached, the recurrent laryngeal nerve can be identified laterally just prior to its entrance in the larynx (Fig. 18.10). Once this nerve is identified, the ligament of Berry can be safely divided, and the lateral attachments of the thyroid released. The isthmus is divided with the Harmonic (Fig. 18.11), and the middle thyroid vein is ligated. The inferior pole is fully mobilized, the inferior parathyroid gland is identified and dissected inferiorly away from the thyroid gland with its blood supply intact, and the inferior thyroid artery and veins are divided with the Harmonic device, completely freeing

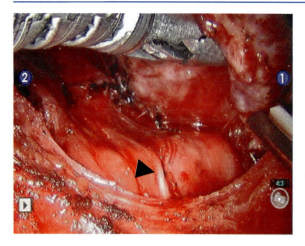

Fig. 18.9 The superior laryngeal nerve (*black arrowhead*) may be seen crossing over the inferior constrictor muscle (Reprinted with permission from Terris et al. (2011b))

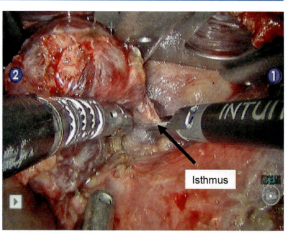

Fig. 18.11 The isthmus is divided with an ultrasonic energy device (Reprinted with permission from Terris et al. (2011b))

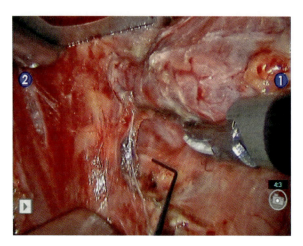

Fig. 18.10 The recurrent laryngeal nerve is identified in its most constant location, just prior to its entrance underneath the inferior constrictor muscle, and is shown being stimulated to confirm its identity (Reprinted with permission from Terris et al. (2011a))

up the thyroid lobe. Any remaining attachments to the trachea are divided, and the specimen is retrieved.

18.3.5 Closure

The wound is irrigated with saline, and absolute hemostasis is assured. A large sheet of Surgicel is placed in the thyroid bed, and the subcutaneous tissues are closed with interrupted sutures of 4-O Vicryl. Cyanoacrylate glue is placed on the skin, and quarter-inch steri-strips are placed on top of the glue to facilitate removal 3 weeks after the operation. The patient is extubated deep and taken to the recovery room.

18.3.6 Postoperative Management

Patients are observed in the recovery room for 60–90 min. Once they are awake and able to protect their airway, and assuming stable vital signs, they are transferred to the same-day surgery area. As long as they are taking liquids adequately and the pain is controlled, they are discharged to home.

Assuming unilateral surgery, patients are given pain medicine and antiemetics as needed and instructed to limit activities for 10–14 days. They may shower the evening of surgery. A return visit is scheduled 3–4 weeks after surgery, at which time the steri-strips are removed (taking with them most of the glue). Residual glue is carefully removed.

Patients who have undergone bilateral or completion surgery are prescribed a 3-week course of oral calcium supplementation beginning on the evening of surgery and counseled regarding the signs and symptoms of hypocalcemia.

Presuming normal postoperative healing, the patients are discharged back to their endocrinologist and instructed to avoid sun exposure for 6 months.

18.4 Clinical Experience

18.4.1 Patient Demographics

In a recently published series, a total of 18 RFT procedures were undertaken in 14 patients (Terris et al. 2011a). There were 13 females and one male with a mean age of 33.7 years. All but one of the patients were female. There were 13 lobectomies, one bilateral thyroidectomy and three completion thyroidectomies.

18.4.2 Results

All but the very first procedure were performed on an outpatient basis and without the use of a drain. There were no conversions to open surgery. The pathology consisted of two papillary cancers and one follicular cancer; the remaining lobes were benign and included four follicular adenomas, one Hurthle cell adenoma, nine cases of nodular hyperplasia, and one normal contralateral lobe. The operative times have ranged from 97 to 193 min, and a comparison of the early robotic axillary cases to the robotic facelift procedures in our center reveals a more favorable learning curve.

18.4.3 Complications

There was one episode of transient vocal fold dysfunction which resolved within 1 month. There were no permanent nerve injuries. There were two seromas which resolved promptly and without treatment. There were no cases of temporary or permanent hypoparathyroidism (in the four patients who underwent staged or simultaneous total thyroidectomy). All patients described temporary periauricular hypesthesia in the distribution of the greater auricular nerve which resolved within several weeks.

18.5 Future Directions

We have cautiously pursued robotic thyroidectomy using a facelift access point with excellent results and favorable patient satisfaction. Because of the limitations of the technology, unilateral surgery remains the preferred approach. As operative times continue to improve, and with advances in the technology, we anticipate routinely offering bilateral surgery. Furthermore, it is conceivable that surgery for low-risk thyroid cancer would be appropriate.

Because of the generous exposure of the lateral and central neck, it is conceivable that lymphadenectomy could be performed using this approach, as has been described for robotic axillary surgery. Prior to embarking on more advanced procedures, further experience at additional centers should be undertaken in order to validate this promising procedure.

References

Choe JH, Kim SW, Chung KW, Park KS, Han W, Noh DY, Oh SK, Youn YK (2007) Endoscopic thyroidectomy using a new bilateral axillo-breast approach. World J Surg 31(3):601–606

Ikeda Y, Takami H, Niimi M, Kan S, Sasaki Y, Takayama J (2001) Endoscopic thyroidectomy by the axillary approach. Surg Endosc 15(11):1362–1364

Kang SW, Jeong JJ, Yun JS, Sung TY, Lee SC, Lee YS, Nam KH, Chang HS, Chung WY, Park CS (2009a) Robot-assisted endoscopic surgery for thyroid cancer: experience with the first 100 patients. Surg Endosc 23(11):2399–2406

Kang SW, Lee SC, Lee SH, Lee KY, Jeong JJ, Lee YS, Nam KH, Chang HS, Chung WY, Park CS (2009b) Robotic thyroid surgery using a gasless, transaxillary approach and the da Vinci S system: the operative outcomes of 338 consecutive patients. Surgery 146(6):1048–1055

Kuppersmith RB, Holsinger FC (2011) Robotic thyroid surgery: an initial experience with North American patients. Laryngoscope 121(3):521–526

Landry CS, Grubbs EG, Morris GS, Turner NS, Holsinger FC, Lee JE, Perrier ND (2011) Robot assisted transaxillary surgery (RATS) for the removal of thyroid and parathyroid glands. Surgery 149(4):549–555

Lee KE, Kim HY, Park WS, Choe JH, Kwon MR, Oh SK, Youn YK (2009) Postauricular and axillary approach endoscopic neck surgery: a new technique. World J Surg 33(4):767–772

Miccoli P, Berti P, Materazzi G, Massi M, Picone A, Minuto MN (2004) Results of video-assisted parathyroidectomy: single institution's six-year experience. World J Surg 28(12):1216–1218

Naitoh T, Gagner M, Garcia-Ruiz A, Heniford BT (1998) Endoscopic endocrine surgery in the neck. An initial report of endoscopic subtotal parathyroidectomy. Surg Endosc 12(3):202–205

Singer MC, Seybt MW, Terris DJ (2011) Robotic facelift thyroidectomy: I. Pre-clinical simulation and morphometric assessment. Laryngoscope 121(8):1631–1635

Terris DJ, Amin SH (2008) Robotic and endoscopic surgery in the neck. Op TechE Otolaryngol Head Neck Surg 19(1):36–41

Terris DJ, Tuffo KM, Fee WE Jr (1994) Modified facelift incision for parotidectomy. J Laryngol Otol 108(7):574–578

Terris DJ, Nettar K, Ciecko S, Haus B, Gourin CG (2004) Prospective evaluation of endoscopic approaches to the thyroid compartment. Laryngoscope 114(8):1377–1382

Terris DJ, Singer MC, Seybt MW (2011a) Robotic facelift thyroidectomy: II. Clinical feasibility and safety. Laryngoscope 121(8):1636–1641

Terris DJ, Singer MC, Seybt MW (2011b) Robotic facelift thyroidectomy: patient selection and technical considerations. Surg Laparosc Endosc Percutan Tech 21(4):237–242

Wang M, Zhang T, Mao Z, Dong F, Li J, Lu A, Hu W, Zang L, Jiang Y, Zheng M (2009) Effect of endoscopic thyroidectomy via anterior chest wall approach on treatment of benign thyroid tumors. J Laparoendosc Adv Surg Tech A 19(2):149–152

Trans-oral Endoscopic Thyroidectomy

Thomas Wilhelm

19.1 Introduction

Since ancient times, surgical procedures were always associated with a laceration of the surface of the human body. The aim of surgeons at all times was to access the targeted area directly to perform proper and fast surgical procedures. This was even more important in times where anaesthesia, electrocautery and aseptic principles were not basic part of surgical procedures. Therefore, our forefathers have had an intimate knowledge about the separating layers of the body since in these layers an almost bloodless and gentle procedure is possible.

Regarding thyroid surgery, the most prominent protagonists were Christian Albert Theodor Billroth (born 26 April 1829 in Bergen, Germany; deceased 6 February 1894 in Abbazia, Istria) who worked in Zurich, Switzerland and later in Vienna, Austria and Emil Theodor Kocher (born 25 August 1841 in Bern, Switzerland; deceased 27 July 1917 in Bern, Switzerland). Billroth reduced the high mortality of thyroid surgery by adopting the principles of asepsis, anaesthesia and electrocautery for coagulation from 40% to 8% (DuBose et al. 2004). By gently developing the surgical technique, Kocher established the standards in thyroid surgery and decreased mortality down to 0.2% in over 7,000 surgeries performed by him.

Furthermore, he increased the knowledge about the endocrine basics of thyroid action and was finally awarded with the Nobel Prize in 1909 (Kocher 1909).

19.1.1 Complication Rate of Conventional Thyroid Surgery

19.1.1.1 Mortality

Due to refined surgical technique, minimized risks of anaesthesia and meanwhile standard use of intraoperative neuromonitoring, thyroidectomy is a safe procedure today. Depending on the underlying disease, the mortality rate in Germany in 2004 ranged from 0.01% to 0.13% (Helios Kliniken 2005). Mortality rate ranges from 0.2% in developed countries (Röher et al. 1999) to 2.4% reported from studie from third-world countries (Sano et al. 1995).

19.1.1.2 Peri- and Postoperative Haemorrhage

Despite these low mortality rates, thyroidectomy is associated with specific risks. These risks include especially peri- and postoperative haemorrhage which is observed in 0.3–4.9% of the cases (Dralle et al. 2004b; Frick and Largiader 1989; Tarafder et al. 2007). An analysis of pro- and retrospective studies published during the past two decades with 43,410 patients totally revealed a postoperative haemorrhage rate of 1.5% (Table 19.1).

19.1.1.3 Hypoparathyroidism

Hypocalcaemia due to resection of the parathyroid glands is reported to be the second most common complication following thyroidectomy: a temporary

---

T. Wilhelm, M.D.
Department of Otolaryngology, Head/Neck & Facial Plastic Surgery, HELIOS Klinikum Borna, Rudolf-Virchow-Straße 2, Borna D-04552, Germany
e-mail: thomas.wilhelm@helios-kliniken.de

Table 19.1 Postoperative local infections and haemorrhage following thyroidectomy (authors are sorted alphabetically)

Authors	Year	N	Local infection (%)	Haemorrhage (%)
Alvarado et al.	2008	1,054	0.6	1.0
Bhattacharyya and Fried	2002	517	0.2	1.0
Diclic et al.	2005	1,478	0.2	0.4
Frick and Largiader	1989	548	0.7	4.9
Gaujoux et al.	2006	5,141	0.3	1.7
Ignjatovic et al.	2003	2,138	0.9	1.1
Lefevre et al.	2007	685	0.2	0.9
Lucha et al.	2000	827	0.6	1.3
Röher et al.	1999	5,961	0.1	1.2
Rosato et al.	2004	14,934	0.3	1.2
Serpell and Phan	2007	336	1.5	0.9
Shaha and Jaffe	1988	200	1.0	
Spanknebel et al.	2005	1,025	0.1	0.5
Tarafder et al.	2007	93	2.2	4.4
Thomusch et al.	2000	7,266	0.6	2.7
Vincent	2008	1,207	1.2	1.5

hypocalcaemia is reported in up to 15.6% and permanent in up to 4.0% of the patients (Dralle et al. 2004b; Röher et al. 1999).

19.1.1.4 Vocal Cord Palsy

The greatest impact on the quality of life after thyroidectomy, however, is caused by vocal cord palsy as a result of a damage to or dissection of the recurrent laryngeal nerve (Rosato et al. 2005). For prevention of postoperative vocal cord palsy, the identification of the nerve during surgery is of great importance; according to a recent literature review (Dralle 2009), vocal cord arrest following thyroidectomy is observed permanently from 0.0% to 12.0% in cases without identification of the recurrent laryngeal nerve during surgery and is reduced to 0.0–3.8% when the nerve is routinely represented.

When pooling the data reported in different studies, temporarily unilateral vocal cord palsy was observed in 4.0% out of 62,784 cases whereas permanent vocal cord palsy occurred in 2.1% of the patients (Dralle et al. 2008; Lombardi et al. 2006; Röher et al. 1999; Rosato et al. 2004; Thomusch et al. 2000; Zornig et al. 1989). The integration of an intraoperative neuromonitoring system reduced the palsy rates dramatically. In a total of 19,250 pooled cases, temporarily vocal cord palsies were observed in 2.7%, and only 0.8% permanent palsies were reported (Brauckhoff et al. 2002; Chan et al. 2006; Dralle et al. 2004a; Robertson et al. 2004; Shindo and Chheda 2007; Yarbrough et al. 2004). In a prospective German multicenter trial, a significant reduction of postoperative vocal cord palsy could be demonstrated with the use of an intraoperative neuromonitoring system (Thomusch et al. 2000).

Unilateral vocal cord palsy results usually with proper compensation following logopaedic therapy only in reduced speech strength; the worst case is the bilateral dissection of the recurrent laryngeal nerve with consecutive acute dyspnoea in rest: this requires in almost all cases a permanent tracheostomy. But fortunately, these outcomes are rare and depend on the surgery performed (partial or total resection); it is reported in 0.1–0.6% of the cases (Rosato et al. 2004).

The additional use of a microscope during thyroidectomy decreased the rate of postoperative vocal cord palsy down to 0.6% which may be attributed to the magnification of the microscope and the therefore better identification of relevant anatomical structures (Nielsen et al. 1998). This will become important with respect to endoscopic techniques of thyroid resection since scopes are naturally associated with a magnified view.

19.1.1.5 Local Infections

When pooling the data of different studies (N=43,410), a local infection rate of 0.4% was observed (Table 19.1). It could have been shown that the rate of postoperative local infections is associated with the use of postoperative wound drainage systems (Tabaqchali et al. 1999); therefore, efficiency of such drainage is interpreted at least as questionable and thus rejected by many authors (Karayacin et al. 1997; Ruark and bdel-Misih 1992; Samraj and Gurusamy 2007).

19.1.1.6 Postoperative Dysphagia

In the direct postoperative course, 80% of the patients report a dysphagia which results from the manipulation during the procedure (Sano et al. 1995). Permanent postoperative dysphagia due to scarring of the cervical fascial layers and/or vocal cord palsy was observed in 1.3% of the patients (Table 19.2).

When discussing postoperative dysphagia caused by postoperative scarring, the rates may be underestimated because a routine follow-up is not performed for patients undergoing thyroidectomy with respect to this issue; additionally long-term follow-up studies are warranted.

Table 19.2 Analysis of reported dysphagia rates following thyroidectomy

Authors	Year	N	Dysphagia (%)
Rosato et al.	2000	300	1.3
Rosato et al.	2004	14,934	1.4
Palestini et al.	2005	1,221	0.1

19.1.2 Conclusion

Rosato et al. published in 2004 their results of a multicenter survey from 42 centres for thyroid surgery in Italy with at least 50 procedures performed per year: an overall incidence of complication was reported in 17.4% of the cases and 7.1% of the 14,934 patients suffered from permanent complications following thyroid surgery.

In conclusion, the surgical technique for thyroidectomy nowadays is safe regarding severe or fatal complications (mortality, postoperative haemorrhage, bilateral vocal cord palsy), and adverse events occur in an acceptable rate. Nevertheless, there is further potential to decrease the complication rate and increase the quality of life of the treated patients.

19.2 Endoscope-Assisted Techniques in the Anterior Neck Region

Improved surgical skills and endoscopic practice brought more negligible aspects of thyroid surgery into the focus in the recent years. The question arose whether an improvement in surgical technique might be associated with a further reduction of complications and other 'side effects' while minimizing the surgical trauma and maintaining the high quality and safety of the procedure itself. Regarding the expectation of patients, the avoidance of visible scars in the anterior neck area can be cited as a primary goal; scars in this area are felt to be particularly bothersome.

The technical developments in video-assisted endoscopic surgery over the past 40 years (Semm 1983, 2001) enabled innovations also in thyroid surgery. With the adoption of the principles of minimally invasive surgery, the cosmetic demands of the patients were for the first time addressed (Miccoli et al. 1999): the incision length was reduced and the procedure was performed as a minimally invasive video-assisted thyroidectomy (MIVAT) under endoscopic vision and control. Reducing the cervical incision length is always associated with a higher tension on the wound edges to expose all parts of the thyroid. By histological examination, there are no alterations of the wound edges, and therefore, the minimized incision length is a minimally invasive procedure (Ezzat et al. 2011).

As early as 1996, Hüscher, a surgeon from Esine, Italy reported a successful hemithyroidectomy performed endoscopically through small incisions that were localized in the less visible lateral neck region (Hüscher et al. 1997). One major aim of the authors was to take advantage from the magnification due to endoscopic control and visualization.

In addition to the MIVAT technique, developed by Miccoli et al. 1999, different extracervical approaches were developed in Asian region: axillary, chest and breast approaches were described (Ikeda et al. 2002, 2003; Ohgami et al. 2000; Shimazu et al. 2003). The primary objective of these approaches was to shift the visible scar from view (Bärlehner and Benhidjeb 2008; Benhidjeb et al. 2006; Miccoli et al. 1999, 2004b; Park et al. 2003; Yamamoto et al. 2002; Yeung et al. 1997). Due to the large amount of subcutaneous dissection in these extracervical approaches, these techniques could not be addressed as being minimally invasive – moreover, they seem maximally invasive. In a recent report (Koh et al. 2009), pain scores following unilateral axillo-breast approach for benign thyroid lesions were rated on the first postoperative day as moderate or severe in 52% of the cases; 4 days following surgery almost 23% of the patients rated these pain scores. Additionally, on the 3-month follow-up, a hypo- or paraesthesia in the dissected area was described in 5.8% and swallowing disorders in 3.8%.

Nevertheless, endoscopic resection techniques in thyroid surgery represent a clear advance. Previously published comparative studies have shown a consistently favourable cosmetic result (Lombardi et al. 2006; Miccoli et al. 1999). When comparing the MIVAT technique with conventional thyroidectomy, postoperative haemorrhage with the need of a return to theatre was observed in 1.04% in conventional and in 0.88% in the endoscopic group (Alvarado et al. 2008). Miccoli et al. reported a local infection rate of 0.7% with the MIVAT technique (Miccoli et al. 2004a, b). A working group from Rome, Italy, described in 521 video-assisted thyroidectomies a 1% rate of temporarily vocal cord palsies; local infections were observed in 0.4%, and haemorrhage in 0.2% of the cases (Lombardi et al. 2006).

The increasing use of video-assisted techniques for thyroidectomies since 1996 reflects the current demands of the patients for good cosmetic results and also expresses the acceptance of these techniques by the acting surgeons. Depending on personal experience of the surgeons, up to 40% of thyroid lesions might be applicable for minimally invasive techniques. Thus, it is only consequent to further improve quality and cosmetic results with minimally invasive techniques by reducing necessary dissection and access the thyroid as near as possible endoscopically. This is the aim of the endoscopic minimally invasive trans-oral approach.

Not at least a visible scar in the neck region is not only a cosmetic problem; it could have been shown that visible scars correlate with different aspects of body esteem in 381 survivors of burn wounds. Self-satisfaction with appearance, perception of others' reaction to the own appearance, and perceived stigmatization were significantly correlated to visible scaring (Lawrence et al. 2004).

19.3 Natural Orifice Translumenal Endoscopic Surgery (NOTES) and Natural Orifice Surgery (NOS)

Natural orifice translumenal endoscopic surgery (NOTES) utilizes a natural orifice as the access point but is limited to truly endoscopic procedures. These techniques were established by Anthony Kalloo and his team in 2000 (Kalloo et al. 2000, 2004), and meanwhile different surgical procedures like appendectomies, cholecystectomies and nephrectomies have been performed by this technique (Bernhardt et al. 2008; Hochberger et al. 2009). NOTES procedures are always performed with a flexible scope with its inherent limitations: small working channels, great diameters and sometimes difficult handling especially in resections and wound closure.

The concept of natural orifice surgery (NOS) is based on the principle of reaching the pathology to be treated by passing also through natural entries of the human body (oral cavity, vagina, anus, or urethra) and act with rigid rather than flexible endoscopes. This should minimize access trauma, spare working time and therefore be gentler than standard surgical procedures. NOS principles in patient's procedures were followed in resections of tumours of the rectum and in endoscopic transvaginal appendectomies as well as cholecystectomies (Bernhardt et al. 2008; Hochberger et al. 2009; Hogan et al. 2009; Sodergren et al. 2009; Palanivelu et al. 2008).

19.3.1 Endoscopic Neck Surgery

Regarding neck surgery, several endoscopic approaches have been described during the past years especially for thyroid gland resections including cervical and extracervical approaches (Papaspyrou et al. 2011). Other endoscopic approaches tested experimentally the harvesting of sentinel nodes (Malloy et al. 2007; Sesterhenn et al. 2008; Werner et al. 2004) as well as endoscopic submandibular gland resection (Guyot et al. 2005; Hong and Yang 2008; Kessler et al. 2006; Terris et al. 2004). All those techniques as well as the minimally invasive approaches for thyroidectomy are not really NOS procedures because they always depend on skin incisions to reach the working area by endoscopic view and instruments; thus they are hybrid procedures and not pure endoscopic approaches.

19.3.2 The Single-Port Trans-oral Approach for Thyroidectomy

In 2008, Witzel and colleagues published an NOS approach for thyroidectomy. In order to minimize surgical trauma, they presented an experimental trans-oral access to the thyroid gland using a single-port access via an axilloscope (Witzel et al. 2008). However, this approach was also a hybrid one because an additional 3.5-mm skin incision, 15 mm below the level of the larynx, was necessary (Witzel and Benhidjeb 2009). The working group of Witzel et al. did not progress with this approach past the experimental phase.

Karakas et al. started another attempt in this direction by placing this scope in the lateral sublingual floor of the mouth (Karakas et al. 2010a, b) to gain access to the thyroid gland. In contrast to Witzel and colleagues, they entered the cervical spaces through the lateral floor of the mouth and the submandibular triangle; there they passed the larynx laterally and were able to reach the thyroid gland unilateral. The upper pole vessels could be identified as well as the recurrent laryngeal nerve. A major disadvantage of this technique is the mandatory working through the scope, which results in a limited triangulation of the working instruments. Lateral approaches near the larynx also limit the procedure to a hemithyroidectomy.

From an anatomical point of view, using the lateral endoscopic approach when dissecting the upper pole vessels of the thyroid may result in lacerations of the cricothyroid muscle. Also due to the complicated anatomical situation in the submandibular triangle, there are a lot of possible complications following this approach. This was shown too by the first clinical application of this endoscopic approach through the lateral floor of the mouth; lingual and hypoglossal nerve paresis were observed (Karakas et al. 2010a, b). Lastly, the use of a scope limits the resected specimen in volume and size, as also described for other endoscopic techniques (Duh 2003).

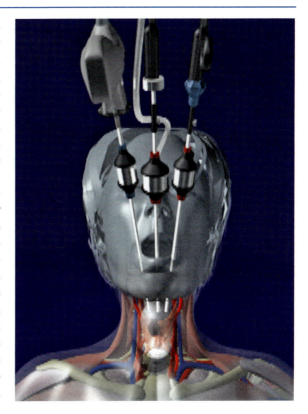

Fig. 19.1 Vision of a trans-oral endoscopic and minimally invasive thyroidectomy

19.3.3 Endoscopic Minimally Invasive Thyroidectomy (eMIT): A Vision for Trans-oral Thyroid Gland Resection

Based on the previous experiences and communications from Witzel et al. (2007, personal communication, 2008), the idea came up to reach the anterior neck region on a trans-oral endoscopic route by a three-point access through the floor of the mouth (Fig. 19.1). The aim was to reduce the necessary amount of dissections for reaching the anterior neck region and create an endoscopic access nearby the targeted area, act totally endoscopically and enhance triangulation of instruments for a comfortable handling during thyroid resection. This should result in a safe and fast endoscopic procedure respecting anatomically predefined surgical layers and therefore reduce the rate of postoperative complications, especially swallowing disorders and dysphagia. Additionally, this approach would not leave any visible scar either cervical or extracervical.

19.4 Anatomical Foundations for Trans-oral Neck Surgery

To act in the sublingual and submandibular region or through the floor of the mouth, an intimate knowledge about the anatomical relationships is mandatory. By dissections of human bodies at the Anatomical Skills Laboratory of the Erasmus University at Rotterdam, the Netherlands, safe and risky areas of access could be identified (Wilhelm et al. 2010).

Aim of this study was to define anatomical spaces, surgical planes and related neural and vascular structures to create a safe and reproducible trans-oral access and pathway to the cervical spaces especially to the more distant thyroid gland. This access should guide an easy and safe way to preformed anatomical spaces between different fascial layers of the neck. In these 'sliding' layers, a preparation without any bleeding should be possible, and neural structures can be spared. The space to be reached is the subplatysmal layer

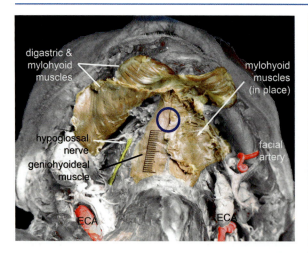

Fig. 19.2 Muscles of the floor of the oral cavity and relevant neural and vascular structures. *Blue circle* indicating entry point for the median sublingual trocar (*ECA* external carotid artery) (From Wilhelm et al. (2010). Copyright by Springer; permission for reproduction has to be obtained)

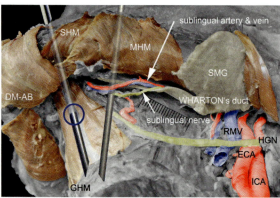

Fig. 19.3 Muscles of the floor of the oral cavity. *Blue circle* indicating pass through of the optical trocar, optical trocar in the midline and working trocar on the *left side* in place (*MHM* mylohyoid muscle, *SHM* sternohyoid muscle, *DM-AB* anterior belly of the digastric muscle, *GHM* genohyoid muscle, *ICA* internal carotid artery, *ECA* external carotid artery, *RMV* retromandibular vein, *HGN* hypoglossal nerve, *SMG* submandibular gland – lift up) (From Wilhelm et al. (2010). Copyright by Springer; permission for reproduction has to be obtained)

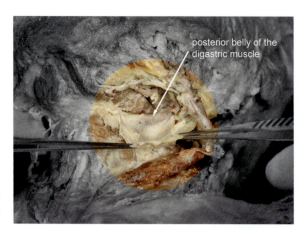

Fig. 19.4 "Submandibular bag." Part of the superficial fascia covering the submandibular spatium, the submandibular gland and relevant vascular and neural structures (*left side*, submandibular gland removed) (From Wilhelm et al. (2010). Copyright by Springer; permission for reproduction has to be obtained)

above the pretracheal strap muscles. Here the linea alba colli can easily be identified, transected, and the thyroid gland visualized, mobilized and resected. For minimally invasive thyroid resection, the principal access to this working space was executed with standard instruments with a diameter of 2.7 and 3.5 mm used in general abdominal surge endoscopic minimally invasive ry for minimally invasive procedures (Karl Storz GmbH, Tuttlingen, Germany).

To access the working space by a trans-oral manner, a trocar for optical information with a 3-mm Hopkins endoscope (Karl Storz GmbH, Tuttlingen, Germany) should be placed in the midline between and before the papillae of Wharton's duct. The scope then passes the muscles of the floor of the oral cavity easily in the midline (linea alba) without damage to relevant anatomical structures. The muscles of the floor of the oral cavity are separated bilaterally in the midline. No vessels or nerves are present in this area, and hence there are no structures at risk (Fig. 19.2).

19.4.1 The Submandibular Triangle

To get access for the working trocars, we aimed to pass the floor of the oral cavity sublingually on both sides through the submandibular triangle. The submandibular triangle can be divided into two compartments: the sublingual and the submandibular space. In the sublingual spatium, it is possible to localize the duct of the submandibular gland, the sublingual glands and the lingual nerve as well as the sublingual artery and vein (Fig. 19.3). The submandibular space includes the submandibular gland, the hypoglossal nerve, the facial artery and parts of the lingual nerve. The two spaces are partially divided by the mylohyoid muscle. The complete submandibular triangle is covered with a shield of the superficial cervical fascia, originating from the premandibular subplatysmal plane, enveloping the gland totally and running to its attachment at the posterior belly of the digastric muscle. This results in a 'bag', carrying the sublingual and the submandibular gland (Fig. 19.4).

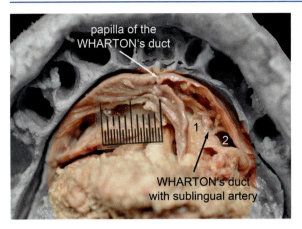

Fig. 19.5 Cranial view of a dissection of the sublingual lateral area (*1* Sublingual spatium, *2* submandibular spatium) (From Wilhelm et al. (2010). Copyright by Springer; permission for reproduction has to be obtained)

Superficial to the submandibular gland, the facial vein crosses the superficial fascia to reach the anterior border of the mandible. The facial artery enters the triangle under the posterior belly of the digastric and stylohyoid muscle; it ascends to emerge above or through the upper border of the gland (Fig. 19.3). The marginal mandibular branch of the facial nerve courses through the triangle under the platysma muscle and under the superficial fascia but outside the submandibular 'bag.' It courses over the facial vessels as it travels upward to supply the peri-oral muscles.

The hypoglossal nerve enters the triangle deep to the posterior belly of the digastric muscle. It lies on the surface of the hypoglossus muscle and runs deep to the mylohyoid muscle to supply motor function to the tongue. The lingual nerve, a branch of the mandibular nerve, is found under the border of the mandible on the hypoglossus muscle superficial to the hypoglossal nerve. It is attached to the submandibular gland by the submandibular ganglion and courses deep to the mylohyoid muscle to provide sensation to the anterior tongue and floor of the oral cavity (Fig. 19.3).

Finally, when passing the sublingual gland and the Wharton's duct medially and proceeding forward to the submandibular gland (Fig. 19.5), it is possible to reach the submandibular triangle safely. In this region, we have to carefully avoid damage to the lingual and hypoglossal nerve and leave the submandibular 'bag' to reach the working space through the mylohyoid muscle. Therefore, these structures are at risk when performing an approach through the lateral floor of the mouth.

19.4.2 Exclusively Sublingual Versus Sublingual Bi-vestibular Access

A major disadvantage of this exclusively sublingual access was the minimal triangulation of the working instruments which only reaches 5.8° (Fig. 19.6a). Beside this, the surrounding superficial fascia of the submandibular gland is injured when the submandibular spatium is left; here the hypoglossal and lingual nerves are at risk for injury. To improve triangulation of instruments, either special instruments with bendable tips have to be developed or a modified approach has to be established.

For these reasons, the trans-oral exclusively sublingual approach was changed to a combined bi-vestibular and sublingual access. The optical access port is also placed in the midline sublingually, but the working trocars are moved to the vestibule of the mouth bilaterally beneath the incisive teeth of the mandible (Fig. 19.7). Through a 5-mm incision in the mucosa of the vestibule, we can reach the edge of the mandible directly and pass under the attachment of the platysma muscle and the superficial fascia to get access to the infrahyoidal working space. Because of the anterior approach by entering the plane under the superficial fascia, it is possible to avoid damage to the marginal branch of the facial nerve as well as damage to the facial vein (Fig. 19.8). The only structure at risk is the mental nerve, but blunt submucosal dissection helps to secure intact function of the nerve after surgery (Fig. 19.9). The triangulation of instruments with this combined bi-vestibular and sublingual access reached acceptable 20–30° (Fig. 19.6b).

Therefore, in the described anatomical dissections, the trans-oral sublingual and bi-vestibular access route proofed to be safe since no relevant vascular or neural structures are at risk.

19.5 Preclinical Studies

19.5.1 First Successful Application of the Trans-oral Endoscopic Approach in an Anatomical Study

On 14 May 2008, a successful trans-oral endoscopic hemithyroidectomy was performed for the first time ever by Benhidjeb and Wilhelm at the Anatomical Skills Laboratory of the Erasmus University at Rotterdam, the Netherlands (Benhidjeb et al. 2009).

Fig. 19.6 Possible triangulation of instruments in different endoscopic approaches. (**a**) Exclusively sublingual approach. (**b**) Sublingual bi-vestibular approach (From Wilhelm et al. (2010). Copyright by Springer; permission for reproduction has to be obtained)

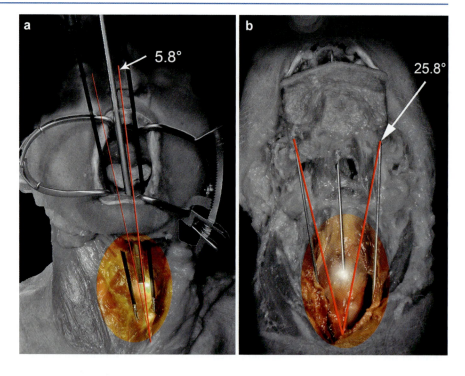

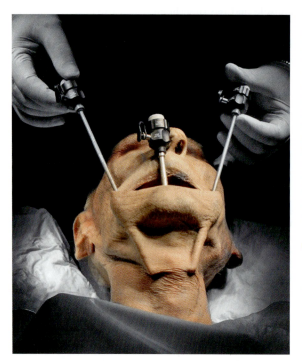

Fig. 19.7 Sublingual bi-vestibular endoscopic approach. The two working and the midline optic trocars are in place under the platysma muscle without carbon dioxide insufflation (From Wilhelm et al. (2010). Copyright by Springer; permission for reproduction has to be obtained)

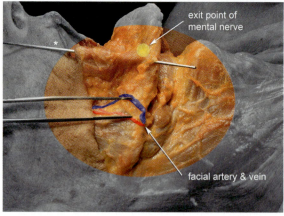

Fig. 19.8 Position of the lateral working trocar (*) placed in the oral vestibule – no relevant structures are under risk (From Wilhelm et al. (2010). Copyright by Springer; permission for reproduction has to be obtained)

The access for the 'optical' trocar was placed sublingually in the midline between the papillae of the Wharton's duct added by a bi-vestibular placement of additional working trocars. By this approach, the structures under risk in the submandibular groove could be spared, and a direct access to the working space under the platysma muscle could be created. By

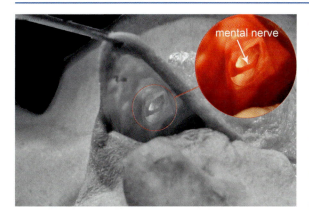

Fig. 19.9 Vestibular access on the *left side*. Under the mucosa, the mental nerve can be easily identified and spared (From Wilhelm et al. (2010). Copyright by Springer; permission for reproduction has to be obtained)

this fast and safe approach, the anterior neck region could be reached and the left hemithyroid resected. Therefore, feasibility could be proven in human cadaver experiments.

19.5.2 Ultrasound Studies on the Shift of Cervical Tissues in Different Head and Neck Positions

During trans-oral endoscopic procedures, the patient is positioned in a supine position, flat on the operation table in contrast to conventional and endoscopic approaches. Standard positioning of the patients in conventional thyroid surgery is the so-called beach chair position with an extended neck (Gemsenjaeger 2009).

When comparing the positioning of the patient, the following questions arise:
- Is there a relevant shift of the cervical tissues, especially the thyroid gland, with respect to different head and neck positions?
- Are there differences with respect to gender or body mass index?
- Do the distances from the floor of the mouth to the thyroid differ from that in conventional thyroid surgery dissected areas?

To assess the access route and the distances to be overcome by a trans-oral approach, an ultrasound study in healthy volunteers was performed (Wilhelm and Krüger 2011). The distances between the submandibular gland, hyoid bone and thyroid gland were measured, and the change in these distances in different head and neck positions (normal, reclined and reclined with open mouth position) were documented.

A lengthening of the distance from the submandibular gland to the hyoid bone was found when the head was reclined, but this almost returned to the measured distances when the mouth was opened in this reclined position. This is mainly attributed to a fascial bag which covers the submandibular gland which keeps the gland in position despite the head and neck position. The distance from the hyoid bone to the thyroid gland was shortened when the head was reclined; this fact can be attributed to the fixation of the thyroid gland to the cricothyroid cartilage by means of the suspensory ligament of the thyroid gland. Therefore, the entire distance from the submandibular gland to the thyroid gland in the various head positions studied did not change substantially. These findings were not affected by age or gender. Only in greater body weights (BMI ≥ 25), longer distances compared to the normal weighted subjects were found. The average distance between the submandibular gland and the thyroid gland (36.5 ± 7.4 to 37.8 ± 9.2 mm) was comparable to the dissected areas in conventional open thyroid surgery. Therefore, the trans-oral endoscopic approach for thyroidectomy meets the criteria of minimally invasive surgery regarding the distance from entry point to target area.

19.5.3 Feasibility and Safety in a Porcine Model with Short-Time Survival

The development of innovative surgical procedures was described most recently by the IDEAL concept, published by the Balliol collaboration (Barkun et al. 2009; Ergina et al. 2009; McCulloch et al. 2009): it includes the innovation itself, the development and exploration as well as the assessment and long-term study of the new method. This concept was also adopted for innovations in endoscopic surgery (Neugebauer et al. 2010).

After finishing the development and the anatomical studies for the endoscopic minimally invasive thyroidectomy (eMIT), the next consecutive step was to

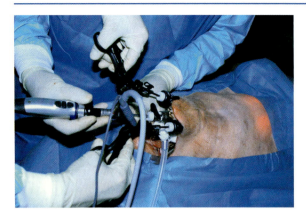

Fig. 19.10 View of a surgical procedure during the experimental series in a porcine model – all trocars in place (From Wilhelm and Benhidjeb (2011). Copyright by Springer; permission for reproduction has to be obtained)

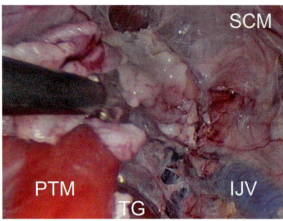

Fig. 19.11 Endoscopic view (*SCM* sternocleidomastoid muscle, *PTM* pretracheal muscle, *IJV* internal jugular vein, *TG* thyroid gland under PTM) (From Wilhelm and Benhidjeb (2011). Copyright by Springer; permission for reproduction has to be obtained)

evaluate feasibility and safety in an animal experiment with short-time survival (Wilhelm and Benhidjeb 2011). The study was undertaken in five pigs under general anaesthesia. The surgical approach was transoral and totally endoscopic; due to the anatomy of the animal model, a partial thymectomy was performed (Wilhelm and Metzig 2010b). Perioperative antibiotics were administered, but no analgesics were given in the postoperative course. Oral intake as well as the behaviour was observed during the 2 days following surgery. After necropsy, examination of the access route took place by dissections on the third postoperative day. The tissue surrounding the working trocar was examined histologically.

The pretracheal region could be reached without problems, and the procedure was performed almost 'bloodless' in an anatomically defined layer (Figs. 19.10 and 19.11). The interventional time decreased successively. Postoperative awaking was inconspicuous; already after 2–3 h, a regular oral intake was observed. Pain reactions were not to be registered in the whole postoperative phase. After necropsy, all relations appeared inconspicuous (no infections, fresh or old haematoma), but two local capsuled seromas were observed. This was attributed to the action of the bipolar devices used during resection. Histologically, only a mild tissue reaction was noted (Fig. 19.12).

So this experimental series with a short-time survival proved the safety and feasibility of an endoscopic trans-oral approach for minimally invasive neck surgery in an animal model.

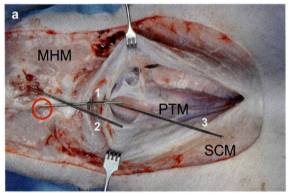

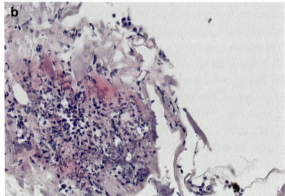

Fig. 19.12 (a) Dissection view with probes in place of the original trocars. (*Red circle*: histology taken; *SCM* sternocleidomastoid muscle, *MHM* mylohyoid muscle, divided in the *midline*, *PTM* pretracheal muscle, 1/2 channels of the working trocars, 3 channel of the trocar for the endoscope). (b) Histology. (Staining: HE) (From Wilhelm and Benhidjeb (2011). Copyright by Springer; permission for reproduction has to be obtained)

19.6 The Trans-oral Endoscopic Approach Surgical Procedures in the Anterior Neck Region

After finishing all preclinical studies, an intensive discussion about the ethical aspects of a possible first clinical application of this new endoscopic approach took place (Wilhelm and Metzig 2010b). We decided that the eMIT technique could be stated a safe and feasible procedure, and after getting a full informed consent, the procedure was performed on a 53-year-old male patient with a single nodular change in the right thyroid gland on 18 March 2009 for the first time ever (Wilhelm and Metzig 2010a).

19.6.1 Setup

The setup for the procedure is orientated at endoscopic procedures performed in head and neck surgery. The acting surgeon stands above the head of the patient, the assisting surgeon and 'cameraman' next to him on his left side. The scrub nurse is positioned on the right side. The anaesthesia team has its place on the left side of the patient positioned in leg height. To the right side of the patient, the video tower including the electronic Endoflator® (Karl STORZ Company, Tuttlingen, Germany) and the control unit for the harmonic scalpel (Ultracision©, Ethicon Endosurgery, Norderstedt, Germany) are positioned; at the foot end, the suction and electrosurgery unit are positioned (Figs. 19.13 and 19.14).

19.6.2 Instruments and Patient Preparation

The instruments used for this trans-oral endoscopic approach are standard instruments (3.7 mm diameter) for laparoscopic procedures as well as HOPKINS endoscopes of 2.7 (0°) and 5.0 mm (30°) diameter, (Karl STORZ Company, Tuttlingen, Germany, Fig. 19.15). Trocars were adapted to the special needs of this type of endoscopic surgery; they had a diameter of 6.0 mm and a working length of 200 mm.

Endocrine staging regarding the underlying disease is performed as routinely done in thyroid disease. A B-mode ultrasound study as well as a scintigraphy is performed. Preoperatively, a direct laryngoscopy for evaluation of vocal cord function is done; also the upper airways are examined by anterior rhinoscopy since there have to be sufficient space for a nasotracheal intubation.

After oral premedication (dormicum, fortecortin), the patients' airways are secured by means of a nasotracheal tube. The patient is positioned in a supine position, flat on the operating table without reclination of the head (Fig. 19.16). Surface electrodes for the neuromonitoring of the recurrent laryngeal nerve (NeMo Neuromonitor, Inomed Medizintechnik GmbH, Teningen, Germany) are placed above the cuff of the inspiration tube. The correct position of the electrodes at the level of the vocal cords is checked by direct laryngoscopy. We administer local anaesthesia using Xylocaine 1% with adrenaline, 3.0 ml at every incision site. After use of skin and mucosal disinfectant (Octenisept®, Schülke & Mayr GmbH, Norderstedt, Germany; Betaisadona®, Mundipharma GmbH, Limburg a. d. Lahn, Germany), the patient is covered with sterile dressing.

19.6.3 Surgical Technique

On the basis of the previous studies, a roadmap for endoscopic minimally invasive thyroidectomy was established. The surgical steps are as follows:

1. A sublingual sagittal mucosal incision, 10.0 mm in length, is made between the papillae of Wharton's duct in the midline.
2. The muscles of the floor of the mouth (geniohyoid muscle, mylohyoid muscle and anterior belly of the digastric muscle) are then divided directly in the midline by Metzenbaum scissors in order to reach the plane under the superficial fascia of the neck and the platysma muscle. This plane is characterized as a sliding plane and can be easily identified by palpation (Fig. 19.17).
3. Then the hyoid bone is palpated, and the upper third of the ligaments that keep the subcutaneous tissue fixed to the hyoid bone are transected with the scissors.
4. The first trocar is then inserted into the subplatysmal layer, anterior to the thyroid cartilage. After endoscopic control, air with a pressure of 6–8 mmHg is insufflated. The air forms a tent over the pretracheal strap muscles through 'gas dissection' (Fig. 19.18).

Fig. 19.13 Setup during the procedure

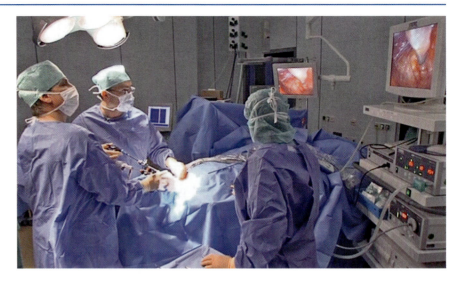

Fig. 19.14 Schematic drawing of the setup

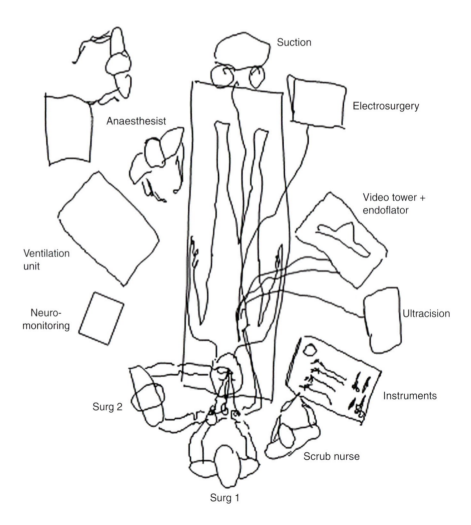

Fig. 19.15 Standard instruments for laparoscopic surgery were used for endoscopic minimally invasive thyroidectomy (*1* suction/irrigation, *2* trocars, *3* scalpel with no. 15 blade, *4* laparoscopic instruments [dissector, grasping forceps, scissor], *5* 30° scope 5 mm, *6* probe for active stimulation of the recurrent laryngeal nerve, *7* mouth gag, *8* suction tube, *9* hooks, forceps, Metzenbaum scissor, and needle holder, *10* Ultracision©)

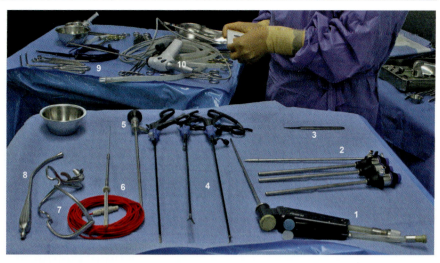

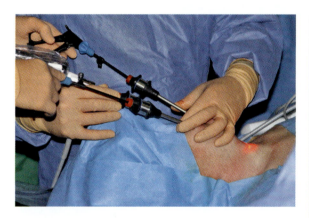

Fig. 19.16 Setup during surgical procedure and positioning of the patient – all trocars in place

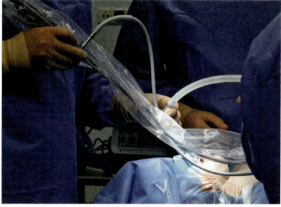

Fig. 19.18 The pretracheal working space is created by air dissection and optical scissor

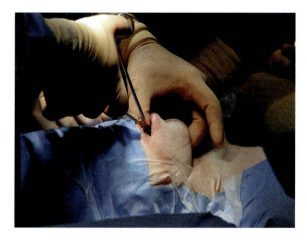

Fig. 19.17 Creation of the midline access with palpation of the sliding layer of the submental region (*left hand*)

5. Under the view of a scope, the pretracheal space can now be created with an 'optical scissor', usually used for bronchoscopic procedures in children (Karl STORZ Company, Tuttlingen, Germany).
6. As a next step, the mucosa is incised bilaterally in the vestibule of the mouth, one centimetre or more lateral to the buccal fold at the level of the canine teeth (Fig. 19.19). Care had to be taken not to injure the mental nerve, which runs very superficially. This nerve is easily visible and can therefore be preserved.
7. With a Metzenbaum scissor, a pocket down to the edge of the mandible is created where both bilateral 'working' trocars are guided straight below the platysma muscle. As proved in previous

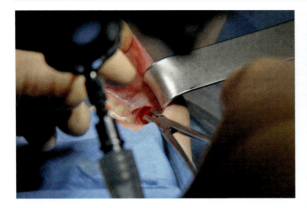

Fig. 19.19 Creation of the vestibular entry for the working trocar on the *right side*

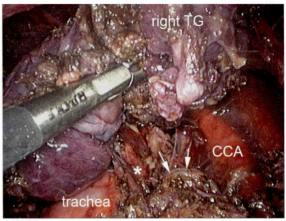

Fig. 19.21 Endoscopic view of the Berry ligament (*), the right thyroid gland (*TG*), the common carotid artery (*CCA*), and the recurrent laryngeal nerve (*white arrows*)

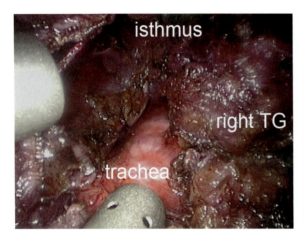

Fig. 19.20 Endoscopic view of the transected isthmus of the thyroid gland (TG) in the *midline*

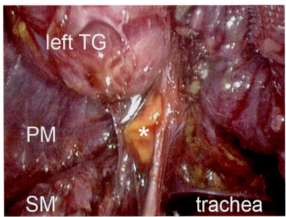

Fig. 19.22 Endoscopic view of the left thyroid gland (*TG*), the platysma (*PM*) and sternocleidomastoid muscle (*SM*) and the left upper parathyroid gland (*)

anatomical studies, there are no vascular or neural structures at risk in this trans-oral route (Wilhelm et al. 2010).

8. With both working trocars in place, the strap muscles are divided in the midline and the thyroid gland becomes visible. The fibrous capsule of the thyroid has to be identified, and strap muscles are loosened on both sides.
9. First, an attempt is made to display the upper pole of the thyroid gland. This is sometimes difficult as it runs under the cricothyroid muscle.
10. In these cases, a 'reverse resection' is performed: the isthmus of the thyroid gland is displayed in full length and transected with the harmonic scalpel (Ultracision©, Ethicon Endosurgery, Norderstedt, Germany; Fig. 19.20).
11. After identifying the trachea and displaying the recurrent laryngeal nerve, as well as the upper parathyroid gland, the suspensory ligament of the thyroid (Berry's ligament) is divided with the harmonic scalpel (Figs. 19.21 and 19.22).
12. After transecting this ligament, the upper pole could be dislocated caudally and the vessels of the thyroid gland become visible; they are divided with the harmonic scalpel.
13. Following the adjacent lamella downward, the lateral thyroid vein comes into the surgical field and can be divided.

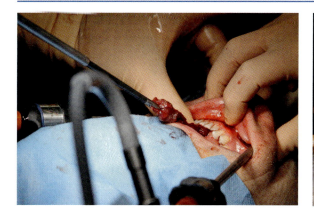

Fig. 19.23 Harvesting of the specimen through the midline tunnel

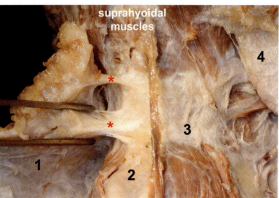

Fig. 19.24 Attaching ligaments of the hyoid bone. (*1* Skin and subcutaneous tissues, *2* upper end of the thyroid cartilage, *3* hyoid bone, *4* submandibular gland, * indicating the ligaments that attach the subcutaneous tissues to the hyoid bone)

14. The recurrent laryngeal nerve can be identified by means of direct stimulation with a probe. The intact vocal cord function can be verified by direct stimulation of the recurrent laryngeal nerve and the vagal nerve by a probe.
15. Then the lower pole vessels of the thyroid are separated and divided with the Ultracision©. Now the hemithyroid is freely movable. If necessary, the other hemithyroid can be dissected in the same way.
16. The scope is then switched to the left working trocar, and the specimen harvested through the midline tunnel with grasping forceps (Fig. 19.23).
17. Finally, the surgical field is once again checked for active bleeding or residual thyroid tissues, and the trocars are removed.
18. Intraoral incision sites are closed with absorbable sutures (Vicryl©, Ethicon, Norderstedt, Germany), and a plaster tape is applied on the cervical skin to attach the cervical tissues in their correct anatomical position and prevent postoperative swelling of the soft tissues. This plaster tape is removed 2 days after surgery.

19.6.3.1 Hints and Pitfalls

- Be sure to palpate the sliding layer of the superficial fascia during separation of the suprahyoidal muscles to avoid lacerations of the muscles and end up in the right layer.
- Separate the suprahyoidal muscles strictly in the midline and from the mentum down to the hyoid bone to get a sufficient width of the midline tunnel.
- When reaching the hyoid bone, turn the scissor by 90° and transect the ligament attaching the skin and subcutaneous tissues to the hyoid bone (Fig. 19.24) in the anterior third of the hyoid.
- Identify the linea alba of the pretracheal muscles properly – keep the head of the patient in the midline and do not turn it at the side.
- Be sure to dissect on the fibrous capsule of the thyroid gland.
- Dissect the isthmus of the thyroid gland strictly in the midline. Further dissection on the posterior aspect of the thyroid have to be strictly at the fibrous capsule to prevent damage to the parathyroids as well as to the recurrent laryngeal nerve at the suspensory ligament of the thyroid.
- Avoid extensive action of the harmonic scalpel at the Berry's ligament since damage to the recurrent laryngeal nerve may occur.
- First, identify and separate the upper pole vessels of the thyroid gland – a supine head position facilitates the displacement of the upper pole downwards.

19.6.4 Postoperative Management

We administer oral antibiotics (sulbactam + ampicillin) for 6 days and recommend month rinses with chlorhexidine three times daily for a week. A routine analgetic treatment with paracetamol and NSAID is performed for 5 days. Oral intake can be normal direct postoperatively. Plaster tape of the neck is removed

2 days after surgery. On the first postoperative day, a direct laryngoscopy to check the vocal cord function is performed.

Routine treatment principles regarding substitution of thyroidin and calcium (where necessary) are performed according to conventional thyroid surgery.

19.6.5 Advantages of the Trans-oral Endoscopic Approach for Thyroidectomy

After the first successful clinical application, a prospective proof-of-concept study was performed in eight patients (Wilhelm and Metzig 2011a). Within this study, we did not select the patients a priori regarding the size of the thyroid changes. Therefore, three conversions to open surgery were necessary, and size criteria could be established:
- Endoscopic minimally invasive thyroidectomy is limited to thyroid pathologies with a maximum volume of 30–40 ml and
- A maximum nodule size of approximately 20 mm

In one case, a permanent palsy of the recurrent laryngeal nerve (unilateral) occurred. The patient complained of no restriction in voice function after logopaedic therapy, and there was no postoperative dyspnoea. Palsy of the recurrent laryngeal nerve is one of the typical complications of thyroidectomy. Whether the palsy observed in our study was due to the surgical technique itself or whether we were unlucky enough to experience the first paresis in 100 within our first eight procedures remains unclear. Definitive information about the effective palsy rate can only be given in a prospective comparative study.

Certainly, attention has to be paid to the recurrent laryngeal nerve, particularly regarding the surgical technique. Difficulties may occur with the release of Berry's ligament and thus the conservation of the recurrent nerve. The harmonic scalpel, with a branch length of 10 mm, appears to be perfectly suited neither to maintaining haemostasis in this sensitive area nor to sparing the nerve. When working with the harmonic scalpel near the recurrent nerve, the heat during vessel sealing can be a potential cause of postoperative nerve dysfunction or even palsy.

The main advantage for the patients was the total absence of postoperative swallowing pain or disorders, even in the direct postoperative course. This is attributed to the concept of entering anatomically defined layers and planes directly, therefore avoiding lacerations of the cervical muscle layers, especially the platysma muscle. The final cosmetic result was also excellent (Fig. 19.25), and even the access sites in the floor and vestibule of the mouth healed without visible scaring (Fig. 19.26). And last but not least, the procedure is a minimally invasive one because the access point and the approach route are nearby the targeted thyroid gland.

Due to the endoscopic approach, we have had a magnified display of the anatomical structures facilitating a more gentle and bloodless procedure. Therefore, in comparison to conventional thyroid surgery, the eMIT approach is at the same time minimally invasive and cosmetically optimal. For estimation of the procedure-associated complications especially in comparison to other minimally invasive procedures with transcervical approaches like the MIVAT technique, prospective comparative studies are needed (Wilhelm and Metzig 2011b).

19.7 Robotic-Assisted Trans-oral Endoscopic Thyroidectomy

Robotic-assisted and telerobotic surgery date back to the mid-1980s of the last century and were mainly supported by the Ministry of Defence of the United States; several systems like the AESOP, ZEUS and da Vinci have been developed and got approval of the FDA for different indications (Ballantyne 2002). During the past 10 years, indications for telerobotic surgery have expanded even in head and neck surgery. Most of the procedures represent trans-oral endoscopic procedures for oncological indications (tumour resections in the hypopharynx or larynx) and robotic parathyroid and thyroid resections (Arora et al. 2011). The endoscopic trans-oral procedures are a common head and neck procedure since they are performed in otolaryngology since decades, endoscopically by microscope and micro instruments through specula, for example as microlaryngoscopy or endolaryngeal microsurgery. With respect to our NOTES/NOS classification, these surgeries have to be classified as pure NOTES procedures.

Due to the approval of the da Vinci system by the American FDA, a lot of studies and case series have been published in the United States. Major concerns in Europe are the lack of haptic feedback by these systems

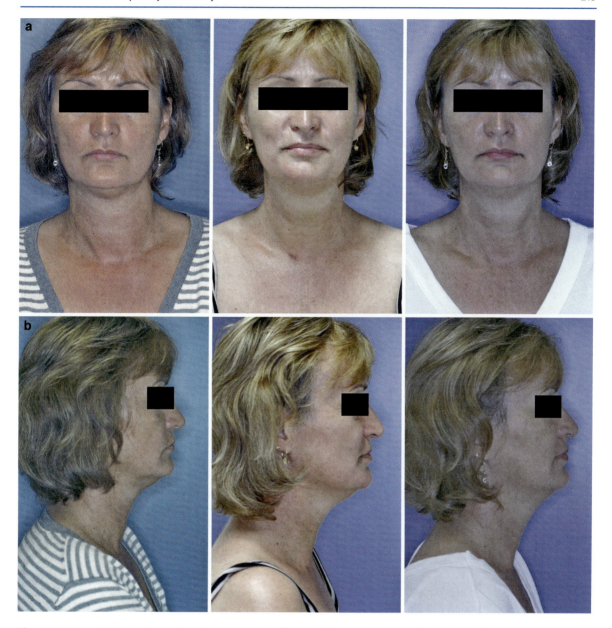

Fig. 19.25 Frontal (**a**) and oblique view (**b**) preoperatively (*1st row*), 7 days postoperative (*2nd row*) and 14 days postoperative (*3rd row*) (From Wilhelm and Metzig (2011a). Copyright by Springer; permission for reproduction has to be obtained)

and the cost-effectiveness (Arora et al. 2011). Evidence of cost-effectiveness in head and neck surgery has not been published till now. On the other hand, telerobotic systems are limited to patients with suitable anatomical conditions. If the pathology could not be well exposed, this reflects a contraindication for the use of a robotic system. Additionally, longer operating times, a steep learning curve and the time taken to dock the robot as well as the space required in the operating theatre limit the use of robotic systems in head and neck surgery.

In a more recent study, Lee et al. (2011) reviewed the value of robotic thyroidectomy for thyroid carcinoma retrospectively in a multicenter setting. The robotic thyroidectomy was performed by a transaxillary gasless approach with the da Vinci surgical robot. They found the use of the robotic system to be feasible, safe and with good outcomes for the treated patients.

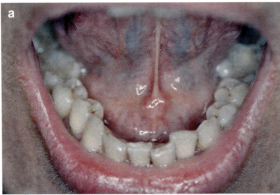
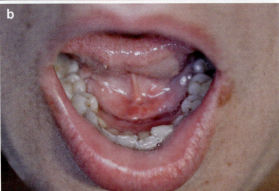
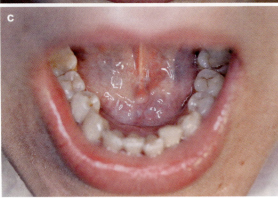

Fig. 19.26 Sublingual incision site. (**a**) Preoperatively, (**b**) 14 days after surgery, (**c**) follow-up at 7 months (From Wilhelm and Metzig (2011a). Copyright by Springer; permission for reproduction has to be obtained)

Major postoperative complications were only reported in 1% of the cases.

Richmon et al. (2011) published their results with the use of a robotic-assisted trans-oral thyroidectomy in two human cadavers. They utilized the trans-oral endoscopic approach as described in this chapter and state that the 'trans-oral robotic-assisted thyroidectomy (TRAT) provides an attractive approach to the central compartment for thyroidectomy in a field of "minimally invasive" and "scarless" techniques'. No further details about setup time, handling and discussion about cost-effectiveness are mentioned in their communication.

So, in conclusion, robotic-assisted techniques for trans-oral, natural orifice surgery procedures are in a very early and experimental stadium. Further developments have to be awaited.

19.8 Applications of the eMIT Technique Beyond the Current Scope: Trans-oral Endoscopic Mediastinal Surgery

Shortly after the development of the trans-oral endoscopic approach for surgical procedures in the anterior neck region and the proven feasibility, the question about other possible indications of this approach arose. One consequent further development was seen in the access to the middle mediastinum at this stage. It remained unclear at this time, whether:

- The trans-oral endoscopic approach to the mediastinum is feasible.
- The intrathoracic vessels and nerves could be identified and protected.
- A 'working space' within the mediastinum for lymph node dissection and resection could be created.
- The method is feasible and safe in an animal study.
- Respiration and gas exchange in an animal model may be affected by mediastinal CO_2 insufflation.

Therefore, at the beginning of 2009, another series of anatomical experiments for the application of the trans-oral endoscopic approach for mediastinal surgery were performed at the Anatomical Skills Laboratory of the Erasmus University at Rotterdam, the Netherlands (Wilhelm et al. 2011a). It could be shown that a working space could be established within the middle mediastinum and all relevant anatomical structures could be displayed and spared.

Following the anatomical development and application of the procedure, an animal experiment in a porcine model was conducted in autumn 2009; this study in five pigs with a short-time survival demonstrated the feasibility and safety of the method (Wilhelm et al. 2011a).

Meanwhile, the method has been applied on the 16 September 2010 successfully for the first time in a 47-year-old man with suspect lymph nodes of the mediastinum (Wilhelm et al. 2011b).

19.9 Conclusion

In conclusion, with this trans-oral endoscopic minimally invasive approach to the anterior neck region and the mediastinum, a new approach for endoscopic minimally invasive thyroidectomy and mediastinal surgery within natural orifice surgery has been established. Preclinical studies, animal experiments, the first clinical applications and a proof-of-concept study in humans for thyroidectomy have shown possible advantages for patients, namely faster recovery, decreased postoperative pain and dysphagia, and of course, no visible scars. The actual complication rate can only be estimated in the context of a prospective comparative study. In such a study, the method also has to prove its possible superiority to alternative minimally invasive surgical procedures.

References

Alvarado R, McMullen T, Sidhu SB, Delbridge LW, Sywak MS (2008) Minimally invasive thyroid surgery for single nodules: an evidence-based review of the lateral mini-incision technique. World J Surg 32:1341–1348

Arora A, Cunningham A, Chawdhary G, Vicini C, Weinstein GS, Darzi A, Tolley N (2011) Clinical applications of Telerobotic ENT-Head and Neck surgery. Int J Surg 9(4):277–284. doi:10.1016/j.ijsu.2011.01.008, Epub 2011 Jan 27

Ballantyne GH (2002) Robotic surgery, telerobotic surgery, telepresence, and telementoring. Review of early clinical results. Surg Endosc 16:1389–1402

Barkun JS, Aronson JK, Feldman LS, Maddern GJ, Strasberg SM, For the Balliol Colloboration (2009) Surgical innovation and evaluation 1: evaluation and stages of surgical innovation. Lancet 374(9695):1089–1096

Bärlehner E, Benhidjeb T (2008) Cervical scarless endoscopic thyroidectomy: axillo-bilateral breast approach (ABBA). Surg Endosc 22:154–158

Benhidjeb T, Anders S, Bärlehner E (2006) Total video-endoscopic thyroidectomy via axillo-bilateral-breast-approach (ABBA). Langenbecks Arch Surg 391:48–49

Benhidjeb T, Wilhelm T, Harlaar J, Kleinrensink G-J, Schneider TAJ, Stark M (2009) Natural orifice surgery on thyroid gland: totally transoral video-assisted thyroidectomy (TOVAT): report of first experimental results of a new surgical method. Surg Endosc 23(5):1119–1120

Bernhardt J, Gerber B, Schober H-C, Kähler G, Ludwig K (2008) NOTES-case report of a unidirectional flexible appendectomy. Int J Colorectal Dis 23:547–550

Bhattacharyya N, Fried MP (2002) Assessment of the morbidity and complications of total thyroidectomy. Arch Otolaryngol Head Neck Surg 128:389–392

Brauckhoff M, Walls G, Brauckhoff K, Thanh PN, Thomusch O, Dralle H (2002) Identification of the non-recurrent inferior laryngeal nerve using intraoperative neurostimulation. Langenbecks Arch Surg 386:482–487

Chan WF, Lang BH, Lo CY (2006) The role of intraoperative neuromonitoring of recurrent laryngeal nerve during thyroidectomy: a comparative study on 1000 nerves at risk. Surgery 140:866–872

Diklic A, Zivaljevic V, Paunovic I, Kalezic N, Tatic S (2005) Surgical procedures in patients with thyroid autoimmune disease. Srp Arh Celok Lek 133(Suppl 1):77–83

Dralle H (2009) Rekurrens- und Nebenschilddrüsenpräparation in der Schilddrüsenchirurgie. Chirurg 80:352–363

Dralle H, Sekulla C, Haerting J, Timmermann W, Neumann HJ, Kruse E, Grond S, Muhlig HP, Richter C, Voss J, Thomusch O, Lippert H, Gastinger I, Brauckhoff M, Gimm O (2004a) Risk factors of paralysis and functional outcome after recurrent laryngeal nerve monitoring in thyroid surgery. Surgery 136:1310–1322

Dralle H, Sekulla C, Lorenz K, Grond S, Irmscher B (2004b) Ambulante und kurzstationäre Schilddrüsen- und Nebenschilddrüsenchirurgie. Chirurg 75:131–143

Dralle H, Sekulla C, Lorenz K, Brauckhoff M, Machens A (2008) Intraoperative monitoring of the recurrent laryngeal nerve in thyroid surgery. World J Surg 32:1358–1366

DuBose J, Barnett R, Ragsdale T (2004) Honest and sensible surgeons: the history of thyroid surgery. Curr Surg 61:213–219

Duh Q-Y (2003) Presidential address: minimally invasive endocrine surgery – standard of treatment or hype? Surgery 134:849–857

Ergina PL, Cook JA, Blazeby JM, Boutron I, Clavien P-A, Reeves BC, Seiler CM, For the Balliol Colloboration (2009) Surgical innovation and evaluation 2: challenges in evaluating surgical innovation. Lancet 374(9695):1097–1104

Ezzat WH, O'Hara BJ, Fisher KJ, Rosen D, Pribitkin EA (2011) The minimally-invasive thyroidectomy incision: a histological analysis. Med Sci Monit 17:SC7–SC10

Frick T, Largiader F (1989) Perioperative Komplikationsrate von Schilddrüseneingriffen. Helv Chir Acta 56:503–505

Gaujoux S, Leenhardt L, Tresallet C, Rouxel A, Hoang C, Jublanc C, Chigot JP, Menegaux F (2006) Extensive thyroidectomy in Graves' disease. J Am Coll Surg 202:868–873

Gemsenjaeger E (2009) Part 1 – Chapter 1: Notes on positioning the patient. In: Atlas of thyroid surgery. Principles, practise, and clinical cases. Thieme, Stuttgart/New York, p 2

Guyot L, Duroure F, Richard O, Lebeau J, Passagia J-G, Raphael B (2005) Submandibular gland endoscopic resection: a cadaveric study. Int J Oral Maxillofac Surg 34:407–410

Helios Kliniken GmbH (2005) Medizinischer Jahresbericht 2005. http://www.helios-kliniken.de/ueber-helios/publikationen/medizinischer-jahresbericht.html

Hochberger J, Menke D, Matthes K, Lamadé W, Köhler P (2009) Transluminale Interventionen ("NOTES") – aktueller Stand. Dtsch Med Wochenschr 134:467–472

Hogan S, Cullen JP, Talamini MA, Mintz Y, Ferreres A, Jacobsen GR, Sandler B, Bosia J, Savides T, Easter DW, Savu MK, Ramamoorthy SL, Whitcomb E, Agarwal S, Lukacz E, Dominguez G, Ferraina P (2009) Natural orifice surgery: initial clinical experience. Surg Endosc 23:1512–1518

Hong KH, Yang JS (2008) Surgical results of the intraoral removal of the submandibular gland. Otolaryngol Head Neck Surg 139:530–534

Hüscher CSG, Chiodini S, Napolitano C, Recher A (1997) Endoscopic right thyroid lobectomy. Surg Endosc 11:877

Ignjatovic M, Cuk V, Ozegovic A, Cerovic S, Kostic Z, Romic P (2003) Rane komplikacije operativnog lecenja oboljenja stitaste zlezde: analiza 2100 bolesnika. Acta Chir Iugosl 50:155–175

Ikeda Y, Takami H, Niimi M, Kan S, Sasaki Y, Takayama J (2002) Endoscopic thyroidectomy and parathyroidectomy by the axillary approach. A preliminary report. Surg Endosc 16:92–95

Ikeda Y, Takami H, Sasaki Y, Takayama J, Niimi M, Kan S (2003) Clinical benefits in endoscopic thyroidectomy by the axillary approach. J Am Coll Surg 196:189–195

Kalloo AN, Kantsevoy SV, Singh VK, Magee CA, Vaughn CA, Hill SL (2000) Flexible transgastric peritoneoscopy: a novel approach to diagnostic and therapeutic interventions in the peritoneal cavity. Gastroenterology 118:A1039

Kalloo AN, Singh VK, Jagannath SB, Niiyama H, Hill SL, Vaughn CA, Magee CA, Kantsevoy SV (2004) Flexible transgastric peritoneoscopy: a novel approach to diagnostic and therapeutic interventions in the peritoneal cavity. Gastrointest Endosc 60(1):114–117

Karakas E, Steinfeldt T, Gockel A, Sesterhenn A, Bartsch DK (2010a) Transorale partielle Parathyreoidektomie. Chirurg 81:1020–1025

Karakas E, Steinfeldt T, Gockel A, Westermann R, Kiefer A, Bartsch DK (2010b) Transoral thyroid and parathyroid surgery. Surg Endosc 24:1261–1267

Karayacin K, Besim H, Ercan F, Hamamci O, Korkmaz A (1997) Thyroidectomy with and without drains. East Afr Med J 74:431–432

Kessler P, Bloch-Birkholz A, Birkholz T, Neukam FW (2006) Feasibility of an endoscopic approach to the submandibular neck region – Experimental and clinical results. Br J Oral Maxillofac Surg 44:103–106

Kocher ET (1909) Concerning pathological manifestations in low-grade thyroid diseases. Nobel Lecture, Stockholm, December 11 1909. http://www.helios-kliniken.de/ueber-helios/publikationen/medizinischer-jahresbericht.html

Koh YW, Kim JW, Lee SW, Choi EC (2009) Endoscopic thyroidectomy via a unilateral axillo-breast approach without gas insufflation for unilateral benign thyroid lesions. Surg Endosc 23:2053–2060

Lawrence JW, Fauerbach JA, Heinberg L, Doctor M (2004) Visible vs hidden scars and their relation to body esteem. J Burn Care Rehabil 25:25–32

Lee J, Yun JH, Nam KH, Choi UJ, Chung WY, Soh E-Y (2011) Perioperative clinical outcomes after robotic thyroidectomy for thyroid carcinoma: a multicenter study. Surg Endosc 25:906–912

Lefevre JH, Tresallet C, Leenhardt L, Jublanc C, Chigot JP, Menegaux F (2007) Reoperative surgery for thyroid disease. Langenbecks Arch Surg 392:685–691

Lombardi CP, Raffaelli M, Princi P, De Crea C, Bellantone R (2006) Video-assisted thyroidectomy: report of a 7-year experience in Rome. Langenbecks Arch Surg 391:174–177

Lucha PA Jr, Wallace D, Pasque C, Brickhouse N, Olsen D, Styk S, Dortch M, Beckman WA Jr (2000) Surgical wound morbidity in an austere surgical environment. Mil Med 165:13–17

Malloy KM, Cognetti DM, Wildemore BM, Cunnane MF, Keane WM, Pribitkin EA, Rosen D (2007) Feasibility of endoscopic sentinel node biopsy in the porcine neck. Otolaryngol Head Neck Surg 136:806–810

McCulloch P, Altman DG, Campbell WB, Flum DR, Glasziou P, Marshall JC, Nicholl JCM, For the Balliol Colloboration (2009) Surgical innovation and evaluation 3: no surgical innovation without evaluation: the IDEAL recommendations. Lancet 374(9695):1105–1112

Miccoli P, Berti P, Conte M, Bendinelli C, Marcocci C (1999) Minimally invasive surgery for small thyroid nodules: preliminary report. J Endocrinol Invest 22:849–851

Miccoli P, Berti P, Materazzi G, Minuto M, Barellino L (2004a) Minimally invasive video-assisted thyroidectomy: five years of experience. J Am Coll Surg 199:243–248

Miccoli P, Minuto MN, Barellini L, Galleri D, Massi M, D'Agostino J, Materazzi G, Berti P (2004b) Tiroidectomia video-assistita minimamente invasiva (Mivat)–cenni di tecnica an e risultati di 4 anni di esperienza (Analisi della casistica 1999–2002). Ann Ital Chir 75:47–51

Neugebauer EAM, Becker M, Buess GF, Cuschieri A, Dauben H-P, Fingerhut A, Fuchs KH, Habermalz B, Lantsberg L, Morino M, Reiter-Theil S, Soskuty G, Wayand W, Welsch T, EAES (2010) EAES recommendations on methodology of innovation management in endoscopic surgery. Surg Endosc 24(7):1594–1615

Nielsen TR, Andreassen UK, Brown CL, Balle VH, Thomsen J (1998) Microsurgical technique in thyroid surgery – a 10-year experience. J Laryngol Otol 116:556–560

Ohgami M, Ishii S, Arisawa Y, Ohmori T, Noga K, Furukawa T, Kitajima M (2000) Scarless endoscopic thyroidectomy: breast approach for better cosmesis. Surg Laparosc Endosc Percutan Tech 10:1–4

Palanivelu C, Rajan PS, Rangarajan M, Parthasarathi R, Senthilnathan P, Prasad M (2008) Transvaginal endoscopic appendectomy in humans: a unique approach to NOTES-world's first report. Surg Endosc 22:1343–1347

Palestini N, Tulletti V, Cestino L, Durando R, Freddi M, Sisti G, Ribecchi A (2005) Post-thyroidectomy cervical hematoma. Minerva Chir 60:37–46

Papaspyrou G, Ferlito A, Silver CE, Werner JA, Genden E, Sesterhenn AM (2011) Extracervical approaches to endoscopic thyroid surgery. Surg Endosc 25:995–1003

Park YL, Han WK, Bae WG (2003) 100 cases of endoscopic thyroidectomy. Breast approach. Surg Laparosc Endosc Percutan Tech 13:20–25

Richmon JD, Pattani KM, Benhidjeb T, Tufano RP (2011) Transoral robotic-assisted thyroidectomy: a preclinical feasibility study in 2 cadavers. Head Neck 33:330–333

Robertson ML, Steward DL, Gluckman JL, Welge J (2004) Continuous laryngeal nerve integrity monitoring during thyroidectomy: does it reduce risk of injury? Otolaryngol Head Neck Surg 131:596–600

Röher HD, Goretzki PE, Hellmann P, Witte J (1999) Risiken und Komplikationen der Schilddrüsenchirurgie. Häufigkeit und Therapie. Chirurg 70:999–1010

Rosato L, Mondini G, Ginardi A, Clerico G, Pozzo M, Raviola P (2000) Incidence of complications of thyroid surgery. Minerva Chir 55:693–702

Rosato L, Avenia N, Bernante P, De Palma M, Gulino G, Nasi PG, Pelizzo MR, Pezzullo L (2004) Complications of thyroid surgery: analysis of a multicentric study on 14,934 patients operated on in Italy over 5 years. World J Surg 28:271–276

Rosato L, Carlevato MT, De TG, Avenia N (2005) Recurrent laryngeal nerve damage and phonetic modifications after total thyroidectomy: surgical malpractice only or predictable sequence? World J Surg 29:780–784

Ruark DS, bdel-Misih RZ (1992) Thyroid and parathyroid surgery without drains. Head Neck 14:285–287

Samraj K, Gurusamy KS (2007) Wound drains following thyroid surgery. Cochrane Database Syst Rev 17:CD006099

Sano D, Ouoba K, Wandaogo A, Sanou A, Soudre BR (1995) Problemes poses par la chirurgie du corps thyroide au Burkina Faso, a propos de 83 cas. Med Trop (Mars) 55:51–54

Semm K (1983) Endoskopische Intraabdominalchirurgie in der Gynakologie. Wien Klein Wochenschr 95:353–367

Semm K (2001) Operationen ohne Skalpell. Ein Gynäkologe als Wegbereiter der Minimal Invasiven Medizin. Ecomed, Landsberg

Serpell JW, Phan D (2007) Safety of total thyroidectomy. ANZ J Surg 77:15–19

Sesterhenn AM, Folz BJ, Werner JA (2008) Surgical technique of endoscopic sentinel lymphadenectomy in the N0 neck. Oper Tech Otolaryngol 19:26–32

Shaha A, Jaffe BM (1988) Complications of thyroid surgery performed by residents. Surgery 104:1109–1114

Shimazu K, Shiba E, Tamaki Y, Takiguchi S, Taniguchi E, Ohashi S, Noguchi S (2003) Endoscopic thyroid surgery through the axillo-bilateral-breast approach. Surg Laparosc Endosc Percutan Tech 13:196–201

Shindo M, Chheda NN (2007) Incidence of vocal cord paralysis with and without recurrent laryngeal nerve monitoring during thyroidectomy. Arch Otolaryngol Head Neck Surg 133:481–485

Sodergren MH, Clark J, Athanasou T, Teare J, Yang G-Z, Darzi A (2009) Natural orifice translumenal endoscopic surgery: critical appraisal of applications in clinical practice. Surg Endosc 23:680–687

Spanknebel K, Chabot JA, Di Giorgi M, Cheung K, Lee S, Allendorf J, Logerfo P (2005) Thyroidectomy using local anesthesia: a report of 1,025 cases over 16 years. J Am Coll Surg 201:375–385

Tabaqchali MA, Hanson JM, Proud G (1999) Drains for thyroidectomy/parathyroidectomy: fact or fiction? Ann R Coll Surg Engl 81:302–305

Tarafder KH, Rahman SH, Hossain MA, Alauddin M, Islam MA, Hadi IA (2007) Outcome of management of differentiated thyroid carcinoma. Mymensingh Med J 16(Suppl):S46–S52

Terris DJ, Haus BM, Gourin CG (2004) Endoscopic neck surgery: resection of the submandibular gland in a cadaver model. Laryngoscope 114:407–410

Thomusch O, Machens A, Sekulla C, Ukkat J, Lippert H, Gastinger I, Dralle H (2000) Multivariate analysis of risk factors for postoperative complications in benign goiter surgery: prospective multicenter study in Germany. World J Surg 24:1335–1341

Vincent G (2008) Thyroidectomy over a quarter of a century in the Belgian ardennes: a retrospective study of 1207 patients. Acta Chir Belg 108:542–547

Werner JA, Sapundzhiev NR, Teymoortash A, Dunne AA, Behr T, Folz BJ (2004) Endoscopic sentinel lamphadenectomy as a new diagnostic approach in the N0 neck. Eur Arch Otorhinolaryngol 261:463–468

Wilhelm T, Benhidjeb T (2011) Trans-oral endoscopic neck surgery: feasibility and safety in a porcine model based on the example of thymectomy. Surg Endosc 25:1741–1746

Wilhelm T, Krüger J (2011) Ultrasound studies on the shift of cervical tissues in different head and neck positions – impact on trans-oral endoscopic, minimally invasive and conventional thyroid surgery. Ultrasound Med Biol 37(9):1430–1435. doi:10.1016/j.ultrasmedbio.2011.05.015, Epub 2011 Jul 7

Wilhelm T, Metzig A (2010a) Endoscopic minimal-invasive thyroidectomy: first clinical experience. Surg Endosc 24:1757–1758

Wilhelm T, Metzig A (2010b) Endoscopic minimally invasive thyroidectomy (eMIT): some clarifications regarding the idea, development, preclinical studies and the application in humans. Surg Endosc 24. doi:10.1007/s00464–010–1312–7, Epub 2010 Aug 24

Wilhelm T, Metzig A (2011a) Endoscopic minimally invasive thyroidectomy (eMIT): a prospective proof-of-concept study in humans. World J Surg 35:543–551

Wilhelm T, Metzig A (2011b) Proof-of-Concept study on the endoscopic minimally invasive thyroidectomy (eMIT) in humans – a realistic assessment is desired. World J Surg. doi:10.1007/s00268–011–1110–y

Wilhelm T, Harlaar J, Kerver A, Kleinrensink G-J, Benhidjeb T (2010) Surgical anatomy of the floor of the oral cavity and the cervical spaces as a rationale for trans-oral, minimal-invasive endoscopic surgical procedures: results of anatomical studies. Eur Arch Otorhinolaryngol 267:1285–1290

Wilhelm T, Klemm W, Leschber G, Harlaar JJ, Kerver ALA, Kleinrensink G-J, Nemat A (2011a) Development of a new trans-oral endoscopic approach for mediastinal surgery based on "natural orifice surgery": preclinical studies on surgical technique, feasibilitiy and safety. Eur J Cardiothorac Surg 39:1001–1008

Wilhelm T, Klemm W, Nemat A (2011b) Erste klinische Anwendung der trans-oral endoskopischen Mediastinalchirurgie. GMS Curr Posters Otorhinolaryngol Head Neck Surg 7:Doc02 (20110414) http://www.egms.de/static/pdf/journals/cpo/2011-7/cpo000591.pdf

Witzel K, Benhidjeb T (2009) Monitoring of the recurrent laryngeal nerve in totally endoscopic thyroid surgery. Eur Surg Res 43(2):72–76

Witzel K, von Rahden BHA, Kaminski K, Stein HJ (2008) Transoral access for endoscopic thyroid resection. Surg Endosc 22:1871–1875

Yamamoto M, Sasaki A, Asahi H, Shimada Y, Saito K (2002) Endoscopic versus conventional open thyroid lobectomy for benign thyroid nodules: a prospective study. Surg Laparosc Endosc Percutan Tech 12:426–429

Yarbrough DE, Thompson GB, Kasperbauer JL, Harper CM, Grant CS (2004) Intraoperative electromyographic monitoring of the recurrent laryngeal nerve in reoperative thyroid and parathyroid surgery. Surgery 136:1107–1115

Yeung HC, Ng WT, Kong CK (1997) Endoscopic thyroid and parathyroid surgery. Surg Endosc 11:1135

Zornig C, de Heer K, Koenecke S, Engel U, Bay V (1989) Darstellung des Nervus recurrens bei Schilddrüsenoperationen – Standortbestimmung. Chirurg 60:44–48

Intraoperative Nerve Stimulation in Minimally Invasive Thyroidectomy

20

Michal Mekel and Gregory W. Randolph

The recurrent laryngeal nerve (RLN) was discovered by Galen in the second century (Dedo 1970). In the seventh century, it was suggested by Paulus Aeginata that the nerve could be avoided during surgical treatment of the thyroid; however, toward the end of the nineteenth century, rates of RLN injury were still high with rates of 30% nerve paralysis revealed in a review of 44 of Billroths' patients (Randolph 2002). Current reported incidence of RLN injury varies considerably, with rates of permanent paralysis ranging from 0.5% to 2.4% and temporary paresis ranging from 2.6% to 5.9% (Myssiorek 2004). However, these reports may underestimate the true incidence of RLN injury, because most surgeons do not routinely perform preoperative and postoperative laryngoscopy. In addition, although the rate of RLN in expert hand may be low, many reports document rates in the 6–8% range.

20.1 RLN Neural Anatomy and Function

The right RLN branches from the vagus and courses up and behind the subclavian artery. The left RLN branches from the vagus and curves up under the aortic arch. On its pass upward the neck, the RLN has several meaningful anatomic landmarks. The first is the crossing of the RLN with the inferior thyroid artery which has large variability. Above the crossing point, the nerve travels superiorly in close proximity with the thyroid midpole region, and more superiorly it relates to the ligament of berry (Fig. 20.1). As the nerve travels upward to enter the larynx, it gives off multiple branches; the majority of these are sensory to the trachea, esophagus, hypopharynx, and larynx.

The RLN plays a major role in the function of the larynx and pharynx. It carries branchial efferents to the inferior constrictor muscle of the pharynx, cricopharyngeus muscle, and all intrinsic laryngeal muscles except for the cricothyroid muscle. The RLN consists of both sensory and motor fibers, and the bulk of sensory fibers are given off before laryngeal entry. The adductor fibers, adducting the vocal cords to the midline, outnumber the abductor fibers within the RLN. Paralysis of the RLN causes significant morbidity with voice changes, dysphagia, and aspirations with unilateral cord injury and airway distress with a need for tracheotomy in the case of bilateral vocal cord paralysis.

20.2 RLN Monitoring

Intraoperative neural monitoring (IONM) of the RLN during thyroid surgery has gained widespread acceptance as an adjunct to the gold standard of visual nerve identification. Lahey helped to introduce the routine dissection and demonstration of the RLN during thyroid surgery (Lahey and Hoover 1938). Since his publication in 1938, routine visual identification of the RLN has been shown to result in a lower incidence of

M. Mekel, M.D.
Endocrine Surgery Service, The Department of General Surgery, Rambam - Health Care Campus, Haifa, Israel
e-mail: m_mekel@rambam.health.gov.il

G.W. Randolph, M.D. (✉)
Division of Thyroid and Parathyroid Surgery,
Department of Otology and Laryngology,
Massachusetts Eye and Ear Infirmary,
243 Charles Street, Boston, MA 02114-3002, USA
e-mail: gregory_randolph@meei.harvard.edu

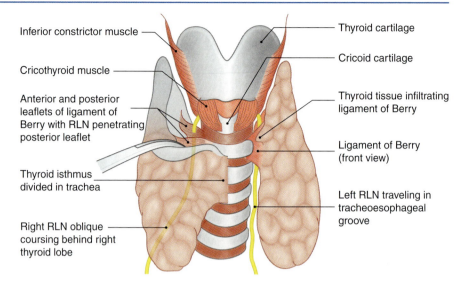

Fig. 20.1 Anterior view of the thyroid and airway, detailing RLN pass in relation to anterior and posterior leaflets of the ligament of Berry

RLN injury in multiple studies. Neural monitoring does not replace the need for surgical skill or the need for detailed anatomic knowledge. Rather, it is an adjunct to the visual identification of the nerve.

The basics of RLN monitoring technology involve two components: a method of stimulating the RLN intraoperatively and a method of assessing vocal cord response to the stimulation (Angelos 2009). IONM may be used for identification of the RLN, aid in the dissection of the RLN, and be used to anticipate postoperative neural function. For first visualization, the neural monitoring may be used to map out the nerve and finding its trajectory, and then dissection can be targeted. The nerve is first viewed as a white region in the dissection field, and additional dissection should then be done to identify the trajectory of the nerve. With the neural monitoring, the RLN is provocatively stimulated with a sterile stimulation probe, resulting in depolarization of the RLN with ipsilateral vocal cord measurement. This probe stimulation facilitates neural identification because non-neural tissue stimulation results in no electromyographic activity whereas neural stimulation does (Fig. 20.2). Electrical stimulation and electric confirmation add to the progressively obtained visual information, especially in cases where the visual information is problematic. The dissection of the RLN through difficult fields of dissection such as the ligament of Berry and a scarred revision field can be aided with stimulation. Finally, the neural monitoring can be used to prognosticate the function of an ipsilateral nerve in cases where a bilateral procedure is planned. This is of great significance in the prevention of bilateral nerve paralysis. In the case of nerve injury, the IONM may be used to identify the exact segment of nerve injured. This is done by first stimulating the most distal point of the RLN (at laryngeal entry point) and progressively running down. The point where the EMG falters is the point of injury. This allows the surgeon to treat the injured segment, depending of the nature of injury.

Even though IONM yields the greatest advantage in difficult thyroid cases, neural monitoring should be considered routinely given that difficult cases cannot always be predicted preoperatively. In addition, routine application has shown to steepen learning curves through greater experience in interpretation of the signal and troubleshooting system malfunction (Dionigi et al. 2008).

20.2.1 RLN Neural Monitoring in Minimally Invasive Thyroid Surgery

With several institutions now performing minimally invasive video-assisted thyroidectomy (MIVAT) in selected cases, there is increased interest in techniques that will maintain reduced morbidity and low complication rate. Laryngeal palpation, often times used in open procedures to assist in RLN identification, is not feasible in MIVAT. In addition, the potential for reduced visual information during minimally invasive thyroid and parathyroid surgery procedure has led to

Fig. 20.2 Stimulation artifact (**a**) and normal recurrent laryngeal nerve waveform (**b**)

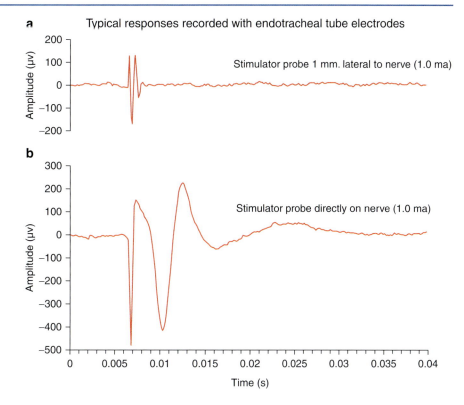

the great application of neural monitoring in those cases. IONM was shown to be feasible, easy, safe, and effective in minimally invasive and video-assisted thyroidectomies (Terris et al. 2007; Dionigi et al. 2009; Kandil et al. 2009). Terris et al. (2007) demonstrated in a prospective analysis that IONM serves as an adjunct to the visual identification in minimal access thyroid surgery. Kandil et al. (2009) found that though the operating space in these endoscopic surgeries was relatively narrow, there was no difficulty using the IONM simulator probe. The use of a flexible tip of a monopolar stimulation probe allows good access to neural structures in areas outside the surgeon's field of view. This stimulator was helpful in detecting the plane of dissection. The small operative space and the possible problems linked to the specific endoscopic instrumentation do not appear to constitute important obstacles to the utilization of this technique (Dionigi et al. 2009). Dionigi et al. (2009) prospectively compared video-assisted thyroidectomy with and without the use of IONM. The vagus nerve and the RLN were correctly localized and monitored in all cases where the IONM was used. There were no permanent RLN injuries. The incidence of temporary RLN injury in the IONM group was 2.7% versus 8.3% in the non-IONM group; however, the difference was not statistically significant. In other minimally invasive techniques using a full endoscopic extracervical approach, such as axillary or breast access, longer stimulator probes are required due to the greater distance from the trocar insertion to the neck.

IONM in minimally invasive technique probably enables surgeons to feel more confident, indicates the correct plane of dissection, and may reduce the conversion rate to an open technique.

20.3 Superior Laryngeal Nerve Neural Monitoring

The superior laryngeal nerve (SLN) arises immediately beneath the nodose ganglion of the upper vagus and descends medial to the carotid sheath. Its external branch descends to the region of the superior pole and extends medially along the inferior constrictor fascia to enter the cricothyroid muscle (Fig. 20.3). The external branch of the superior laryngeal nerve (EBSLN) has a close association with the superior thyroid pedicle. With external

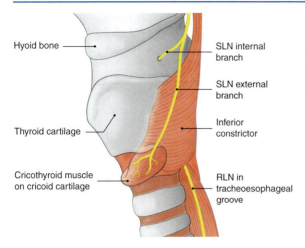

Fig. 20.3 Side view of recurrent and superior laryngeal nerve innervation of the larynx

branch injury, there is loss of vocal cord tensing, manifested by increased vocal tiredness and a loss of higher registers. The superior thyroid pole vessels should therefore be taken as low as possible at the level of the capsule of the thyroid to avoid injury to the EBSLN. In the study of Dionigi et al. (2009), the EBSLN was localized and monitored in 84% of cases in the IONM group. The EBSLN was first identified and exposed under optical magnification guidance and signaled by an audible signal and a corresponding contraction of the cricothyroid muscle using the neural monitoring.

20.4 Monitoring Equipment

Variation of equipment is found across different centers (Randolph et al. 2011). Nerve monitoring equipment is composed of three main components (Fig. 20.4):

1. The recording electrodes. A variety of different recording electrodes are available. These include vocal cord surface electrodes, vocal cord needle electrodes, and postcricoid paddle electrodes. Needle electrodes have a possibility of trauma, including vocal cord and laryngeal hematoma, vocal cord laceration, infection, and cuff deflation. Systems that rely on endotracheal tube–based surface electrodes represent the most common monitoring equipment format in use to date.
2. The stimulating electrodes include monopolar and bipolar neural stimulators. There is insufficient data in the literature as to which of these is preferable; however, when using a bipolar electrode, the utility of mapping the nerve may be compromised.
3. The monitoring system. This component includes a monitor depicting the laryngeal EMG waveform and others that only provide an audio tone. Systems that provide a visual waveform add the information of waveform morphology, amplitude, threshold, and latency. This information may be extremely important in differentiating between a true signal and an artifact. In addition, a visual waveform adds the information of signal quantification which is important in cases where

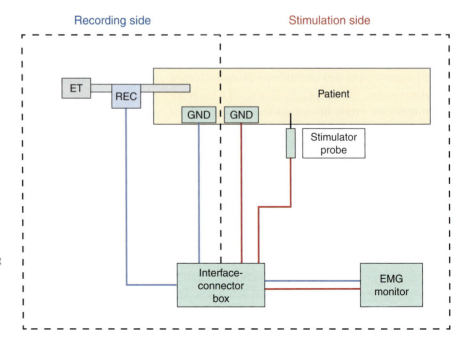

Fig. 20.4 Basic monitoring equipment setup. *ET* endotracheal tube, *REC* recording electrodes, *GND* ground electrodes, *EMG* electromyography

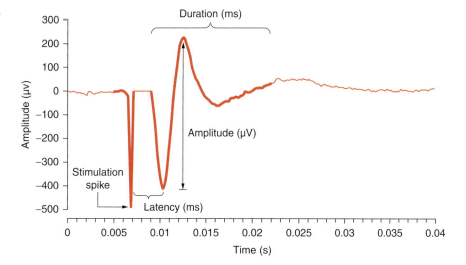

Fig. 20.5 RLN stimulation-induced waveform

there is loss of signal. It may also assist in surgical planning and is available for documentation of response.

20.5 Definitions and Terminology

The basic evoked waveform for the human RLN or vagus nerve is typically biphasic or triphasic (Fig. 20.5).

Amplitude: Vocal cord depolarization amplitudes typically range from 100 to 800 μV during normal awake speech. Monitoring amplitude is measured from the lowest deflection point to the next opposite waveform peak. Amplitudes during intraoperative monitoring vary among patients.

Threshold: Threshold is the minimal level of current that triggers an EMG activity. The RLN will first begin to stimulate at approximately 0.3–0.4 mA on a dissected free nerve. The amplitude will increase as the stimulation level increases to a maximum of approximately 0.8 mA. Beyond this point, increased current will depolarize a greater sphere of tissue with no increase in amplitude. It is therefore recommended that the bulk of intraoperative neural stimulation be performed at 1 mA. When searching for the nerve, a current of 2 mA may be used as this will stimulate a wider diameter sphere.

Latency: The speed of stimulation-induced depolarization. The latency depends on the distance of stimulation point to the ipsilateral vocal cords. It is measured from the stimulation spike to the first evoked waveform peak.

True positive test: Loss of signal during surgery combined with postoperative vocal cord paralysis.

False-positive test: Loss of signal with intact postoperative vocal cord mobility.

True-negative test: Good EMG with intact postoperative vocal cord mobility.

False-negative test: Good EMG with postoperative vocal cord paralysis.

20.6 Practical Steps in Monitoring

- Preoperative laryngoscopy should be done in all cases – it is essential to know the preoperative glottic function in order to accurately monitor the RLN function during surgery (Randolph and Kamani 2006). One cannot rely on the patient's vocal symptoms to predict glottis function. There are variations in vocal cord position with vocal cord paralysis, and there may also be contralateral compensation.
- RLN neuromonitoring should be discussed with the anesthesiologist before the beginning of the operation. The neuromonitoring tube should be prepared. Proper placement of the tube at the beginning of surgery is one of the most important steps and may reduce many technical problems. No muscle relaxation should be used during anesthesia. It is essential to have full muscular activity return within several minutes subsequent to intubation. A short-acting neuromuscular blocking agent such as succinylcholine or a small dose of nondepolarizing muscle relaxant, such as rocuronium, may be used. However, the depth of anesthesia should be deeper than usually employed with neuromuscular blockage in order to avoid spontaneous activity of the vocal cords.
- Stimulation of the vagus at the beginning of the case before surgical dissection should be done to ensure IONM system function. Only with a positive

vagal stimulation, a negative RLN stimulation can be relied on.
- The IONM is used to map out the nerve in the paratracheal region.
- IONM is used to assist in tracing the nerve and all its branches by stimulation of the nerve versus adjacent non-neural tissue.
- Stimulation of the vagus at the end of the dissection allows prognostication of postoperative glottis function. Vagal stimulation is superior to RLN stimulation in predicting vocal cord paralysis by testing the entire neural circuit (Dralle et al. 2004). Stimulating the RLN distal to the site of injury may give a false-negative result. Studies have shown postoperative neural function predictive with IONM associated with high negative prediction values of 92–100%. Positive predictive value, however, varies greatly 10–90% (Dralle et al. 2008).
- In the case of nerve injury, mapping the exact point of injury using the IONM.

20.7 Problem Solving

Technical problems can originate from the recording equipment including the recording electrodes, its connections, or from the stimulation probe and associated connections. The majority of equipment problems originate from malpositioning of the endotracheal tube recording electrodes (Randolph et al. 2011). Any change in larynx position relative to the endotracheal tube may result in malpositioned tube. In these cases, the tube should be repositioned by the anesthesiologist with either advancement or pulling back of the tube during vagal stimulation. The endotracheal tube may also rotate. Rechecking monitor settings for correct impedance values may be helpful in detecting a rotational error. Other possible problems include a misplaced ground electrode. The interface-connector box should be checked for the connection of the recording and ground electrodes.

20.8 Loss of Signal

Only after receiving a signal by vagal stimulation at the beginning of the operation can one trust an absent signal. Loss of signal can also represent a degradation of a satisfactory signal >100 µV to a signal <100 µV with suprathreshold level of stimulation. When a signal is lost, the first step is to assess whether there is laryngeal twitch upon stimulation of the vagus (Fig. 20.6). This is done with an index finger behind the posterior plate of the cricoid cartilage to palpate the twitch of the

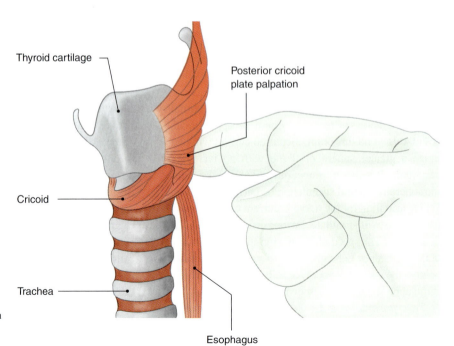

Fig. 20.6 Side view of the larynx, demonstrating position of finger to palpate laryngeal twitch

posterior cricoarytenoid muscle. A positive twitch ensures a functioning nerve and the presence of a technical error. If the twitch is not present, a stimulation error is present. The connections at the interface-connector box should be checked, and if no disconnection, the stimulator probe should be checked on a muscle to identify a twitch. A probe malfunction is considered if current delivery is not confirmed, and a new probe should be obtained. Another option is to stimulate the contralateral vagus nerve (side not yet dissected). If the contralateral vagus does not give a normal signal, one can assume a technical stimulation problem. If there is a normal stimulation from the contralateral vagus and other stimulation errors have been ruled out, nerve injury is suspected. In this setting, the nerve monitor can be used to precisely identify the point of injury. This is done by stimulation of the RLN from distal (laryngeal entry site) to proximal. Identification of a nonstimulated segment may reveal a clip or suture entrapping the nerve. Probably, the most important role for the nerve monitor is deciding on the timing of contralateral surgery when signal is lost in the first side in order to avoid the potential of bilateral nerve paralysis. Neuropraxia cannot be detected visually but can be detected electrically.

20.9 Summary

IONM is being increasingly used in the conventional open thyroid surgery approach. The principals of its use in minimally invasive techniques are no different than those applied in the open approach. It is easy to use. The regular flexible stimulator probe is suitable for use in many of the minimally access and video-assisted operations. Minimal modification in the stimulating equipment should be employed with total external minimally invasive approach. The use of a nerve monitor seems to provide the surgeon with greater confidence and improve the quality of minimally invasive thyroid and parathyroid surgery.

References

Angelos P (2009) Recurrent laryngeal nerve monitoring: state of the art, ethical and legal issues. Surg Clin North Am 89(5): 1157–1169

Dedo HH (1970) The paralyzed larynx: an electromyographic study in dogs and humans. Laryngoscope 80(10):1455–1517

Dionigi G, Bacuzzi A, Boni L, Rovera F, Dionigi R (2008) What is the learning curve for intraoperative neuromonitoring in thyroid surgery? Int J Surg 6(Suppl 1):S7–S12

Dionigi G, Boni L, Rovera F, Bacuzzi A, Dionigi R (2009) Neuromonitoring and video-assisted thyroidectomy: a prospective, randomized case–control evaluation. Surg Endosc 23(5):996–1003

Dralle H, Sekulla C, Haerting J, Timmermann W, Neumann HJ, Kruse E et al (2004) Risk factors of paralysis and functional outcome after recurrent laryngeal nerve monitoring in thyroid surgery. Surgery 136(6):1310–1322

Dralle H, Sekulla C, Lorenz K, Brauckhoff M, Machens A (2008) Intraoperative monitoring of the recurrent laryngeal nerve in thyroid surgery. World J Surg 32(7):1358–1366

Kandil E, Wassef SN, Alabbas H, Freidlander PL (2009) Minimally invasive video-assisted thyroidectomy and parathyroidectomy with intraoperative recurrent laryngeal nerve monitoring. Int J Otolaryngol 2009:739798

Lahey FH, Hoover WB (1938) Injuries to the recurrent laryngeal nerve in thyroid operations: their management and avoidance. Ann Surg 108(4):545–562

Myssiorek D (2004) Recurrent laryngeal nerve paralysis: anatomy and etiology. Otolaryngol Clin North Am 37(1):25–44, v

Randolph GW (2003) Surgical anatomy of the recurrent laryngeal nerve. In: Randolph GW (ed) Surgery of the thyroid and parathyroid glands. Elsevier Science, Philadelphia

Randolph GW, Kamani D (2006) The importance of preoperative laryngoscopy in patients undergoing thyroidectomy: voice, vocal cord function, and the preoperative detection of invasive thyroid malignancy. Surgery 139(3):357–362

Randolph GW, Dralle H, Abdullah H, Barczynski M, Bellantone R, Brauckhoff M et al (2011) Electrophysiologic recurrent laryngeal nerve monitoring during thyroid and parathyroid surgery: international standards guideline statement. Laryngoscope 121(Suppl 1):S1–S16

Terris DJ, Anderson SK, Watts TL, Chin E (2007) Laryngeal nerve monitoring and minimally invasive thyroid surgery: complementary technologies. Arch Otolaryngol Head Neck Surg 133(12):1254–1257

Complications of Minimally Invasive Thyroidectomy

David Soonmin Kwon and Nancy Dugal Perrier

In recent years, minimally invasive thyroid (MIT) surgery has become a well-recognized adjunct to the traditional standard cervicotomy for thyroid diseases. It has been postulated that this procedure potentially could achieve the same results as those obtained with traditional surgery in the setting of less trauma, earlier hospital discharges, less postoperative pain, and better cosmetic results.

A variety of minimal invasive thyroid techniques have been introduced since Gagner et al. first introduced the minimally invasive technique in 1996 (Gagner 1996). Multiple variations on the minimally invasive approach to thyroid surgery have been endorsed. These techniques can generally be grouped into two major categories: minimally invasive thyroidectomy with or without video assistance, or a pure endoscopic approach, known as minimal access thyroidectomy (MAT). Others have attempted MIT through axillary approaches, axillo-breast approaches, and, most recently, robot-assisted thyroid surgery (RATS). It is thought these procedures facilitate accurate and stable dissection with superior three-dimensional visualization of vital structures, including the superior laryngeal nerve, the recurrent laryngeal nerve, and parathyroid glands, and avoid the cervical incision.

The minimally invasive video-assisted thyroidectomy (MIVAT) technique, pioneered by Miccoli et al. (1999), combines endoscopic visualization and Harmonic technology along with a series of departures from conventional steps in thyroid surgery to achieve a minimally invasive thyroidectomy that has been readily adopted by surgeons (Terris et al. 2008). A multi-institutional North American study (Terris et al. 2008) validated previous reports (Miccoli et al. 1999, 2001, 2009) that MIVAT is readily feasible with low complication rates and low conversion rates to open surgery in those patients who fit inclusion criteria for MIT.

While MIVAT has shown promising results, there has been a surging interest in RATS (Kang et al. 2009a, b, c, d; Landry et al. 2010, 2011). Proponents for this procedure argue that the advanced articulation resolves the difficulties of conventional endoscopic instrumentation and the difficulty manipulating in tight operative spaces. In addition, because the operator controls the entire operative procedure, there are fewer problems associated with assistant-dependent movements or camera instability (Kang et al. 2009b). Hand tremor is eliminated, and the fine motion scaling of the robot system provides for more accurate dissection (Gutt et al. 2004; Savitt et al. 2005; Link et al. 2006).

Although thyroid operations are considered safe procedures, complications in thyroid surgery are not uncommon and account for significant malpractice claims in the United States. Recurrent laryngeal nerve (RLN) injury accounts for the majority of malpractice suits after thyroid surgery, although compromised airway, hematoma formation, perforated esophagus, parathyroid injury, and inadequate surgery have been cited as other reasons for malpractice suits (Abadin et al. 2010). The reported risk of complications in MIT ranges from 0% to 7.4% (Terris et al. 2008;

D.S. Kwon, M.D. • N.D. Perrier, M.D. (✉)
Department of Surgical Oncology, University of Texas
MD Anderson Cancer Center,
PO Box 301402, Houston, TX 77230, USA
e-mail: dkwon1@hfhs.org; nperrier@mdanderson.org

Lombardi et al. 2005; Terris et al. 2006), and robotic thyroid surgery currently ranges from 8% to 28.5% of patients (Kang et al. 2009d; Landry et al. 2011). Therefore, the surgeon undertaking the minimally invasive approach must be mindful of the risks associated with the inherent thyroid dissection. For those undertaking RATS, additional factors such as patient positioning, longer planes of dissection, and the potential for significant bleeding must be taken into consideration.

21.1 Preoperative Considerations

Appropriate preoperative patient selection and technical considerations are the first steps to avoiding complications associated with MIT. Patients interested in pursuing MIT must first meet eligibility criteria (Table 21.1), including a single nodule or goiter that does not exceed 3.5 cm or a total thyroid volume over 25 ml. A small (maximum 2 cm) differentiated carcinoma without lymph node involvement is not a contraindication to MIT.

For those undergoing RATS, preoperative workup must first exclude a known malignancy. Potential candidates are those who require thyroid lobectomy for diagnostic purposes (based on fine needle aspiration suggestive of follicular neoplasm) or for symptomatic reasons (i.e., enlarged solitary symptomatic nodule). Resections are limited to a unilateral thyroid lobe less than 6.5 cm in size. Body habitus is also very important. Based on the MD Anderson experience, copious subcutaneous fat or large body frames make the operation more technically challenging. Ideal body mass index (BMI) is less than 35, and the distance from the sternal notch to the axillary incision should be 18 cm or less (Fig. 21.1).

A thorough musculoskeletal history and physical must be documented prior to surgery. Any previous shoulder or cervical operations or prior injury are noted, and exclude eligibility. A cervical examination should be performed to document neck extension and to assess preoperative ipsilateral, upper extremity range of motion. If a female patient wishes to undergo RATS, she should have a recent documented mammogram, as postoperative changes such as fluid tracking may hinder immediate postoperative or future mammogram readings.

Table 21.1 Inclusion and exclusion criteria for minimally invasive thyroid surgery

	Indications	Relative contraindications
MIT	Single nodules or goiter < 3.5 cm	History of thyroiditis
	Total thyroid volume < 25 ml	History of prior neck irradiation
	Small, differentiated carcinoma (<2 cm) without LN involvement	History of prior neck surgery
		Large, multinodular goiter
		LN metastasis
		Reoperative surgery
RATS	Lobectomy required for diagnostic purposes	Diagnosis of malignancy
	Thyroid lobe < 6.5 cm	History of prior cervical or shoulder surgery
	BMI < 35	Large, multinodular goiter
	Distance from incision to sternal notch < 18 cm	Reoperative surgery

MIT minimally invasive thyroidectomy (includes MIVAT and MAT), *RATS* robot-assisted thyroid surgery, *LN* lymph node

21.2 Intraoperative Complications

21.2.1 Patient Positioning

Care must be taken to avoid cervical injury in MIT or RATS due to the hyperextension of the neck that is required for surgery. Brachial plexus injury, which causes significant postoperative pain or temporary paralysis, is a known intraoperative complication associated with RATS. Pain with decreased range of motion, temporary ulnar nerve paresthesia, and temporary arm paralysis have been reported (Kang et al. 2009d; Landry et al. 2011).

To assure that brachial plexus stretch and injury is avoided, several key steps must be taken at the time of arm positioning. When the patient is brought into the operating suite and placed supine on the operating room table, a wedge is placed horizontally under the patient's shoulder blades to allow for slight hyperextension of the neck. The patient's comfort with arm placement is the most important aspect of positioning and should be achieved with the patient awake and alert. The patient's ipsilateral arm is first raised with

Fig. 21.1 In the proposed planes of dissection for RATS, the distance from the sternal notch (*SN*) to the axillary incision should be 18 cm or less

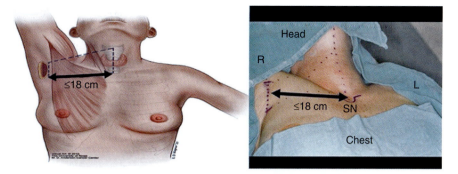

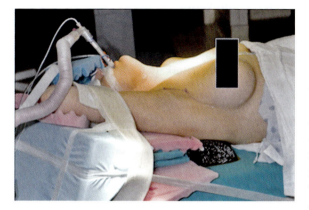

Fig. 21.2 During patient positioning, the forearm is placed above the head, and the arm is secured on an arm board and padded to avoid hyperextension

the bicep parallel to the jawbone. For most patients, the shoulder is then flexed to approximately 160° and internally rotated. The elbow is flexed to approximately 90°. The forearm is placed superior to the head, and the arm is secured on an arm board and padded to avoid pressure points or hyperextension (Fig. 21.2). After wrapping the arm in gauze to prevent a change in position during the operation, the patient is intubated.

21.2.2 Hemorrhage

A clear understanding of the cervical anatomy is critical to prevent bleeding. In MIVAT, there is a significant risk for bleeding at the time the thyroidal vessels are ligated due to the limited space in the operative field. At particular risk is the superior pole vessel; if it is not properly ligated, there can be significant bleeding, and controlling the blood loss may require converting to a traditional cervicotomy for optimal visualization.

When performing RATS, it is essential that the surgeon understand the lateral cervical anatomy, especially the relationship between the clavicle, the carotid artery, internal jugular vein, and sternocleidomastoid muscle as visualized from the axilla. Familiarity of the axillary anatomy, including the location of the axillary vein, relative to the lateral border of the pectoralis muscle is necessary to avoid injury to the vein during the initial dissection. As the dissection courses toward the lateral border of the strap muscles, careful attention must also be given to an unnamed tributary of the external jugular vein near the superior-most portion of the dissection. Suction, a laparoscopic clip applier, and a sponge on a stick are important instruments to facilitate the dissection. During the development of the avascular plane between the sternal and clavicular heads of the sternocleidomastoid muscle, care must be taken also to identify and avoid injury to the carotid artery and internal jugular vein. These vessels are at highest risk for injury when the planes between the two heads of the sternocleidomastoid muscle are separated. Attention to the carotid pulse and keen attention to fascia is important since it is difficult to palpate the vessels at this level of dissection. Injury to either of these vessels could cause significant blood loss and would require immediate conversion to a formal cervical excision and exploration.

21.2.3 Nerve Injury

Damage to the recurrently laryngeal nerve (RLN) may cause unilateral paralysis of the ipsilateral vocal cord. Symptoms can include hoarseness of voice as well as difficulty swallowing or aspiration of liquids. RLN injury is often temporary and resolves over days to

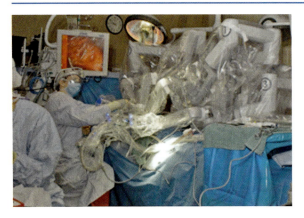

Fig. 21.3 Robotic arms are docked during RATS. The thyroid parenchyma has been rotated medially and anteriorly

months. The 30°, 5-mm endoscope used in MIVAT affords improved visualization of the RLN. Although the nerve may be more readily identified and seen, the imprecise movements of the surgical instrumentation (14-cm-long Harmonic scalpel) may cause iatrogenic RLN injury. Data suggest that temporary nerve palsy may occur in upward of 5% of patients, with permanent injury that has been reported up to 2% of the time (Kandil et al. 2009; Dionigi et al. 2010; Snissarenko et al. 2009). In a series of 581 patients undergoing RATS, 13 (2%) experienced transient hoarseness; 2 patients experienced permanent nerve injury (Kang et al. 2009c).

During a robotic procedure, after the robotic arms have been docked (Fig. 21.3) and the console-directed portion of the procedure has started, the thyroid parenchyma must be rotated medially and anteriorly as in a standard open procedure. During this elevation, the superior and inferior parathyroid glands are identified, and the RLN is identified as it courses in the tracheoesophageal groove. Care must be taken to protect the nerve when dissecting the thyroid and ligating vessels. Due to the limited haptic feedback associated with robotic surgery, injury to the RLN may occur inadvertently when excessive traction is applied or with overaggressive dissection. This is also applicable to the external branch of the superior laryngeal nerve, where injury may occur when the upper pole of the thyroid is drawn downward to isolate the superior thyroid vessels.

Nerve injury may also occur secondarily during dissection with the Harmonic scalpel, which is utilized in both MIVAT and RATS. Although less heat is generated than with conventional unipolar or bipolar electrocautery, the space constraints of these procedures may transmit inadvertent thermal energy to be to the surrounding tissue, which may cause injury to the nerve. Therefore, utilizing intraoperative nerve monitoring may be a useful adjunct for precautionary measures.

21.3 Postoperative Complications

21.3.1 Hematoma

In open cervical procedures, a neck hematoma requiring reoperative intervention occurs in about 1 of every 150 thyroid cases (Burkey et al. 2001; Abbas et al. 2001). Symptoms of hematoma, including neck swelling, increased pain, hoarseness of voice, or difficulty breathing, often indicate the need for emergent decompression. This is a relative rare complication in open thyroid surgery, and most recent data suggest that significant blood loss requiring reoperative intervention in MIVAT is extremely low, similar to the open procedure (Sgourakis et al. 2008; Fan et al. 2010; El-Labban 2009).

However, due to the complex anatomy associated with RATS, there has been significant concern for blood loss and hematomas. A significantly larger operative field is created during the subcutaneous dissection leading to the thyroid, and care must be taken to identify and cauterize or ligate perforating vessels arising from the pectoralis muscle during the development of skin flaps to access to the cervical region. In addition, care must be taken to avoid traction injuries to the anterior jugular vein during the placement of the bladed robotic thyroid retractor. The vascular pedicles supplying the thyroid must be hemostatically secured under direct visualization with the Harmonic scalpel. At a single-center experience in South Korea, where the most RATS have been performed, the incidence of postoperative hematoma was less than 1% (Kang et al. 2009c, d).

21.3.2 Seroma

Seromas have not been readily recognized as a complication of MIVAT. However, due to the extensive operative field created by the flap dissection from the axilla to the anterior neck in RATS, the risk for seroma formation may be greater than either MIVAT or an open thyroid procedure. A seroma may be recognized by a patient complaint of chest or supraclavicular fullness. Accumulated fluid collections at the sight of the ipsilateral chest wall can often be palpated. As a preventive method, a drain is routinely placed in the inferior portion of the field of dissection to drain any accumulating fluid. This drain is routinely removed on either postoperative day number 1 or 2.

21.3.3 Postoperative Pain

Unlike a standard cervical incision, MIT incisions are generally smaller, ranging from 2 to 3.5 cm in length (Miccoli et al. 1999, 2001, 2008, 2010a, b; Ruggieri et al. 2005, 2003) and have been associated with less postoperative pain and less narcotic use (Miccoli et al. 2010b; Ujiki et al. 2006). However, RATS entails at least a 5–6-cm longitudinal incision along the outer border of the pectoralis major muscle. In addition, there is significantly more dissection required to perform the operation safely and adequately. Unfortunately, in some patients, this may equate to more postoperative pain, requiring more analgesics than would be required in a standard cervical procedure. Often the pain is the result of irritation from the axillary drain. Patients may also note tingling and burning or numbness in the area of the supraclavicular dissection in the months following the procedure as the cutaneous nerves reinnervate.

21.3.4 Hypoparathyroidism

Devascularization of the parathyroid glands is a well-known complication of thyroid surgery. In open cases, temporary hypocalcemia may occur in approximately 10% of patients after total thyroidectomy, and permanent hypocalcemia in about 1% of the population (Doherty 2005). This can occur with either arterial or venous devascularization of the parathyroid glands or with inadvertently removal. The endoscopic view and the three-dimensional optics of the robotic system offer magnified views and should decrease the risk for hypoparathyroidism. However, the inability to perform precision dissection with the MIVAT instrumentation or the lack of haptic feedback during robotic dissection of the thyroid gland may contribute to injury of the parathyroid gland. When the parathyroid is dissected free from the thyroid, excessive traction or overaggressive dissection causes damage to the blood supply of the parathyroid, rendering it transiently ischemic, which may cause symptomatic hypocalcemia. Medial dissection and avoidance of disrupting the lateral vascular pedicle is likely to prevent this type of injury from occurring.

Postoperative serum calcium levels and parathyroid hormone levels are obtained to monitor for hypoparathyroidism if the thyroid lobectomy is being performed as a completion thyroidectomy. Patients may complain of numbness and tingling if the patients are rendered temporarily hypoparathyroid. More severe symptoms of hypocalcemia such as severe muscle cramping at rest or tetany are possible but rare. An elicitable Chvostek's or Trousseau's sign means that treatment with both intravenous calcium supplements and oral supplementation is required. The duration and aggressiveness of replacement are guided by the severity of symptoms. If the PTH levels are low, supplementing with vitamin D will facilitate the gastrointestinal absorption of calcium.

21.4 Conclusion

Minimally invasive thyroid surgery is increasingly being utilized as an adjunct in the armamentarium of options for the patient requiring thyroid gland removal. Although popularized in Europe and Asia, these novel techniques are becoming more commonplace in the United States. Robot-assisted thyroid surgery is still in its infancy, and its role in thyroid surgery will be defined in the future.

Minimally invasive surgery has compared favorably to the conventional open surgical approach, and many proponents note advantages in terms of postoperative cosmesis, pain, and earlier hospital discharges in comparison to the traditional open technique. However, there are still considerable drawbacks to these procedures. Despite the improved visualization with the minimally invasive techniques, careful attention must be made to the cervical and axillary anatomy to prevent unwanted effects of hemorrhage or nerve injury. Avoidance of iatrogenic thermal injury to the recurrent laryngeal nerve is necessary.

Little has been documented regarding the complications of robot-assisted thyroid surgery. Careful preoperative workup must include thorough documentation of cervical musculoskeletal issues and range of motion, as well as documentation of preoperative mammographic imaging, if the patient is female. In addition to the aforementioned risks associated with MIT, optimal patient positioning of the ipsilateral arm and neck is key in preventing stretch of the brachial plexus or range of motion injuries. Drain placement avoids seroma formation. Vigilant postoperative observation must be ensured to avoid a missed hematoma.

References

Abadin SS, Kaplan EL, Angelos P (2010) Malpractice litigation after thyroid surgery: the role of recurrent laryngeal nerve injuries, 1989–2009. Surgery 148:718–722; discussion 722–713

Abbas G, Dubner S, Heller KS (2001) Re-operation for bleeding after thyroidectomy and parathyroidectomy. Head Neck 23: 544–546

Burkey SH, van Heerden JA, Thompson GB et al (2001) Reexploration for symptomatic hematomas after cervical exploration. Surgery 130:914–920

Dionigi G, Boni L, Rausei S (2010) Minimally invasive video-assisted thyroidectomy and parathyroidectomy with intraoperative recurrent laryngeal nerve monitoring. Int J Otolaryngol 2010:834913

Doherty G (2005) Complications of thyroid and parathyroid surgery. In: Mulholland MW (ed) Complications in surgery. Lippincott and Williams, Philadelphia

El-Labban GM (2009) Minimally invasive video-assisted thyroidectomy versus conventional thyroidectomy: a single-blinded, randomized controlled clinical trial. J Minim Access Surg 5:97–102

Fan Y, Guo B, Guo S et al (2010) Minimally invasive video-assisted thyroidectomy: experience of 300 cases. Surg Endosc 24:2393–2400

Gagner M (1996) Endoscopic subtotal parathyroidectomy in patients with primary hyperparathyroidism. Br J Surg 83:875

Gutt CN, Oniu T, Mehrabi A et al (2004) Robot-assisted abdominal surgery. Br J Surg 91:1390–1397

Kandil E, Wassef SN, Alabbas H, Freidlander PL (2009) Minimally invasive video-assisted thyroidectomy and parathyroidectomy with intraoperative recurrent laryngeal nerve monitoring. Int J Otolaryngol 2009:739798

Kang SW, Jeong JJ, Nam KH et al (2009a) Robot-assisted endoscopic thyroidectomy for thyroid malignancies using a gasless transaxillary approach. J Am Coll Surg 209:e1–e7

Kang SW, Jeong JJ, Yun JS et al (2009b) Robot-assisted endoscopic surgery for thyroid cancer: experience with the first 100 patients. Surg Endosc 23:2399–2406

Kang SW, Jeong JJ, Yun JS et al (2009c) Gasless endoscopic thyroidectomy using trans-axillary approach; surgical outcome of 581 patients. Endocr J 56:361–369

Kang SW, Lee SC, Lee SH et al (2009d) Robotic thyroid surgery using a gasless, transaxillary approach and the da Vinci S system: the operative outcomes of 338 consecutive patients. Surgery 146:1048–1055

Landry CS, Grubbs EG, Perrier ND (2010) Bilateral robotic-assisted transaxillary surgery. Arch Surg 145:717–720

Landry CS, Grubbs EG, Stephen Morris G et al (2011) Robot assisted transaxillary surgery (RATS) for the removal of thyroid and parathyroid glands. Surgery 149(4):549–555

Link RE, Bhayani SB, Kavoussi LR (2006) A prospective comparison of robotic and laparoscopic pyeloplasty. Ann Surg 243:486–491

Lombardi CP, Raffaelli M, Princi P et al (2005) Safety of video-assisted thyroidectomy versus conventional surgery. Head Neck 27:58–64

Miccoli P, Berti P, Conte M et al (1999) Minimally invasive surgery for thyroid small nodules: preliminary report. J Endocrinol Invest 22:849–851

Miccoli P, Berti P, Raffaelli M et al (2001) Comparison between minimally invasive video-assisted thyroidectomy and conventional thyroidectomy: a prospective randomized study. Surgery 130:1039–1043

Miccoli P, Berti P, Ambrosini CE (2008) Perspectives and lessons learned after a decade of minimally invasive video-assisted thyroidectomy. ORL J Otorhinolaryngol Relat Spec 70:282–286

Miccoli P, Pinchera A, Materazzi G et al (2009) Surgical treatment of low- and intermediate-risk papillary thyroid cancer with minimally invasive video-assisted thyroidectomy. J Clin Endocrinol Metab 94:1618–1622

Miccoli P, Materazzi G, Berti P (2010a) Minimally invasive thyroidectomy in the treatment of well differentiated thyroid cancers: indications and limits. Curr Opin Otolaryngol Head Neck Surg 18:114–118

Miccoli P, Rago R, Massi M et al (2010b) Standard versus video-assisted thyroidectomy: objective postoperative pain evaluation. Surg Endosc 24:2415–2417

Ruggieri M, Straniero A, Pacini FM et al (2003) Video-assisted surgery of the thyroid diseases. Eur Rev Med Pharmacol Sci 7:91–96

Ruggieri M, Straniero A, Mascaro A et al (2005) The minimally invasive open video-assisted approach in surgical thyroid diseases. BMC Surg 5:9

Savitt MA, Gao G, Furnary AP et al (2005) Application of robotic-assisted techniques to the surgical evaluation and treatment of the anterior mediastinum. Ann Thorac Surg 79:450–455; discussion 455

Sgourakis G, Sotiropoulos GC, Neuhauser M et al (2008) Comparison between minimally invasive video-assisted thyroidectomy and conventional thyroidectomy: is there any evidence-based information? Thyroid 18:721–727

Snissarenko EP, Kim GH, Simental AA Jr et al (2009) Minimally invasive video-assisted thyroidectomy: a retrospective study over two years of experience. Otolaryngol Head Neck Surg 141:29–33

Terris DJ, Gourin CG, Chin E (2006) Minimally invasive thyroidectomy: basic and advanced techniques. Laryngoscope 116:350–356

Terris DJ, Angelos P, Steward DL, Simental AA (2008) Minimally invasive video-assisted thyroidectomy: a multi-institutional North American experience. Arch Otolaryngol Head Neck Surg 134:81–84

Ujiki MB, Sturgeon C, Denham D et al (2006) Minimally invasive video-assisted thyroidectomy for follicular neoplasm: is there an advantage over conventional thyroidectomy? Ann Surg Oncol 13:182–186

Minimally Invasive Thyroidectomy for Thyroid Carcinoma

22

Roy Phitayakorn

22.1 Introduction

The incidence of thyroid cancer around the world has been steadily rising over the last several decades for many reasons including the increase in imaging of the thyroid gland and therefore the detection of small papillary thyroid cancers, as well as rising body mass index, insulin-resistance syndrome, and the use of fertility medications (Goodman et al. 1992; Engeland et al. 2006; Davies and Welch 2006; Hannibal et al. 2008; Rezzonico et al. 2008). Thyroid cancer typically occurs in women and is most commonly diagnosed in the third to fourth decades of life (Sherman 2003). Therefore, minimally invasive thyroidectomy (MIT) may be well suited to the treatment of certain types of thyroid carcinoma.

This chapter is an evidence-based review of the current medical literature on the use of MIT techniques for thyroid carcinoma. Specifically, we will review various guidelines from different organizations for the treatment of well-differentiated and medullary thyroid carcinoma and compare these guidelines to results with MIT in the literature. The classification level for the different types of medical literature evidence was based on recommendations by Sackett with Heinrich et al.'s modification, as detailed in Table 22.1. This review is structured around several themes or controversies including the use of MIT techniques for the surgical management of:

1. Indeterminate thyroid nodules
2. Papillary thyroid carcinoma that is <1 cm and >1 cm including postoperative staging and surveillance
3. Medullary thyroid carcinoma
4. Prophylactic and therapeutic central neck compartment lymphadenectomy
5. Lateral neck compartment lymphadenectomy

22.2 MIT and Indeterminate Thyroid Nodules

Thyroid nodules that are indeterminate on FNA (i.e., follicular neoplasm or Hürthle cell neoplasm) comprise 15–30% of all FNA diagnoses (Haugen et al. 2002; Hegedus 2004). Approximately 20–30% of these indeterminate nodules will contain a follicular carcinoma, follicular variant of papillary carcinoma, or Hürthle cell carcinoma (McHenry and Phitayakorn 2011; Baloch et al. 2008). Thyroid nodules that are classified as atypia or follicular lesion of undetermined significance (FLUS) have a 5–10% risk of malignancy. The optimal initial extent of surgery for these lesions is unclear. Certain clinical features such as marked atypia, history of external beam or ionizing radiation as a child, male gender, nodule size >4 cm, family history of thyroid cancer, older patient age, and FDG-PET positivity may all increase the overall chance that these types of thyroid nodules are malignant (Tuttle et al. 1998; Tyler et al. 1994; Kelman et al. 2001). A diagnostic thyroid lobectomy ± intraoperative frozen section may be the preferred approach in patients without any of these features and a solitary follicular lesion. However, a total thyroidectomy is also reasonable as the initial operation in patients with bilateral thyroid

---

R. Phitayakorn, M.D., MHPE
Endocrine Surgery Unit, The Massachusetts
General Hospital, Harvard Medical School, WACC Suite 460,
15 Parkman Street, Boston, MA 02114, USA
e-mail: rphitayakorn@partners.org

Table 22.1 Sackett's classification of level of evidence with Heinrich's modification (Sackett (1989) and Heinrich et al. (2006))

Level of evidence	Type of trial	Criteria for classification
I	Large randomized trials with clear-cut results (and low risk of error)	Sample size calculation provided and fulfilled, study endpoint provided
II	Small randomized trials with uncertain results (and moderate to high risk of errors)	Matched analysis, sample size calculation not provided, convincing comparative studies
III	Nonrandomized, contemporaneous controls	Noncomparative, prospective
IV	Nonrandomized, historical controls	Retrospective analysis, cohort studies
V	No control, case series only, opinion of experts	Small series, review articles

nodules, an increased risk of malignancy, or patients who do not wish to return to the operating room for a possible completion thyroidectomy.

Since many patients with follicular lesions of the thyroid will not have malignant disease, several different surgical groups have endeavored to apply minimally invasive thyroidectomy techniques for diagnostic thyroid lobectomy. Two of these studies are small randomized studies without sample size calculations (level II evidence), two studies are nonrandomized and prospective (level III evidence), and three studies are nonrandomized and retrospective (level IV evidence).

For example, the University of Rome surgical group in Rome, Italy (Bellantone et al. 2002), conducted a randomized prospective study of 62 patients (31 MIVAT lobectomy and 31 conventional lobectomy) with a solitary thyroid nodule that was not malignant on FNA. Four patients in the MIVAT group required conversion to a conventional operation because the recurrent laryngeal nerve could not be identified. Patients in the MIVAT group were significantly more satisfied with their scars, as well as experienced less postoperative pain, and a decreased number of hospitalization days.

In addition, the Mansoura University surgical group in Mansoura, Egypt (Hegazy et al. 2007), performed a prospective randomized study of 74 patients undergoing thyroidectomy. Patients were randomized to either MIVAT ($n=41$) or conventional thyroidectomy via the Sofferman technique ($n=33$). Six patients in the MIVAT group required conversion to conventional thyroidectomy for frozen section positive for follicular carcinoma ($n=3$), technical reasons ($n=2$), and underestimated thyroid gland size ($n=1$) and were excluded from analysis. Although a specific subgroup analysis was not performed for patients with follicular neoplasm, it appeared that both groups had similar mean operating times, complication rates, and patient satisfaction with cosmetic result. The MIVAT group had significantly less pain at 6, 24, and 48 h postsurgery.

Similarly, the Chang Gung Memorial Hospital surgical group in Taoyuan, Taiwan (Chao et al. 2004a, b), randomized 116 patients with either follicular neoplasm and/or benign nodular thyroid disease to MIVAT ($n=52$) or conventional thyroidectomy ($n=59$). Interestingly, they found a decreased rate of external branch of the superior laryngeal nerve injuries ($p=0.03$) and similar rates of temporary recurrent laryngeal nerve palsy in the MIVAT group compared to conventional thyroidectomy groups.

Also, the University of Sydney surgical group in Sydney, Australia (Lundgren et al. 2007), conducted a retrospective cohort study of 201 patients who underwent minimally invasive thyroidectomy using a lateral mini-incision approach for a preoperative FNA of atypical or inconclusive follicular pattern. These patients were matched to 819 patients who underwent conventional thyroidectomy during the same time period (2002–2006). There was no difference in postoperative complications between the two groups.

The Northwestern University surgical group in Chicago, Illinois, USA (Ujiki et al. 2006), performed a nonrandomized prospective study of 22 patients with at least one indeterminate nodule on FNA. Eighteen MIVAT lobectomies and 4 total thyroidectomies were then matched to 26 patients who underwent traditional open thyroidectomy (23 thyroid lobectomies and 3 total thyroidectomies). On final analysis, MIVAT appeared to be as safe as conventional thyroidectomy with comparable usage in postoperative narcotics but significantly less usage of a COX-2 anti-inflammatory medication. However, MIVAT required an extra 56 min for total thyroidectomy and 16 min for thyroid lobectomy compared to conventional thyroidectomy, but operative costs were believed to be similar.

The Mount Sinai surgical group in New York City, New York, USA (Gagner and Inabnet 2001), described the use of endoscopic thyroidectomy with CO_2 insufflation on 15 patients with indeterminate thyroid nodules compared to conventional thyroidectomy in 18 patients. Mean operating time for endoscopic thyroidectomy was 220 min (range = 120–330 min), but the patients in the endoscopic thyroidectomy group had improved overall self-reported cosmesis and faster return to normal activity (5 ± 4 versus 11 ± 8 days).

The Soonchunhyang University surgical group in Bucheon, Korea (Koh et al. 2009), described 52 consecutive patients who underwent a unilateral axillobreast approach endoscopic thyroidectomy for a solitary thyroid nodules that was less than 6 cm and benign or indeterminate on FNA. There were no conversions to open, but postoperative complications including transient moderate or severe pain in their neck or anterior chest wall on postoperative day 1 ($n = 27$), seroma ($n = 5$), mild hypoesthesia or paresthesia at operative sites ($n = 3$), swallowing difficulty 3 months postoperatively ($n = 2$), RLN palsy ($n = 1$), and minimal hematoma that was drained at the bedside ($n = 1$).

The University of Texas M.D. Anderson surgical group in Houston, Texas, USA (Kuppersmith and Holsinger 2011), published their early results of a nonrandomized retrospective review of 31 consecutive robotic thyroidectomies. Only six of these patients had a follicular neoplasm on preoperative FNA. Total surgical times were 132–328 min, and three postoperative complications were recorded. One patient had a temporary distal radial nerve neuropraxia likely secondary to positioning on the operating room table, and two patients had significant blood loss related to anterior jugular vein injuries. There were no conversions to conventional thyroidectomy.

As a note of caution, Hur et al. (2011) described the case report of a 61-year-old woman who presented to another institution with a 4.4-cm left thyroid mass that was described as a follicular neoplasm on FNA. The patient underwent left thyroidectomy via bilateral breast/axillary technique. Thirty-one months later, the patient presented with numerous bean-sized lesions along her sternum, anterior neck, anterior chest wall, and thyroid bed. These tumors and the right thyroid lobe were resected using conventional thyroidectomy and were follicular carcinomas on final pathology.

In summary, in small randomized and nonrandomized studies, nonendoscopic MIT, such as the lateral mini-incision and hybrid endoscopic procedures, such as the MIVAT, appear to be at least as safe as conventional thyroidectomy for indeterminate thyroid nodules with likely improved cosmesis and less postoperative pain. On the other hand, purely endoscopic thyroidectomy procedures offer improved cosmesis compared to conventional thyroidectomy but require significantly more operative time with increased complications and expense. Pure endoscopic techniques may also not be suitable for large follicular neoplasms due to complications of tumor spillage in case of malignancy.

22.3 MIT and Micropapillary Thyroid Carcinoma

The World Health Organization defines micropapillary thyroid carcinoma as papillary thyroid carcinoma in a thyroid nodule that is ≤1 cm in greatest dimension (Lloyd et al. 2004). The overall incidence of micropapillary thyroid carcinoma has dramatically increased in the last several decades likely due to the development of high-resolution ultrasonography and ultrasound-guided fine needle aspiration techniques. The management of micropapillary thyroid carcinoma is controversial in the medical literature, although it is generally agreed that it has an excellent prognosis as death from disease is very rare. The American Thyroid Association (ATA), Latin American Thyroid Society (LATS), European Thyroid Association (ETA), British Thyroid Association (BTA), and the National Cancer Center Network (NCCN) guidelines all state that thyroid lobectomy may be sufficient for micropapillary thyroid carcinoma in patients with low risk for recurrence. However, multifocal micropapillary carcinoma (≥2 tumors) or lymph node involvement has been associated with an increased risk of recurrence (Roti et al. 2008), and these patients would likely benefit from total thyroidectomy and/or postoperative radioactive iodine.

Several surgical groups, primarily in Asia, have used various types of purely endoscopic MIT techniques in patients with micropapillary carcinoma. We did not find any articles that focused on the use of MIVAT for micropapillary carcinoma. Unfortunately, there are no randomized prospective studies and only two large retrospective studies using purely endoscopic techniques (level IV evidence).

For example, the Seoul National University surgical group in Seoul, Korea (Chung et al. 2007), reviewed the records of 198 patients who underwent conventional thyroidectomy versus 103 patients who underwent bilateral axillo-breast (BAB) approach for micropapillary carcinoma from 2003 to 2006. The BAB approach was associated with significantly increased operative times (165 versus 111 min) and transient recurrent laryngeal nerve palsies (2.5% versus 25.2%). One patient in the BAB group had an operative site infection that was associated with a tracheoesophageal injury. A subset analysis of 146 patients who underwent conventional thyroidectomy versus 72 endoscopic surgery patients demonstrated no difference in postoperative thyroglobulin (Tg) levels after levothyroxine withdrawal and a similar recurrence rate. Mean follow-up time was not provided.

Similarly, the Yonsei University surgical group also in Seoul, Korea (Jeong et al. 2009), reviewed the records of 224 patients who underwent conventional thyroidectomy versus 275 patients who underwent a gasless endoscopic transaxillary approach for micropapillary carcinoma from 2005 to 2007. This group also noted that the endoscopic approach was associated with increased operative times (139±49 versus 106±42 min) and increased postoperative complications including temporary hypocalcemia, transient RLN palsies, and tracheoesophageal injuries. A subset analysis of 35 patients in the endoscopic group and 117 patients in the conventional thyroidectomy group demonstrated comparable levels of RAI uptake 4–6 weeks after surgery. Interestingly, the mean thyroid-stimulating hormone (TSH) suppressed serum Tg levels and recurrence rates were higher in the conventional thyroidectomy group, but it is unclear if these results are statistically significant. The mean follow-up period of 18.4 months was very short (range=4–37 months).

Given the limited available evidence, it does not appear that purely endoscopic MIT techniques are an ideal treatment method for micropapillary carcinoma. Further randomized trials will be needed to see if there are any advantages to using MIT for this disease.

22.4 MIT and Papillary Thyroid Carcinoma

The guidelines from the ATA, LATS, and ETA agree that total (or near total) thyroidectomy is indicated in patients with papillary thyroid cancer (PTC) >1 cm. However, the BTA and the NCCN guidelines state that thyroid lobectomy may be acceptable for well-differentiated carcinomas in patients with low risk factors for recurrence (see Table 22.2 for definitions of risk). All of the above guidelines use the Union for International Cancer Control (UICC) or American Joint Committee on Cancer (AJCC) postoperative TNM staging system for differentiated thyroid cancer (DTC) (Table 22.3). In addition, radioactive iodine (RAI) for remnant ablation should be used selectively

Table 22.2 Definitions of risk by different thyroid organizations

Categories	ATA	BTA	ETA	LATS
Very low risk	N/A	N/A	T1 ≤ 1 cm, no extension beyond the thyroid capsule, and N0M0	T1 ≤ 1 cm, no extension beyond the thyroid capsule, and N0M0
Low risk	N0M0, no residual tumor, no tumor invasion, no aggressive histology or vascular invasion, no I131 uptake outside of thyroid bed on 1st WBS after RAI ablation	Any T, any N, M0 in patient <45 years or T1, N0, M0 in patient ≥45 years	Unifocal T1 or T2, N0M0, or multifocal T1N0M0	T1 > 1 cm, multifocal T1 or T2, N0M0, no extracapsular extension or vascular invasion, no I131 uptake outside the thyroid bed on first posttreatment WBS, and nonaggressive histological features
Intermediate risk	Microscopic tumor invasion, N1, aggressive histology or vascular invasion, or I131 uptake outside of thyroid bed	N/A	N/A	N/A
High risk	Macroscopic tumor invasion, incomplete tumor resection, M1, thyroglobulinemia out of proportion to posttreatment RAI scan	Age >40, male gender, aggressive histology, extrathyroidal tumor extension, N1, or M1	Any T3 or T4 or any T1N1 or any M1	>45 years of age, T3 or T4, N1, M1, persistent disease, extracapsular extension or vascular invasion, and aggressive histology

ATA American Thyroid Association, *BTA* British Thyroid Association, *ETA* European Thyroid Association, *LATS* Latin America Thyroid Society, *NCCN* National Cancer Center Network

Table 22.3 TNM classification system for DTC

T1	Tumor diameter 2 cm or smaller
T2	Primary tumor diameter >2–4 cm
T3	Primary tumor diameter >4 cm limited to the thyroid or with minimal extrathyroidal extension
T4a	Tumor of any size extending beyond the thyroid capsule to invade subcutaneous soft tissues, larynx, trachea, esophagus, or recurrent laryngeal nerve
T4b	Tumor invades prevertebral fascia or encases carotid artery or mediastinal vessels
TX	Primary tumor size unknown but without extrathyroidal invasion
N0	No metastatic nodes
N1a	Metastases to level VI (pretracheal, paratracheal, and prelaryngeal or Delphian lymph nodes)
N1b	Metastasis to unilateral, bilateral, contralateral cervical or superior mediastinal nodes
NX	Nodes not assessed at surgery
M0	No distant metastases
M1	Distant metastases
MX	Distant metastases not assessed
	Patient age <45 years
Stage I	Any T, any N, M0
Stage II	Any T, any N, M1
Stage III	N/A
Stage IV	N/A
	Patient age 45 years or older
Stage I	T1, N0, M0
Stage II	T2, N0, M0
Stage III	T3, N0, M0
	T1–3, N1a, M0
Stage IVa	T4a, N0–N1a, M0
	T1–4a, N1b, M0
Stage IVb	T4b, Any N, M0
Stage IVc	Any T, Any N, M1

in patients with DTC. The benefits of RAI ablation include the presumed eradication of remaining thyroid and thyroid cancer cells which improves overall sensitivity of Tg measurement and may decrease risk of recurrence and improve overall survival. However, RAI is also associated with early side effects of nausea, dry mouth, neck discomfort, and sialadenitis. Late side effects of RAI have also been reported to include a small risk of secondary malignancy (leukemia, bladder, colorectal, breast, and salivary glands), increased risk of miscarriage up to 1 year postablation, and infertility in men. A summary of the RAI recommendations from the various thyroid organizations is listed in Table 22.4. TSH suppressive therapy should be offered as summarized in Table 22.5. Finally, serum Tg measurements are an important aspect of the long-term follow-up for patients with DTC (Table 22.6). Due to differences in assay techniques, these measurements should be performed by the same laboratory over time if possible. Antithyroglobulin antibodies (anti-TgAbs) are present in approximately 25% of thyroid cancer patients and may falsely elevate or suppress serum Tg levels. Since anti-TgAb levels typically decline to undetectable levels over a period 2–3 years, the persistence of recurrence of anti-TgAbs may be an indicator of recurrent disease (Chiovato et al. 2003 and Spencer et al. 1998).

Several research groups have examined the usage of MIVAT specifically in patients with papillary thyroid carcinoma. There is one small prospective randomized study (level II evidence) and one nonrandomized prospective study (level III evidence) in the recent medical literature.

The randomized study was from the University of Pisa surgical group in Pisa, Italy (Miccoli et al. 2002). They conducted a prospective randomized study where 33 patients with FNA-proven PTC received total thyroidectomy either via MIVAT (16 patients) or conventional surgery (17 patients). There were no statistical differences between the two surgical techniques in terms of final tumor size, postoperative mean I-131 uptake, or mean serum Tg levels. However, critics noted that this study was underpowered to detect any true differences and also did not describe any final oncologic outcomes. Therefore, a follow-up prospective study was published in 2009 (Miccoli et al. 2009) which examined 221 patients with PTC smaller than 3 cm. One hundred and eighty-four patients underwent MIVAT and 50 patients had conventional thyroidectomy and then all patients received ablative dosages of RAI. After 1 year, TSH-stimulated serum Tg levels were 25.3 ± 118.4 ng/mL (range 15–1322 ng/mL) in the MIVAT group versus 8.3 ± 9.5 ng/mL (range = 1–38 ng/mL). Patients with a TSH-stimulated serum Tg > 1 ng/mL underwent repeated RAI treatment. The patients in the MIVAT group required statistically more RAI treatments than the conventional thyroidectomy group, but there was no difference in the number of patients who were disease-free versus persistent disease in either group. The mean follow-up time was 3.6 ± 1.5 years (range 1–8 years).

The University of Rome surgical group (Lombardi et al. 2007a, b) also performed a retrospective study of 271 patients with papillary thyroid carcinoma (215T1,

Table 22.4 Summary of RAI recommendations from thyroid organizations

Factors	Description	ATA	BTA	ETA	LATS	NCCN
T1	≤1 cm	No	Selective	No	No	Selective
	1–2 cm	Selective	Selective	Selective	Selective	Selective
T2	>2–4 cm	Selective	Selective	Selective	Selective	Selective
T3	>4 cm	Yes	Yes	Yes	Yes	Selective
T4	Gross extrathyroidal extension	Yes	Yes	Yes	Yes	Selective
NX, N0	No metastatic nodes	No	No	Selective	No	Selective
N1	Metastatic to local/regional nodes	Selective	Selective	Yes	Yes	Selective
M1	Distant metastasis present	Yes	Yes	Yes	Yes	Selective
Unfavorable histology	Tall cell, columnar, diffuse sclerosing, insular, solid, and poorly differentiated	Selective	Selective	Selective	Yes	Selective

Yes RAI indicated, *No* RAI not indicated, *Selective* RAI may be indicated, *ATA* American Thyroid Association, *BTA* British Thyroid Association, *ETA* European Thyroid Association, *LATS* Latin America Thyroid Society, *NCCN* National Cancer Center Network

Table 22.5 Recommendations for TSH levels based on risk

Categories	ATA	BTA	ETA	LATS
Very low risk	N/A	N/A	Not specified	Supplemental dosages only
Low risk	Equal to or slightly below lower limit of normal (0.1–0.5 mU/L)	<0.5 mU/L	Initially <0.1 mU/L and then <0.5 mU/L once confirmed to be in remission	0.4–1.0 mU/L
Intermediate risk	<0.1 mU/L	N/A	N/A	N/A
High risk	<0.1 mU/L	<0.1 mU/L	≤0.1 mU/L	<0.1 mU/L

ATA American Thyroid Association, *BTA* British Thyroid Association, *ETA* European Thyroid Association, *LATS* Latin America Thyroid Society, *NCCN* National Cancer Center Network

Table 22.6 Recommendations for thyroglobulin measurements

	Recommendation	Supporting organization
Logistics	Should use the same laboratory each time	ATA, BTA, ETA, LATS, NCCN
	TSH and anti-Tg antibody levels should be checked with each serum Tg	ATA, BTA, ETA, LATS, NCCN
Initial Tg check	Initial Tg measurement should be >3 months after surgery	ETA
	Initial Tg measurement should be >6 weeks after surgery	BTA
	Initial Tg measurement should be 6–12 months after surgery	LATS
	If anti-TgAb is positive, then should recheck at 6 month intervals	BTA
Subsequent Tg checks	Check serum Tg every 6–12 months	ATA, LATS
	Check serum Tg every 12 months if patient is in remission	BTA
	If patient is low risk for recurrence, check TSH-stimulated Tg 12 months after surgery	ATA, ETA, LATS
Long-term follow-up	Rising consecutive Tg levels may warrant diagnostic WBS	ETA
	Tg > 2 ng/mL following TSH stimulation indicates persistent/recurrent disease	ATA, LATS
	Tg > 10 ng/mL requires empiric I-131 treatment	NCCN
	Ig Tg positive, but WBS negative consider other forms of imaging	ATA, ETA, LATS, NCCN

ATA American Thyroid Association, *BTA* British Thyroid Association, *ETA* European Thyroid Association, *LATS* Latin America Thyroid Society, *NCCN* National Cancer Center Network

23T2, 33 with T3 tumors) who underwent MIVAT from 1998 to 2006. Nineteen of the 102 patients who had a video-assisted central neck lymph node dissection had positive lymph node metastases. Follow-up data was available for only 85.2% of these patients with a mean follow-up time of only 19.5±5.7 months (range=3–40 months). One hundred fifty-two patients (79 low risk and 73 high risk) were subsequently followed with postoperative cervical ultrasound (U/S), whole-body scans (WBS), radioactive iodine uptake (RAIU), and TSH-stimulated Tg levels. Postoperative U/S demonstrated no residual thyroid tissue in any patient, but post-RAI WBS demonstrated residual thyroid tissue in 66 (90.4%) of the high-risk patients and coexisting lymph node metastases in one high-risk patient. Mean RAIU and TSH-stimulated Tg levels were 2.1±3.3% (range=0–22.6%) and 5.5±6.2 ng/mL (range=<0.1–25.3 ng/mL), respectively. The number of patients with anti-Tg antibodies was not described. Fifty-four of the 73 high-risk patients were reevaluated 6–10 months after initial RAI administration, and successful ablation was noted in 49 patients (90.7%).

In addition, the Changhua Christian Hospital surgical group in Changhua, Taiwan (Wu et al. 2010), offered 44 patients with FNA-proven PTC the choice between MIVAT ($n=21$) and conventional total thyroidectomy ($n=23$). Median tumor size was 1.5 cm (range=1.0–2.5 cm) for the MIVAT group and 1.7 cm (range=1.0–3.0 cm) for the conventional group. Ten patients in the MIVAT group required central neck lymphadenectomy with 60% positive for malignancy. Fifteen patients in the conventional group had central neck lymph node dissection with only 33% positive for PTC. All patients had serum Tg levels and anti-Tg antibody levels measured prior to receiving 120 mCi of RAI 4 weeks after surgery. Interestingly, levothyroxine withdrawal serum Tg levels were significantly lower in the MIVAT group (<0.5 ng/mL, range=<0.5–15.8 ng/mL) versus the conventional thyroidectomy group (5.4 ng/mL, range=<0.5–60.3 ng/mL). The authors state that this result is due to the superior visualization offered by the endoscope during MIVAT. No ultrasound results were provided regarding the lateral neck lymph node status and amount of residual thyroid tissue.

The University of Parma surgical group in Parma, Italy (Del Rio et al. 2009), performed a retrospective case–control study of 16 patients who underwent MIVAT versus 26 patients who underwent traditional total thyroidectomy and had papillary carcinomas on final pathology. Mean tumor size was similar in both groups (1.33±0.63 cm in MIVAT versus 1.64±0.82 cm in traditional thyroidectomy). No separate subanalysis was performed for patients with papillary microcarcinomas. Postoperative WBS demonstrated residual thyroid tissue in two patients from the MIVAT group and five patients from the traditional total thyroidectomy group ($p=$ns). After 12 months, serum Tg levels in both groups were similar (0.65 in MIVAT versus 0.71 ng/mL in traditional thyroidectomy), but it is unknown if these values were drawn while on levothyroxine or after levothyroxine withdrawal.

The Chang Gung University surgical group in Taoyuan, Taiwan (Chao et al. 2004a, b), performed a nonrandomized prospective study of MIVAT in seven patients with papillary thyroid carcinoma. Tumor size was from 0.7 to 3.8 cm, and postoperative serum Tg levels ranged from <1.0 in three patients to 19.9 µg/L approximately 4 weeks after total thyroidectomy. Postoperative ultrasound findings were not reported. All patients received ablation of thyroid remnants with 1,110 MBq, and 1-year serum Tg levels were <1.0 in one patient with a TSH < 1.0 and were <1.0 in six patients after levothyroxine withdrawal. Total follow-up time was 17–43 months with a median of 34 months.

One must follow standard oncological surgery principles when using MIT for patients with thyroid carcinoma. These principles include meticulous dissection technique with minimal direct contact with the tumor to avoid rupturing the thyroid capsule and possibly spilling malignant cells into the thyroid bed. One of the potential disadvantages of using MIT for thyroid carcinoma is the small working space and the need to remove the tumor through a very small skin opening. In a small randomized study (level III evidence), Lombardi et al. (2005) demonstrated that MIVAT can be associated with no tumor cell spillage or difference in inflammatory markers when compared to conventional thyroidectomy. However, seeding of malignant cells from tumor spillage has been reported after MIT from purely endoscopic techniques. Kim et al. (2008) described the case of a

25-year-old woman who presented with a 3.1-cm solitary right thyroid nodule that was steadily increasing in size but was benign on FNA and ultrasound. A right endoscopic thyroidectomy was performed using the bilateral breast/axillary approach, but during surgery, there was an inadvertent tear of the tumor capsule with spillage of nodular contents. One year later, the patient presented with multiple small nodules in the operative bed, sternocleidomastoid, strap muscles, and subcutaneous tissue within the tunnel in her anterior chest from the endoscopic thyroidectomy. These nodules were positive for PTC on FNA. Two more operations were performed for completion thyroidectomy and excision of the involved tissues.

22.5 MIT and Medullary Thyroid Carcinoma

Medullary thyroid cancer (MTC) accounts for approximately 4% of all thyroid cancers and is a neuroendocrine tumor of the parafollicular thyroid cells (C cells). These cells are typically located in the lateral upper two-thirds of the thyroid gland and produce calcitonin, which helps regulate calcium metabolism. About 20–25% of cases, MTC is an autosomal dominant trait that is part of familial MTC (FMTC) or multiple endocrine neoplasia (MEN) type 2A or 2B. Mutations in the RET (REarranged during Transfection) proto-oncogene on chromosome 10 allows the identification of FMTC/MEN carriers in nearly 100% of cases (De Groot et al. 2006). Various thyroid organizations including the ATA and NCCN state that all patients with a personal or family history consistent with FMTC or MEN 2A/2B should be offered RET testing. Patients with Hirschsprung disease should also be tested. If the RET testing is positive, then these patients should be offered prophylactic total thyroidectomy. Central neck lymphadenectomy should also be done if it will be therapeutic, but prophylactic central neck dissection is controversial (Frank-Raue et al. 2006; Scheuba et al. 2007). The timing of thyroidectomy is based on the type of RET mutation and calcitonin screening results but may occur as early as the first year of life (Machens et al. 2001; Brandi et al. 2001; Al-Rawi and Wheeler 2006). The only surgical group with reported results using MIT for prophylactic thyroidectomy and central neck dissection in RET carriers is from the University of Pisa (Miccoli et al. 2007). They performed a non-randomized prospective study (level III evidence) of MIVAT and central neck dissection on 15 RET carriers with a mean age of 32.5 years (range = 10–56 years). The follow-up period was relatively short (range = 8–44 months). Calcitonin levels were undetectable in the six patients who had follow-up for more than 12 months. Prophylactic thyroidectomy using MIT techniques seems ideal for RET carriers since they are typically young and have normal-sized thyroid volumes. However, there is too little evidence to make any conclusions about its utility over conventional thyroidectomy.

About 80% of cases of MTC are sporadic and typically identified on FNA in a solitary thyroid nodule. Unfortunately, about 50% of sporadic cases have lymph node metastases at the time of diagnosis. Therefore, preoperative evaluation for sporadic MTC should include serum measurements of calcitonin, carcinoembryonic antigen (CEA), albumin corrected calcium or ionized calcium, and RET analysis. These patients should also be excluded for pheochromocytoma. Patients with sporadic MTC and no lymph node metastases should undergo a total thyroidectomy with prophylactic central neck dissection (ATA MTC guidelines, grade B). Patients with sporadic MTC and lateral neck lymph node metastases should undergo a total thyroidectomy, central neck dissection, and lateral compartment-directed neck dissection (ATA MTC guidelines, grade B). Finally, patients with sporadic MTC and local invasive or distant metastatic disease should be offered palliative surgery that minimizes central neck morbidity (ATA MTC guidelines, grade C). Since MTC does not respond to RAI, it is imperative that the primary operation be as complete as possible. Therefore, MIT techniques are not recommended for the treatment of FNA-proven MTC (Miccoli et al. 2010).

22.6 MIT and Central Compartment Lymphadenectomy for DTC

All of the thyroid cancer guidelines recommend consideration of a prophylactic compartment-oriented central lymphadenectomy for patients with tumors >4 cm, high risk of recurrence, or for level, and aggressive histological features. The ETA guidelines add that prophylactic central compartment neck dissection may be done to guide treatment. The ATA guidelines also mention that the surgeon must be very experienced in endocrine surgery to prevent increased risks of hypoparathyroidism and recurrent laryngeal nerve injury. All of the thyroid cancer guidelines agree that a therapeutic central compartment neck dissection at the time of total thyroidectomy may decrease the risk of recurrence and overall mortality in patients with clinically involved level VI lymph nodes. Ideally, at least six lymph nodes should be present in the final specimen to ensure adequate staging. Also, lymph node metastases are frequently found in the central neck compartment even with negative preoperative imaging. Therefore, when operating on patients with DTC via an MIT technique, one must be prepared to also do a central compartment neck dissection via MIT or will have to convert conventional thyroidectomy.

There are very few papers that specifically examine the ability of MIT techniques for a complete central compartment lymphadenectomy. For example, one paper is from several surgical groups in Seoul, Korea (Lee et al. 2010). They examined the use of a robotic BABA approach on 109 patients with mostly micropapillary carcinoma (mean tumor size was 0.7 ± 0.3 cm, range = 0.1–1.8 cm) who underwent total thyroidectomy and ipsilateral central neck dissection. The mean operative time was 206 ± 36 min (range = 145–322 min), and postoperative complications included transient RLN palsy in 16%, transient hypocalcemia in 19%, hematoma in one patient, and chyle leak in one patient. At 1-year follow-up, there was one case of permanent RLN palsy and two cases of permanent hypoparathyroidism. Follow-up time was short with a median of 16 months (range = 1–23 months). Approximately half of the patients received RAI, and their median-stimulated Tg level was 0.2 ng/mL (rage = <0.1–36.4) with 74% of this group with a stimulated Tg < 0.1 ng/mL.

Another paper that examined MIT and central neck lymphadenectomy was the University of Cincinnati surgical group in Cincinnati, Ohio, USA (Neidich and Steward 2011). They retrospectively reviewed 28 patients who underwent MIVAT (25 total thyroidectomies and 3 completion thyroidectomies) and simultaneous prophylactic central neck dissection. Fifteen patients underwent unilateral central neck dissection, and 13 patients had bilateral central neck dissections. On final pathology, 25 patients had PTC, 1 patient had FTC, 1 patient had MTC, and 1 patient had thyroiditis only. There were 145 total lymph nodes resected using MIVAT techniques for a mean of 5.2 nodes per patient (range = 0–16), and 11 patients (28%) had lymph nodes positive for carcinoma. There was no increase in postoperative complications when comparing patients who underwent unilateral versus bilateral central lymphadenectomy. One month postoperatively, 22% of patients had a serum Tg > 1 ng/mL. Further studies should be conducted in this area before any recommendations can be stated about the completeness of central compartment lymphadenectomy via MIT techniques.

22.7 MIT and Lateral Compartment Lymphadenectomy for DTC

All of the thyroid carcinoma guidelines agree that therapeutic lateral compartment neck dissection may decrease the risk of recurrence and overall mortality in patients with biopsy-proven metastatic DTC in the anterior lateral neck (lymph node levels II–IV). Several authors have demonstrated that therapeutic lateral lymph node dissections are possible using MIT techniques (level V evidence). However, there are no studies in the medical literature that compare MIT techniques versus conventional surgery for lateral neck dissection. Several groups have described a MIVAT-based technique (Ikeda et al. 2002; Kitagawa et al. 2003; Miccoli et al. 2008; Lombardi et al. 2007a, b), but only on a few patients (range = 2–4). Other authors have described completely endoscopic lateral neck dissection techniques (Shimizu et al. 2001; Kitano et al. 2002; Kang et al. 2009; Li et al. 2011). These studies also have small groups of patients (range = 1–13 patients) and short follow-up times. Further research is needed to understand if MIT lateral neck dissection techniques offer any advantages over conventional surgery.

22.8 Conclusions

Based on this review of the various guidelines for the management of thyroid carcinoma and current medical literature, the use of MIT techniques for thyroid carcinoma is still uncertain. Many surgical groups have used MIT techniques for differentiated thyroid carcinoma, but these studies are limited by small sample sizes and short follow-up times. We would recommend further research in this area, but the use of MIT for the treatment of DTC should not be done until the surgical team has successfully passed their "learning curve." Although this curve likely varies for each surgeon and MIT technique (Del Rio et al. 2008; Liu et al. 2009; Lee et al. 2010; Papavramidis et al. 2010), careful planning and progression as outlined in a recent paper by Perrier et al. (2010) can help predict intraoperative problems and enhance overall patient safety.

References

Al-Rawi M, Wheeler MH (2006) Medullary thyroid carcinoma: update and present management controversies. Ann R Coll Surg Engl 88:433–438

Baloch ZW, LiVolsi VA, Asa SL et al (2008) Diagnostic terminology and morphologic criteria for cytologic diagnosis of thyroid lesions: a synopsis of the National Cancer Institute Thyroid Fine-Needle Aspiration State of the Science Conference. Diagn Cytopathol 36:425–437

Bellantone R, Lombardi CP, Bossola M et al (2002) Video-assisted vs conventional thyroid lobectomy: a randomized trial. Arch Surg 137(3):301–304

Brandi ML, Gagel RF, Angeli A et al (2001) Guidelines for diagnosis and therapy of MEN type 1 and type 2. J Clin Endocrinol Metab 86:5658–5671

Chao TC, Lin JD, Chen MF (2004a) Video-assisted open thyroid lobectomy through a small incision. Surg Laparosc Endosc Percutan Tech 14(1):15–19

Chao TC, Lin JD, Chen MF (2004b) Gasless video-assisted total thyroidectomy in the treatment of low risk intrathyroid papillary carcinoma. World J Surg 28(9):876–879

Chiovato L, Latrofa F, Braverman LE et al (2003) Disappearance of humoral thyroid autoimmunity after complete removal of thyroid antigens. Ann Intern Med 139(5 Pt 1):346–351

Chung YS, Choe JH, Kang KH et al (2007) Endoscopic thyroidectomy for thyroid malignancies: comparison with conventional open thyroidectomy. World J Surg 31(12):2302–2306

Davies L, Welch HG (2006) Increasing incidence of thyroid cancer in the United States, 1973–2002. JAMA 295(18):2164–2167

de Groot JW, Links TP, Plukker JT et al (2006) RET as a diagnostic and therapeutic target in sporadic and hereditary endocrine tumors. Endocr Rev 27:535–560

Del Rio P, Sommaruga L, Cataldo S et al (2008) Minimally invasive video-assisted thyroidectomy: the learning curve. Eur Surg Res 41(1):33–36

Del Rio P, Sommaruga L, Pisani P et al (2009) Minimally invasive video-assisted thyroidectomy in differentiated thyroid cancer: a 1-year follow-up. Surg Laparosc Endosc Percutan Tech 19(4):290–292

Engeland A, Tretli S, Akslen LA et al (2006) Body size and thyroid cancer in two million Norwegian men and women. Br J Cancer 95(3):366–370

Frank-Raue K, Buhr H, Dralle H et al (2006) Long-term outcome in 46 gene carriers of hereditary medullary thyroid carcinoma after prophylactic thyroidectomy: impact of individual RET genotype. Eur J Endocrinol 155:229–236

Gagner M, Inabnet WB 3rd (2001) Endoscopic thyroidectomy for solitary thyroid nodules. Thyroid 11(2):161–163

Goodman MT, Kolonel LN, Wilkens LR (1992) The association of body size, reproductive factors and thyroid cancer. Br J Cancer 66(6):1180–1184

Hannibal CG, Jensen A, Sharif H et al (2008) Risk of thyroid cancer after exposure to fertility drugs: results from a large Danish cohort study. Hum Reprod 23(2):451–456

Haugen BR, Woodmansee WW, McDermott MT (2002) Towards improving the utility of fine-needle aspiration biopsy for the diagnosis of thyroid tumors. Clin Endocrinol 56:281–290

Hegazy MA, Khater AA, Setit AE et al (2007) Minimally invasive video-assisted thyroidectomy for small follicular thyroid nodules. World J Surg 31(9):1743–1750

Hegedus L (2004) Clinical practice: the thyroid nodule. N Engl J Med 351:1764–1771

Heinrich S, Schafer M, Rousson V et al (2006) Evidence-based treatment of acute pancreatitis: a look at established paradigms. Ann Surg 243:154–168

Hur SM, Kim SH, Lee SK et al (2011) Is a thyroid follicular neoplasm a good indication for endoscopic surgery? Surg Laparosc Endosc Percutan Tech 21(3):e148–e151

Ikeda Y, Takami H, Sasaki Y et al (2002) Minimally invasive video-assisted thyroidectomy and lymphadenectomy for micropapillary carcinoma of the thyroid. J Surg Oncol 80:218–221

Jeong JJ, Kang SW, Yun JS et al (2009) Comparative study of endoscopic thyroidectomy versus conventional open thyroidectomy in papillary thyroid microcarcinoma (PTMC) patients. J Surg Oncol 100(6):477–480

Kang SW, Jeong JJ, Yun JS et al (2009) Gasless endoscopic thyroidectomy using trans-axillary approach; surgical outcome of 581 patients. Endocr J 56:361–369

Kelman AS, Rathan A, Leibowitz J et al (2001) Thyroid cytology and the risk of malignancy in thyroid nodules: importance of nuclear atypia in indeterminate specimens. Thyroid 11:271–277

Kitagawa W, Shimizu K, Akasu H et al (2003) Endoscopic neck surgery with lymph node dissection for papillary carcinoma of the thyroid using a totally gasless anterior neck skin lifting method. J Am Coll Surg 196:990–994

Kitano H, Fujimura M, Kinoshita T et al (2002) Endoscopic thyroid resection using cutaneous elevation in lieu of insufflation. Surg Endosc 16:88–91

Kim JH, Choi YJ, Kim JA, Gil WH, Nam SJ, Oh YL, Yang JH (2008) Thyroid cancer that developed around the operative bed and subcutaneous tunnel after endoscopic thyroidectomy via a breast approach. Surg Laparosc Endosc Percutan Tech 18(2):197–201

Koh YW, Kim JW, Lee SW et al (2009) Endoscopic thyroidectomy via a unilateral axillo-breast approach without gas insufflation for unilateral benign thyroid lesions. Surg Endosc 23(9):2053–2060

Kuppersmith RB, Holsinger FC (2011) Robotic thyroid surgery: an initial experience with North American patients. Laryngoscope 121(3):521–526

Lee KE, Koo do H, Kim SJ et al (2010) Outcomes of 109 patients with papillary thyroid carcinoma who underwent robotic total thyroidectomy with central node dissection via the bilateral axillo-breast approach. Surgery 148(6):1207–1213

Li Z, Wang P, Wang Y, Xu S, Cao L, Que R, Zhou F (2011) Endoscopic lateral neck dissection via breast approach for papillary thyroid carcinoma: a preliminary report. Surg Endosc 25(3):890–896

Liu S, Qiu M, Jiang DZ et al (2009) The learning curve for endoscopic thyroidectomy: a single surgeon's experience. Surg Endosc 23(8):1802–1806

Lloyd R, De Lellis R, Heitz P et al (2004) World Health Organization classification of tumours: pathology and genetics of tumours of the endocrine organs. IARC, Lyon

Lombardi CP, Raffaelli M, Princi P, Lulli P, Rossi ED, Fadda G, Bellantone R (2005) Safety of video-assisted thyroidectomy versus conventional surgery. Head Neck 27(1):58–64

Lombardi CP, Raffaelli M, de Crea C et al (2007a) Report on 8 years of experience with video-assisted thyroidectomy for papillary thyroid carcinoma. Surgery 142(6):944–951

Lombardi CP, Raffaelli M, Princi P et al (2007b) Minimally invasive video-assisted functional lateral neck dissection for metastatic papillary thyroid carcinoma. Am J Surg 193:114–118

Lundgren CI, Stalberg P, Grodski S et al (2007) Minimally invasive thyroid surgery for diagnostic excision of solitary thyroid nodules. Asian J Surg 30(4):250–254

Machens A, Gimm O, Hinze R et al (2001) Genotype–phenotype correlations in hereditary medullary thyroid carcinoma: oncological features and biochemical properties. J Clin Endocrinol Metab 86:1104–1109

McHenry CR, Phitayakorn R (2011) Follicular adenoma and carcinoma of the thyroid gland. Oncologist 16(5):585–593

Miccoli P, Elisei R, Materazzi G et al (2002) Minimally invasive video-assisted thyroidectomy for papillary carcinoma: a prospective study of its completeness. Surgery 132(6):1070–1073

Miccoli P, Elisei R, Donatini G et al (2007) Video-assisted central compartment lymphadenectomy in a patient with a positive RET oncogene: initial experience. Surg Endosc 21(1):120–123

Miccoli P, Materazzi G, Berti P (2008) Minimally invasive video-assisted lateral lymphadenectomy: a proposal. Surg Endosc 22:1131–1134

Miccoli P, Pinchera A, Materazzi G et al (2009) Surgical treatment of low- and intermediate-risk papillary thyroid cancer with minimally invasive video-assisted thyroidectomy. J Clin Endocrinol Metab 94(5):1618–1622

Miccoli P, Materazzi G, Berti P (2010) Minimally invasive thyroidectomy in the treatment of well differentiated thyroid cancers: indications and limits. Curr Opin Otolaryngol Head Neck Surg 18(2):114–118

Neidich MJ, Steward DL (2011) Safety and feasibility of elective minimally invasive video-assisted central neck dissection for thyroid carcinoma. Head Neck. doi:10.1002/hed.21733

Papavramidis TS, Michalopoulos N, Pliakos J et al (2010) Minimally invasive video-assisted total thyroidectomy: an easy to learn technique for skillful surgeons. Head Neck 32(10):1370–1376

Perrier ND, Randolph GW, Inabnet WB et al (2010) Robotic thyroidectomy: a framework for new technology assessment and safe implementation. Thyroid 20(12):1327–1332

Rezzonico J, Rezzonico M, Pusiol E et al (2008) Introducing the thyroid gland as another victim of the insulin resistance syndrome. Thyroid 18(4):461–464

Roti E, degli Uberti EC, Bondanelli M et al (2008) Thyroid papillary microcarcinoma: a descriptive and meta-analysis study. Eur J Endocrinol 159(6):659–673

Sackett DL (1989) Rules of evidence and clinical recommendations on the use of anti-thrombotic agents. Chest 95:2S–4S, 23

Scheuba C, Kaserer K, Bieglmayer C et al (2007) Medullary thyroid microcarcinoma recommendations for treatment – a single-center experience. Surgery 142:1003–1010

Sherman SI (2003) Thyroid carcinoma. Lancet 361(9356):501–511

Shimizu K, Kitagawa W, Akasu H, Tanaka S (2001) Endoscopic hemithyroidectomy and prophylactic lymph node dissection for micropapillary carcinoma of the thyroid by using a totally gasless anterior neck skin lifting method. J Surg Oncol 77(3):217–220

Spencer CA, Takeuchi M, Kazarosyan M et al (1998) Serum thyroglobulin autoantibodies: prevalence, influence on serum thyroglobulin measurement, and prognostic significance in patients with differentiated thyroid carcinoma. J Clin Endocrinol Metab 83(4):1121–1127

Tuttle RM, Lemar H, Burch HB (1998) Clinical features associated with an increased risk of thyroid malignancy in patients with follicular neoplasia by fine-needle aspiration. Thyroid 8:377–383

Tyler DS, Winchester DJ, Caraway NP et al (1994) Indeterminate fine-needle aspiration biopsy of the thyroid: identification of subgroups at high risk for invasive carcinoma. Surgery 116:1054–1060

Ujiki MB, Sturgeon C, Denham D et al (2006) Minimally invasive video-assisted thyroidectomy for follicular neoplasm: is there an advantage over conventional thyroidectomy? Ann Surg Oncol 13(2):182–186

Wu CT, Yang LH, Kuo SJ (2010) Comparison of video-assisted thyroidectomy and traditional thyroidectomy for the treatment of papillary thyroid carcinoma. Surg Endosc 24(7):1658–1662

Conventional Thyroidectomy Versus MIT: An Outcome Analysis

23

Raymon H. Grogan and Quan-Yang Duh

23.1 Introduction

Cristiano Hüscher of Italy published his data on the first completely endoscopic thyroidectomy in 1997 (Huscher et al. 1997). A review of the literature (Linos 2011) shows that at least 20 different minimally invasive thyroidectomy techniques have been proposed since 1997. Various groups from around the world have published hundreds of papers on their clinical experiences regarding these minimally invasive thyroidectomy techniques. Two of these techniques dominate the literature on minimally invasive thyroidectomy and are the best characterized from an evidenced-based viewpoint. First is the minimally invasive video-assisted thyroidectomy (MIVAT) initially developed in 1999 by Paolo Miccoli (Miccoli et al. 1999). Second is the scarless endoscopic thyroidectomy first reported in 2000 by Yoshifumi Ikeda and his Japanese colleagues (Ikeda et al. 2000) and more recently by various groups of Korean surgeons (Tae et al. 2011; Kang et al. 2009). This technique has also been combined with a robot-assisted technique and/or access via multiple sites including the upper chest wall, breast, and axilla. The surgical techniques for these two minimally invasive thyroidectomy procedures are described in detail elsewhere in this book. It is important to note that MIVAT leaves a scar on the neck while the scarless endoscopic thyroidectomy moves the scar from the neck to another site like the axilla. The remainder of this chapter is an overview of the current literature on these two techniques, with a particular focus on any direct, evidence-based comparisons between the two minimally invasive techniques and the traditional open (Kocher incision) thyroidectomy technique.

The true benefit of minimally invasive thyroidectomy has not definitively been answered in a rigorous evidence-based manner. A previously reported power analysis (Dionigi 2009) estimates that to prove a 1% change in morbidity between minimally invasive thyroidectomy and standard thyroidectomy techniques, a study would have to include 1,000 patients in both treatment groups. To date, that type of study has not been done. A large number of case series from individual institutions have been published on this topic. Case series are considered level 4 evidence and, while important, are not very useful for making clear, evidence-based decisions regarding clinical practice unless they show dramatic and unequivocal advancement in a field. In contrast, well-designed systematic reviews with properly executed meta-analysis of multiple homogeneous randomized controlled trials are the highest level of evidence. This chapter will focus on case–control studies (level 3b), cohort studies (level 2b), randomized controlled clinical trials (level 1b), and any systematic review of such data (level 1a–3a).

23.2 Evidence for the MIVAT Procedure

23.2.1 The First Decade, 1997–2007

In 2008, two groups published systematic reviews and/or meta-analysis of the MIVAT procedure and compared it to the standard open thyroidectomy. These two

R.H. Grogan, M.D. • Q.-Y. Duh, M.D. (✉)
Section of Endocrine Surgery, UCSF,
1600 Divisadero Street, Box 1674, San Francisco,
CA 94143, USA
e-mail: rgroganmd@gmail.com; quan-yang.duh@ucsfmedctr.org

D. Linos and W.Y. Chung (eds.), *Minimally Invasive Thyroidectomy*,
DOI 10.1007/978-3-642-23696-9_23, © Springer-Verlag Berlin Heidelberg 2012

papers from Miccoli (Miccoli et al. 2008) and Sgourakis (Sgourakis et al. 2008) do an excellent job of cataloguing, summarizing, and analyzing all the MIVAT data that were published between 1997 and 2007. They represent a focused appraisal of the first decade of worldwide experience and outcomes of the MIVAT procedure, a procedure that has not significantly changed since the writing of these two papers.

The Miccoli systematic review compiled all the studies prior to 2008 that compared the MIVAT procedure to standard thyroidectomy. The main outcomes studied in the review were the safety of MIVAT, the advantages of MIVAT over traditional surgery, and if there were any evidence-based indications for using MIVAT for benign thyroid disease. This was a systematic review that compiled all the previously written papers and graded them based on standard evidence-based medicine criteria. However, there was no attempt at any meta-analysis of the data in this review. In the 10-year period that was analyzed, this systematic review identified only two randomized controlled clinical trials (Miccoli et al. 2001, 2002) that compared MIVAT to traditional surgery. Even if their data were combined, these two studies would only have 41 patients in the MIVAT group and 41 patients in the standard thyroidectomy group. These numbers are clearly short of the estimated 1,000 needed for true statistical significance on the subject. In spite of these low numbers the Miccoli review concluded that MIVAT is indicated for a very select group of patients with benign thyroid disease, it is just as safe as traditional thyroid surgery in this select group of patients (although there is a substantial learning curve), and it offers significant advantages in cosmetic results and postoperative pain. The authors of the review point out that the findings of the two randomized clinical trials are supported by 15 other studies that comprise level III and level IV evidence.

The second systematic review in 2008 was done by Sgourakis and was more specifically focused on the safety, cosmetic results, and postoperative pain of MIVAT compared to standard thyroidectomy. This review identified five randomized controlled trials, combined the data, and performed a rigorous meta-analysis of these data. The meta-analysis found that MIVAT operative times were significantly longer than standard thyroidectomy times (81 vs. 62 min), and patients experienced less pain 6 h after MIVAT compared to standard thyroidectomy. However, at 24 and 48 h after the procedures, there was no difference in pain levels. They also found that patients were significantly more satisfied with the cosmetic outcomes of MIVAT compared to standard thyroidectomy. There were no differences in bleeding, transient hypoparathyroidism, or transient nerve palsy.

23.2.2 2008 to Present

Since 2008, multiple prospective trials comparing MIVAT with conventional thyroidectomy have been reported. These trials focused on the differences in postoperative pain (Alesina et al. 2010; Del Rio et al. 2008), operative time (Wu et al. 2010), hypocalcemia (Del Rio et al. 2010), temporary nerve paralysis (Gal et al. 2008), and cosmetic outcome (El-Labban 2009). The post-2008 studies corroborate the findings from the pre-2008 studies. All the prospective studies after 2008 found that MIVAT can be done through a significantly shorter incision leading to better cosmetic results compared to traditional thyroidectomy. All but one of the post-2008 studies (Dobrinja et al. 2009) found that MIVAT takes longer to perform. The majority of the studies also found that MIVAT patients reported less pain in the first 24 h after surgery. No study found a difference in calcium levels or rates of nerve palsy between MIVAT and traditional thyroidectomy.

23.2.3 MIVAT Conclusions

There is enough evidence in the literature to definitively conclude a few things about the MIVAT procedure. When compared to standard thyroidectomy, the MIVAT procedure can be done through a smaller incision with better cosmetic results. There is also an improvement in immediate postoperative pain when compared to standard thyroidectomy done without a superficial cervical plexus block. However, it warrants noting that a superficial cervical plexus block is a simple procedure that has also been shown to reduce postoperative pain after standard thyroidectomy (Shih et al. 2010; Dieudonne et al. 2001), but no good prospective study has compared MIVAT to standard thyroidectomy with superficial cervical plexus block. The proven negative aspects of MIVAT are that the procedure has a long learning curve and requires longer operative times than standard thyroidectomy even in experienced hands.

There are still questions that have not been definitively answered by the current data. There is mounting evidence that MIVAT is as safe as standard thyroidectomy in terms of parathyroid and laryngeal nerve injury; however, the current evidence is in no way definitive or evidence-based. As stated previously, a prospective trial or meta-analysis will need at least 1,000 patients in each arm to definitively decide if MIVAT is as safe as standard thyroidectomy. Based on the number of studies currently in the literature, it appears that *if* a meta-analysis that included the pre- and post-2008 studies were done *in the future*, it would likely be in position to make a definitive statement on the safety of MIVAT.

In conclusion, MIVAT does offer a cosmetically superior operation and less postoperative pain when compared to standard thyroidectomy done without a superficial cervical plexus block. MIVAT is limited to a small subset of patients (as outlined in previous chapters in this book) who should be well informed of the risks of the procedure, including being told that the true risk to the parathyroid glands and recurrent laryngeal nerves is likely similar to standard thyroidectomy but is currently not known.

23.3 Evidence for the Scarless Endoscopic Thyroidectomy

23.3.1 The First Decade, 1997–2007

The first "scarless" endoscopic thyroidectomy techniques were published 3 years after the first MIVAT publication. The term "scarless" in these procedures means the scar has been moved from the neck to some less visible location. The Ikeda group published their experience using an anterior chest wall approach (Ikeda et al. 2000), and the Ohgami group used a breast approach (Ohgami et al. 2000). Other scarless endoscopic approaches include an axillary approach as well as any combination of anterior chest wall, breast, and axillary techniques. These techniques are further divided based on how much, if any, insufflation is used, and if the procedure is robot-assisted. This large heterogeneity in technique makes a meta-analysis of the literature nearly impossible. Similar to MIVAT, two systematic literature reviews were done in 2008. Studies by Slotema (Slotema et al. 2008) and Tan (Tan et al. 2008) are literature reviews that compile all the papers published on scarless endoscopic thyroidectomy from 1997 to 2007. Because of the heterogeneous nature of the scarless endoscopic thyroidectomy procedures, the two reviews consequently do not contain meta-analysis of the data and should not be considered level I evidence.

The Slotema review identified 22 scarless endoscopic thyroidectomy publications in the first decade of experience. Four of these studies are ranked as level III evidence (385 patients total), and the other 18 studies are ranked as level IV or level V evidence. Because of the lack of high-level evidence in the review, the authors did not draw any definitive evidence-based conclusions. However, some trends were observed, namely, that scarless endoscopic thyroidectomy is feasible from a technical standpoint and it likely offers a cosmetically superior outcome due to the lack of a scar on the neck. Concerns about the procedure included long operative times, a very long learning curve, considerable postoperative pain, and a lack of data regarding the true risks of recurrent laryngeal nerve and parathyroid gland injury.

The review by Tan identified 20 published studies on scarless endoscopic thyroidectomy in the first decade of experience. Four of these studies were graded level IV evidence, and the other 16 were graded level V evidence. Similar to the Slotema review, no evidence-based recommendations were made based on the first decade of experience with scarless endoscopic thyroidectomy because there was a complete lack of significant evidence-based findings. This review also found similar trends, mainly that the procedure is cosmetically superior, but it takes longer to perform, has a long learning curve, is technically challenging, and causes significantly more postoperative pain. The reviewers also point out that this procedure cannot be considered minimally invasive in the strict definition because the plane of dissection is actually more extensive than with standard thyroidectomy and also causes significantly more pain.

23.3.2 2008 to Present

Unfortunately, there has yet to be a single prospective trial comparing standard thyroidectomy to scarless endoscopic thyroidectomy. It is curious that the procedure is at least 12 years old and is an established alternative to standard thyroidectomy in some countries, yet there is no evidence-based proof that it is safe or effective in treating patients with thyroid disease. Since 2008, groups have continued to publish level IV and level V retrospective reviews and case series; however, no level I–III evidence has yet to be established. The biggest study to date was a recently published series by Lee (Lee et al. 2011) that retrospectively compared 570 scarless endoscopic thyroidectomies to 580 robot-assisted scarless thyroidectomies. Unfortunately, this study did not compare either one of these techniques to standard thyroidectomy.

The literature since 2008 shows some interesting trends and changes in the scarless endoscopic thyroidectomy literature. The technique was first developed in Japan, and most of the initial literature in the first decade was from Japanese groups. Since 2008, this has changed, and the majority of the literature is now from Korean surgical groups. The shift to the Korean data has coincided with changes in the technique as well. First, access through the axilla seems to be the most common approach, second, the majority of studies advocate performing the procedure without insufflation, and finally, since 2009 there has been a dramatic increase in publications on robot-assisted scarless thyroidectomy.

23.3.3 Scarless Endoscopic Thyroidectomy Conclusions

There is no solid evidence-based data for the scarless endoscopic thyroidectomy techniques. There are significant numbers of retrospective comparisons as well as case series, but because of the heterogeneity in surgical technique and poor data collection, it has been impossible to use that data for meta-analysis. It is clear that these techniques in their current form have a long learning curve, require a large space of dissection, and cause significant postoperative pain. Some surgeons have suggested that those attributes combined with the fact that the incisions are often larger than standard thyroidectomy incisions make scarless endoscopic thyroidectomy *more* invasive than standard thyroidectomy, and thus these techniques should not be considered minimally invasive. Furthermore, there is concern that the wounds created with these techniques are subject to more postoperative complications like seroma, hematoma, scaring, and surgical site infections (Dionigi et al. 2011). But perhaps most concerning are the multiple case reports of recurrent follicular thyroid cancer at port sites and along the endoscopic access tracts (Hur et al. 2011).

Scarless endoscopic thyroidectomy in its current form cannot be recommended yet as a safe, feasible alternative to standard thyroidectomy. The continued heterogeneity in technique, lack of evidence-based studies, and continued evolution of new techniques are further proof that the current axillary, chest wall, and breast access sites are not ready for mainstream use. Recently, newer techniques have been proposed that include a dorsal approach, a trans-oral approach, a posterior auricular approach, and other robot-assisted approaches.

23.4 Conclusion

Minimally invasive thyroidectomy has made significant advances since its introduction 14 years ago. In its infancy, many surgeons believed that these techniques were mostly "hype" with little evidence to support them as mainstream techniques (Duh 2003). The techniques have proven to have staying power, but it seems that this has been driven more by patient desire for cosmesis, as is seen in the Korean literature, and surgeons desire to push the boundaries of surgical technique. The evidence for the value of these techniques remains unclear at best. Minimally invasive thyroidectomy techniques are not yet ready to replace open thyroidectomy as the standard of care for patients with thyroid pathology.

References

Alesina PF, Rolfs T, Ruhland K, Brunkhorst V, Groeben H, Walz MK (2010) Evaluation of postoperative pain after minimally invasive video-assisted and conventional thyroidectomy: results of a prospective study. ESES Vienna presentation. Langenbecks Arch Surg 395(7):845–849

Del Rio P, Berti M, Sommaruga L, Arcuri MF, Cataldo S, Sianesi M (2008) Pain after minimally invasive video-assisted and after minimally invasive open thyroidectomy – results of a prospective outcome study. Langenbecks Arch Surg 393(3): 271–273

Del Rio P, Iapichino G, De Simone B, Bezer L, Arcuri M, Sianesi M (2010) Is it possible to identify a risk factor condition of hypocalcemia in patients candidates to thyroidectomy for benign disease? Ann Ital Chir 81(6):397–401

Dieudonne N, Gomola A, Bonnichon P, Ozier YM (2001) Prevention of postoperative pain after thyroid surgery: a double-blind randomized study of bilateral superficial cervical plexus blocks. Anesth Analg 92(6):1538–1542

Dionigi G (2009) Evidence-based review series on endoscopic thyroidectomy: real progress and future trends. World J Surg 33(2):365–366

Dionigi G, Boni L, Duran-Poveda M (2011) Evolution of endoscopic thyroidectomy. Surg Endosc 25(12):3951–3952

Dobrinja C, Trevisan G, Makovac P, Liguori G (2009) Minimally invasive video-assisted thyroidectomy compared with conventional thyroidectomy in a general surgery department. Surg Endosc 23(10):2263–2267

Duh QY (2003) Presidential address: minimally invasive endocrine surgery–standard of treatment or hype? Surgery 134(6):849–857

El-Labban GM (2009) Minimally invasive video-assisted thyroidectomy versus conventional thyroidectomy: a single-blinded, randomized controlled clinical trial. J Minim Access Surg 5(4):97–102. doi:10.4103/0972-9941.59307

Gal I, Solymosi T, Szabo Z, Balint A, Bolgar G (2008) Minimally invasive video-assisted thyroidectomy and conventional thyroidectomy: a prospective randomized study. Surg Endosc 22(11):2445–2449

Hur SM, Kim SH, Lee SK, Kim WW, Choi JH, Kim JH, Choe JH, Lee JE, Oh YL, Nam SJ, Yang JH, Kim JS (2011) Is a thyroid follicular neoplasm a good indication for endoscopic surgery? Surg Laparosc Endosc Percutan Tech 21(3):e148–e151

Huscher CS, Chiodini S, Napolitano C, Recher A (1997) Endoscopic right thyroid lobectomy. Surg Endosc 11(8):877

Ikeda Y, Takami H, Sasaki Y, Kan S, Niimi M (2000) Endoscopic neck surgery by the axillary approach. J Am Coll Surg 191(3):336–340

Kang SW, Jeong JJ, Yun JS, Sung TY, Lee SC, Lee YS, Nam KH, Chang HS, Chung WY, Park CS (2009) Gasless endoscopic thyroidectomy using trans-axillary approach; surgical outcome of 581 patients. Endocr J 56(3):361–369

Lee S, Ryu HR, Park JH, Kim KH, Kang SW, Jeong JJ, Nam KH, Chung WY, Park CS (2011) Excellence in robotic thyroid surgery: a comparative study of robot-assisted versus conventional endoscopic thyroidectomy in papillary thyroid microcarcinoma patients. Ann Surg 253(6):1060–1066

Linos D (2011) Minimally invasive thyroidectomy: a comprehensive appraisal of existing techniques. Surgery 150(1):17–24

Miccoli P, Berti P, Conte M, Bendinelli C, Marcocci C (1999) Minimally invasive surgery for thyroid small nodules: preliminary report. J Endocrinol Invest 22(11):849–851

Miccoli P, Berti P, Raffaelli M, Materazzi G, Baldacci S, Rossi G (2001) Comparison between minimally invasive video-assisted thyroidectomy and conventional thyroidectomy: a prospective randomized study. Surgery 130(6):1039–1043

Miccoli P, Elisei R, Materazzi G, Capezzone M, Galleri D, Pacini F, Berti P, Pinchera A (2002) Minimally invasive video-assisted thyroidectomy for papillary carcinoma: a prospective study of its completeness. Surgery 132(6):1070–1073; discussion 1073–1074

Miccoli P, Minuto MN, Ugolini C, Pisano R, Fosso A, Berti P (2008) Minimally invasive video-assisted thyroidectomy for benign thyroid disease: an evidence-based review. World J Surg 32(7):1333–1340

Ohgami M, Ishii S, Arisawa Y, Ohmori T, Noga K, Furukawa T, Kitajima M (2000) Scarless endoscopic thyroidectomy: breast approach for better cosmesis. Surg Laparosc Endosc Percutan Tech 10(1):1–4

Sgourakis G, Sotiropoulos GC, Neuhauser M, Musholt TJ, Karaliotas C, Lang H (2008) Comparison between minimally invasive video-assisted thyroidectomy and conventional thyroidectomy: is there any evidence-based information? Thyroid 18(7):721–727

Shih ML, Duh QY, Hsieh CB, Liu YC, Lu CH, Wong CS, Yu JC, Yeh CC (2010) Bilateral superficial cervical plexus block combined with general anesthesia administered in thyroid operations. World J Surg 34(10):2338–2343

Slotema ET, Sebag F, Henry JF (2008) What is the evidence for endoscopic thyroidectomy in the management of benign thyroid disease? World J Surg 32(7):1325–1332

Tae K, Ji YB, Cho SH, Kim KR, Kim DW, Kim DS (2011) Initial experience with a gasless unilateral axillo-breast or axillary approach endoscopic thyroidectomy for papillary thyroid microcarcinoma: comparison with conventional open thyroidectomy. Surg Laparosc Endosc Percutan Tech 21(3):162–169

Tan CT, Cheah WK, Delbridge L (2008) "Scarless" (in the neck) endoscopic thyroidectomy (SET): an evidence-based review of published techniques. World J Surg 32(7):1349–1357

Wu CT, Yang LH, Kuo SJ (2010) Comparison of video-assisted thyroidectomy and traditional thyroidectomy for the treatment of papillary thyroid carcinoma. Surg Endosc 24(7):1658–1662

Index

A
ABBA. *See* Axillo-Bilateral Breast Approach (ABBA)
Acute thyroiditis, 26, 61
Adenomas, 66
Adenomatoid nodules, 56
Agenesis, 18
Amiodarone, 62
Amplitude, 224, 225
Amyloidosis, 64
Anaesthesia, 199, 208, 209
Anaplastic carcinoma, 28, 51, 57, 67
Anaplastic thyroid tumors, 77
Ansa cervicalis nerve, 146
Anterior approach, 184–185
Antisepsis, 1
Antithyroglobulin antibodies, 239
Asepsis, 199
Aspiraitons, 221
Aspiration technique, 40
Atypia, 235
Atypical follicular adenoma, 67
Autoimmune disease, 68
Autoimmune thyroiditis, 61
Axilla, 149–151, 153
Axillary, 163, 164, 166
Axillary approach, 183, 184, 187, 249
Axillo breast approach, 237
Axillo-Bilateral Breast Approach (ABBA), 183, 186–187
Axilloscope, 202

B
B-flow imaging (BFI), 19
BABA. *See* Bilateral axillo-breast approach (BABA)
BAEA. *See* Bilateral transaxillary endoscopic approach (BAEA)
Berry's ligament, 7, 11, 123, 212, 221, 222
BFI. *See* B-flow imaging (BFI)
BiClamp®, 99
Bilateral axillo-breast approach (BABA), 169–180, 183, 184, 186, 237, 238, 243
Bilateral transaxillary endoscopic approach (BAEA), 187–188
Billroth, 4
Bipolar electrocautery, 98
Brachial plexus, 230, 234
BRAF V600E mutation, 70
Breast, 247, 249, 250

Breast approach, 183, 185–187
Bupivacaine, 106

C
C cells, 47, 59
Calcifications, 23, 24
Calcitonin, 242
Carcinoembryonic antigen (CEA), 242
Cernea, 13
Chronic lymphocytic thyroiditis, 61
Chung's retractor, 150, 151, 157, 162–164
Chvostek's sign, 233
Circumareolar incisions, 176, 180
Classic kocher incision, 2
Clear cell tumors, 76
CO_2 insufflation, 141, 142, 145, 155, 179, 236
Colloid accumulation, 65
Colloid nodules, 56
Color flow, 19
Columnar cell variant, 72
Complex thyroid cysts, 20
Cougard, 114
Cougard anterior endoscopic approach, 115
Cretinoid, 3
Cricothyroid ligament, 8
Cricothyroid muscle, 7–9
Cricothyroid space, 136
Cystic degeneration, 48

D
da Vinci Surgical System robot, 155, 156, 163, 169, 174, 176
De Quervain's thyroiditis, 26
Deep cervical blockade, 107
Deep cervical plexus, 105
Delphian nodes, 11
Differentiated thyroid cancer (DTC), 238, 239, 242–244
Diffuse pattern, 49, 51
Diffuse sclerosis variant, 73
Dissection, 144–147
Docking, 164–166, 176–177
Doppler, 19
DTC. *See* Differentiated thyroid cancer (DTC)
Dyshormonogenetic goiter, 63
Dysphagia, 221

E

Ear forceps, 120
Ectopic thyroid, 60
EJV. See External jugular vein (EJV)
Electrical stimulation, 222
Electrocautery, 120, 199
eMIT. See Endoscopic minimally invasive thyroidectomy (eMIT)
Endoflator®, 209
Endoscope, 128
Endoscopic minimally invasive thyroidectomy (eMIT), 203, 207, 209, 211, 214, 216, 217
Endoscopic thyroidectomy, 113, 155, 156, 158, 183–187, 236, 237, 242
Endoscopic transaxillary thyroidectomy, 141–148
Endoscopically assisted transaxillary approach, 149
Energy device, 95
Epinephrine, 106
Epithelial cysts, 20
Ethanol injection, 32
External jugular vein (EJV), 194

F

Fine-needle aspiration (FNA), 37–39, 235, 237, 239, 240, 242
Flap, 134
Flow pattern, 25
FNA. See Fine-needle aspiration (FNA)
Follicular carcinoma, 73
Follicular cell hyperplasia, 65
Follicular cells, 47
Follicular lesions, 28, 235, 236
Follicular neoplasm, 57, 235–237
Follicular variant of papillary cancer, 71
Frozen section, 81

G

Gagner anterior endoscopic approach, 114
Gagner's technique, 113
GAN. See Greater auricular nerve (GAN)
Gasless technique, 183, 192
Gasless transaxillary approach, 149–154
Goiter, 1, 20
Granulomatous thyroiditis, 61
Graves' disease, 3, 26, 27, 63
Greater auricular nerve (GAN), 193, 194, 197
Guidlines, 235, 237, 238, 242, 243

H

Haemorrhage, 199–201
Halsted, William, 5
Harmonic®, 121, 125, 169, 172, 174, 177, 195
Harmonic ace scalpel, 143
Harmonic curved shears, 163–165
Harmonic scalpel, 95, 98, 134, 151, 152, 185, 188, 209, 212–214
Hashimoto's thyroiditis, 25, 26, 61
Heinrich's modification, 235, 236
Hematoma, 232, 234, 250
Hematoma formation, 229
Hemiagenesis, 18
Hemithyroidectomy, 138
Hemorrhage, 231, 233
Hemorrhagic cysts, 20
Henry lateral endoscopic approach, 115
High-intensity focused ultrasound (HIFU), 32
Hoarseness, 4
Huerthle cell lesions, 54
Hürthle cell, 75
   lesions, 28
   neoplasm, 235
Hyalinizing trabecular neoplasm of the thyroid, 67
Hydrodissection, 171
Hyoid bone, 207, 209, 213
Hyperechoic nodule, 23
Hyperplastic (adenomatous) nodule, 21
Hypocalcemia, 125, 178, 180
Hypoechoic nodules, 22
Hypoglossal nerve, 203–205
Hypoparathyroidism, 4, 199–200, 233
Hypothyroidism, 3

I

Iatrogenic, 64
Immunocytochemistry, 46
Inabnet lateral endoscopic approach, 116
Indeterminate, 235–238
Inferior parathyroid glands, 11, 15, 137, 151, 152, 172–173, 177–178
Inferior pole, 136, 151
Inferior thyroid artery, 10, 11
Inferior thyroid veins, 10
Inflammatory pattern, 48
Insufflation, 142, 145
Insular carcinoma, 76
Internal branch, 13
Intraoperative neural monitoring (IONM), 221–227
Intrathyroidal thymoma-like neoplasms, 78
IONM. See Intraoperative neural monitoring (IONM)
Isoechoic nodules, 22, 23
Isthmectomy, 172, 177
Isthmus, 195, 196

J

Jugular vein, 146

K

Keloids, 149, 150, 153
Kocher incision, 2
Kocher, T., 1, 199
Krischner wire, 184, 185

L

Laser ablation, 32
Latency, 224, 225
Lateral compartment neck dissection, 243

Lateral neck dissection, 172, 177, 180
Lateral neck node metastasis (LNM), 161, 162, 167
Learning curve, 139, 244, 248–250
Lidocaine, 106
Ligament of berry. See Berry's ligament
Ligamentum arteriosum, 13
Ligasure®, 96, 98, 99, 188
Lingual nerve, 204, 205
Lingual thyroid, 60, 80
LNM. See Lateral neck node metastasis (LNM)
Local anesthesia, 40, 105
Local infections, 200, 201
Lymph nodes, 15, 29
Lymphadenectomy, 235, 240, 242, 243
Lymphocytic infiltrate, 56
Lymphocytic thyroiditis, 61
Lymphoma, 80

M
Macrocalcification, 23
Macrofollicular pattern, 48
Malignant neoplasms, 67
Maryland forceps, 177
Maryland grasper, 195
May-Gruenwald-Giemsa (MGG), 45
Mayo, Charles, 5
Medullary carcinoma, 28, 51, 57, 78
Medullary thyroid cancer (MTC), 242, 243
MEN. See Multiple endocrine neoplasia (MEN)
MEN type 2 syndromes, 78
Mepivacaine, 106
Metzenbaum scissor, 209, 211
MGG. See May-Gruenwald-Giemsa (MGG)
MHM. See Mylohyoid muscle (MHM)
Microcalcification, 23, 24
Microfollicular pattern, 48
Micropapillary thyroid carcinoma, 237–238
Middle veins, 10
MINET. See Minimally invasive non-endoscopic thyroidectomy (MINET)
Minimally invasive thyroidectomy techniques, 247, 249, 250
Minimally invasive non-endoscopic thyroidectomy (MINET), 133
Minimally invasive video-assisted thyroidectomy (MIVAT), 119, 127, 183, 184, 201, 214, 229–233, 247–249
Modified radical neck dissection (MRND), 161–167
Monopolar stimulation probe, 223
MRND. See Modified radical neck dissection (MRND)
MTC. See Medullary thryroid cancer (MTC)
Mucoepidermoid carcinoma, 77
Multiple endocrine neoplasia (MEN), 242, 243
Mylohyoid muscle (MHM), 204, 205, 208, 209

N
Natural orifice surgery (NOS), 202–203, 214, 216, 217
Natural orifice translumenal endoscopic surgery (NOTES), 202–203, 214
Nerve injury, 231–233

Nerve of galen, 12
Nodular stage/nodular goiter, 65
Nontoxic goiter, 64
NOS. See Natural orifice surgery (NOS)
NOTES. See Natural orifice translumenal endoscopic surgery (NOTES)

O
Omohyoid muscle (OMO), 7–9, 146, 147, 194
Oncocytic (oxyphilic) metaplasia, 56
Oncocytic cells, 59
Oncocytic follicular (Hürthle) cells, 75
Orphan annie, 68
Oxyphilic cells, 47

P
Palpation thyroiditis, 61
Papanicolaou technique, 45
Papillary CA, 50
Papillary carcinomas, 27, 53, 235, 243
Papillary microcarcinoma (PMC), 71
Papillary pattern, 49
Papillary thyroid carcinoma, 68, 235, 237–242
Parathyroid adenomas, 31
Parathyroid carcinoma, 31
Parathyroid glands, 14, 199, 212
Parathyroid hormone (PTH), 32
Parathyroidal chief or oxyphilic cells, 47
Paratracheoesophageal lymph nodes, 11
PAX8, 74
Pectoralis major muscle, 156
Pigmentation, 64
PMC. See Papillary microcarcinoma (PMC)
Poorly differentiated carcinoma, 57
Postauricular crease, 194
Postauricular region, 191
Postoperative complications, 130
Postoperative dysphagia, 200
Postoperative pain, 229, 230, 233
Power mode, 19
Prelaryngeal lymph nodes, 10
Pretracheal nodes, 11
ProGrasp forceps, 156, 157, 163–165
Psammoma bodies, 69
PTH. See Parathyroid hormone (PTH)
Pyramidal lobe, 7, 17, 138

R
Radiation fibrosis, 64
Radioactive iodine (RAI), 179, 237–240, 242, 243
Radiofrequency Ablation (RFA), 32
Raf/MEK/ERK pathway, 70
RAI. See Radioactive iodine (RAI)
Ras mutations, 75
RATS. See Robot-assisted thyroid surgery (RATS)
Rearranged during transfection (RET), 242

Recurrent laryngeal nerve (RLN), 2, 11, 138, 142, 147, 151, 152, 169, 172–174, 177, 178, 195, 196, 200, 203, 209, 211–214, 221–223, 225–227, 229, 231–233
Regional block, 106
RET. *See* Rearranged during transfection (RET)
RET/PTC, 70
RFA. *See* Radiofrequency Ablation (RFA)
RFT, Robotic facelift thyroidectomy (RFT)
Riedel's disease, 63
Riedel's thyroiditis, 26
RLN. *See* Recurrent laryngeal nerve (RLN)
RLN monitoring, 221–223
Robot, 192, 195
Robot-assisted scarless thyroidectomy, 250
Robot-assisted thyroid surgery (RATS), 229–233
Robotic and endoscopic magnification and maneuverabilit, 192
Robotic arm, 157, 158
Robotic facelift thyroidectomy (RFT), 191, 197
Robotic gasless transaxillary thyroidectomy, 155–159
Robotic MRND, 161–167
Robotic thyroid surgery, 169–180
Robotic thyroidectomy, 191, 193, 197
Robotic-assisted trans-oral endoscopic thyroidectomy, 214–216
Robotically assisted approach, 153

S
Sackett's classification, 235, 236
Salute position, 142–144
Scarless endoscopic thyroidectomy, 247, 249–250
Scarless techniques, 216
SCM. *See* Sternocleidomastoid muscle (SCM)
Seroma, 232–234, 250
Silent thyroiditis, 62
Sipple's syndrome, 78
SLN. *See* Superior laryngeal nerve (SLN)
Smears, 43
Snake retractors, 170, 172
Solid neoplastic pattern, 50
Solid pattern, 49
Solid variant of PTC, 73
Spatulas, 128
Squamous cell carcinoma, 77
Squamous cells:, 47
Steri-strips, 139
Sternocleidomastoid muscle (SCM), 145, 146, 194, 195, 208, 212
Sternothyroid muscle (STM), 7–9, 138, 146, 147
Stimulating electrodes, 224
Stimulator probe, 223, 227
STM. *See* Sternothyroid muscle (STM)
Strap muscles, 7, 134, 172–174, 177, 178
Struma lymphomatosa, 61
Subacute thyroiditis, 26
Sublingual bi-vestibular endoscopic approach, 206
Sublingual gland, 204, 205
Sublingual region, 203
Submandibular gland, 163, 166, 203
Submandibular region, 202, 204, 205, 207, 213
Submandibular triangle, 203–205
Submental region, 211

Suction dissector, 120
Suction-irrigator, 169, 174, 175
Superficial cervical block, 107
Superficial cervical plexus, 105
Superior laryngeal artery, 11
Superior laryngeal nerve (SLN), 11, 13, 151, 152, 195, 196, 223–224
 external branch, 10, 13, 223, 224
 internal branch, 224
Superior parathyroid gland, 11, 14, 136, 137, 151, 152, 195
Superior pole, 135
Superior thyroid artery, 9
Superior thyroid vein, 10
Surgi-Bra®, 174, 178

T
Tall cell variant, 72
Tegaderm®, 120
Telescope, 187, 188
Tetany, 4
Tg. *See* Thyroglobulin (Tg)
Theodor Billroth, 199
Three-dimensional imaging, 18
Threshold, 224–226
Thyroglobulin (Tg), 30, 178, 179, 238, 240, 241, 243
Thyroglossal duct, 17, 18, 80
Thyroglossal tract, 60
Thyrohyoid muscle, 7–9
Thyroid
 cartilage, 9
 cysts, 20
 follicles, 59
 gland, 9
 lymphoma, 29
 nodules, 235–237
 sarcoma, 80
TNM classification system, 239
TNM staging system, 238
Trans-oral endoscopic approach, 205, 207–214, 216
Trans-oral robotic-assisted thyroidectomy (TRAT), 216
Transaxillary, 156
Transaxillary thyroid surgery, 142, 147
Translocation t(2;3), 74
TRAT. *See* Trans-oral robotic-assisted thyroidectomy(TRAT)
Trocars, 142–145, 147, 204–206, 208, 209, 211–213
Trochar, 184–188
Trousseau's sign, 233
TSH levels, 240
Tubercle of zuckerkandl, 11
Tumor cells, 47

U
Ultracision®, 95, 96, 135, 209, 211–213
Ultrasound, 18
Upper pedicle, 121, 125

Index

V
Vagal stimulation, 226
VANS. *See* Video assisted neck surgery (VANS)
Vertical incision, 2
Video assisted neck surgery (VANS), 183–185, 187
Vocal cord palsy, 178, 180, 200, 201
Vocal cords, 7, 9
Voice changes, 221

W
Warthin-like variant, 73
Well-differentiated thyroid carcinoma (WDTC), 161, 162, 167

Z
Zuckerkandl tuberculum, 122, 177

Printing and Binding: Stürtz GmbH, Würzburg